Oncology and Palliative Social Work

Advance Praise for *Oncology and Palliative Social Work: Psychosocial Care for People Coping With Cancer*

"*Oncology and Palliative Social Work: Psychosocial Care for People Coping With Cancer* (*OPSW*) fills an important gap in the serious illness literature. The book illustrates the need for integrating palliative care early in the lives of patients with cancer and illuminates the important role that social workers have in providing psychosocial support services across the cancer trajectory. The authors eloquently discuss the convergence of oncology and palliative care social work, as a specialty practice, in the delivery of comprehensive, culturally congruent, person-centered cancer care. *OPSW* reflects the integrative knowledge, skills, clinical experience, and perspectives of a diverse group of interprofessional contributors with emphasis on best practices, emerging trends, and priorities in psychosocial oncology, as well as the impact of the COVID-19 pandemic on this changing landscape.

Each of the book's four sections is composed of 5–8 thematically connected chapters. Topics go above and beyond the typical discussions of basic treatment and diagnosis to highlight a number of contemporary and critical issues, including but not limited to equitable care. The attention that the authors give to systemic racism, cultural competence, and cultural humility; the vulnerability of diverse patients, including those with severe mental illness and informal caregivers, through a novel collaborative model of care are hallmarks of enlightening and inspiring evidence-based practice. There is so much more to *OPSW* that goes where authors often do not go to challenge clinicians to think critically about what we have learned from the COVID-19 pandemic about oncology and palliative social work. I encourage you to read the book so that you may consider the benefits of incorporating the knowledge gained from these authors into your own ethical practice approaches and professional discourse."

—**Karen Bullock**, PhD, LICSW, FGSA, APHSW-C, Ahearn Endowed Professor in the Boston College School of Social Work

"Nowhere have I seen a more thoughtful convergence of cancer and palliative care social work so well integrated and described as *Oncology & Palliative Care Social Work: Psychosocial Care for People Coping With Cancer*. This is a no-nonsense, clinically astute, and comprehensive textbook that delivers at every level across the spectrum of the cancer experience. Complex and culturally sensitive content at the nexus of oncology, palliative care, and social work, is clearly defined and presented in an engaging manner with clear linkages to a new gold standard of psychosocial care. The authors are all highly skilled, nationally recognized, compassionate experts in the field who are particularly adept at presenting provocative material in a manner that is digestible, wise, and precise."

—**Matthew Loscalzo**, LCSW, APOS Fellow, Executive Director, People & Enterprise Transformation, Emeritus Professor Supportive Care Medicine, Professor Population Sciences

"This inaugural book, *Oncology and Palliative Social Work: Psychosocial Care for People Coping With Cancer*, codifies in exemplary fashion the wisdom, clinical practice, and art of the oncology and palliative social work professions. This outstanding publication highlights the variety of challenges experienced by people living with and undergoing treatment of cancer, cancer survivors, their caregivers, and the bereaved.

It provides an overview of multiple topics, including health care disparities, provider bias, and systemic racism, which the pandemic further underscored. This book presents excellent clinical guidelines for all oncology and palliative care disciplines. I congratulate the editors and authors for their vision in creating this exceptional book, which is an invaluable resource in oncology and palliative social work and for all health care professionals."

—**Edith Peterson Mitchell**, MD, MACP, FCPP, FRCP (London), Clinical Professor of Medicine and Medical Oncology, Department of Medical Oncology, Director, Center to Eliminate Cancer Disparities, Associate Director, Diversity Affairs, Sidney Kimmel Cancer Center at Jefferson, 116th President National Medical Association

"Cancer is not a single disease; some are indolent with little impact on quality or duration of life, while others are aggressive and impose devastating consequences on the patient, family, and loved ones. While clinical care must always bring comfort and hope, it also must authentically reflect the wide spectrum of cancer outcomes and ensure that clinical approach meets the unique needs of the patient and their care givers and loved ones. At the same time we celebrated so many medical advances, we must also continue to advance our knowledge in the value and contributions of palliative care as the authors provide in this book. Addressing and attending to the impact of financial toxicity, psychosocial distress, and the many burdens of care on patients and their nonmedical caregivers are just a few of the contemporary topics that receive the attention they deserve in this authoritative book. I applaud the authors for moving this important field forward."

—**Heidi Nelson**, MD, FACS, Director, Cancer Programs, American College of Surgeons

"This remarkable book reminds us that each patient and their lived experiences are as unique as their cancer. More importantly, it provides a framework for managing each patient as a person as they navigate the diagnosis, treatment, and impact of cancer on their lives and on their families. Thanks to the authors and editors for ensuring that cancer patients everywhere will benefit from an integrated, whole-person approach."

—**Brian Druker**, MD, Physician-Scientist and Professor of Medicine, Oregon Health & Science University, Director of the OHSU Knight Cancer Institute and JELD-WEN Chair of Leukemia Research, Associate Dean for Oncology, OHSU School of Medicine

"This exceptional volume gathers the wisdom and practical advice of pioneers in the field of oncology social work and palliative care. Clinicians will find this an indispensable tool in their practice as they face complex and challenging scenarios in outpatient and inpatient cancer care. The editors have done an amazing job covering concerns of individuals throughout the many phases of cancer care and across the lifespan, bringing the weight of evidence and knowledge and the art of compassionate delivery to inform practice."

—**Lidia Schapira**, MD, FASCO, Professor of Medicine (Oncology), Stanford University School of Medicine, Director Cancer Survivorship Program, Faculty Co-Director for Clinical Research and Clinical Trials, Office of Cancer Health Equity, Stanford Cancer Institute, Associate Editor, *Journal of Clinical Oncology*

"A must-read for anyone working in oncology! Decades of research and clinical expertise by oncology social workers has championed that quality cancer care must include caring for the whole person—and the people who care for them. Health systems have made progress in areas such as distress screening and navigation to support services, but tremendous gaps exist in the implementation of psychosocial services, especially in underserved communities. Too often, addressing the psychosocial health needs of people impacted by cancer has been an afterthought or something care systems say they cannot afford to provide, leading to crises in mental health, poorer health outcomes, inefficient health care utilization, and increased cost of care. This transformational handbook is a vital resource that elevates psychosocial oncology as the key to optimal cancer care delivery—people's lives depend on it!"

—**Vicki Kennedy**, LCSW, Past President of the Association of Oncology Social Work and the American Psychosocial Oncology Society; Executive Director, Oncology Strategy and Patient Engagement, Cullari Communications Global

"It is certainly timely to have the honor of reading this book. Since the outbreak of the pandemic, people generally developed fear of infection and became reluctant to go to health care facilities. Thus, health tests or checkups were deferred or physical symptoms ignored, leading to a long delay in cancer diagnosis. The growing disparities in society created stress on those who cannot afford treatment and palliative care.

This book provides most important knowledge, wisdom, and insights on oncological and palliative intervention for social workers, care providers, and policymakers in addressing cancers for different target populations along their trajectory of illness. The authors are all experts in their respective areas of oncology and palliative care, their chapters are full of touching stories, research evidence, and rich clinical experience that can empower readers in their day-to-day practice in collaboration with the multidisciplinary team, family members, and community partners. I would strongly recommend this invaluable book to all health social workers, educators, and policymakers."

—**Professor Cecilia L. W. Chan**, PhD, RSW, FHKPCA, FHKASW, FAOSW, JP, Professor Emeritus, Department of Social Work and Social Administration, Founding Director and Associate Director, Centre on Behavioral Health, The University of Hong Kong, Fellow, Hong Kong Professional Counselling Association, Founding Fellow, Hong Kong Academy of Social Work, Fellow, Association of Oncology Social Work

"*Oncology & Palliative Social Work: Psychosocial Care for People Coping With Cancer* (*OPSW*) is a long-awaited book and is a major contribution to enhancing skilled care for the breadth of patients and families seen at all times in oncology practice. Oncology social work, nursing, and medicine all began formally around the same time. All have continued to grow together in scope and expertise and have become increasingly interdependent. Supportive care and palliative care are integrated into excellent cancer care just as this new book demonstrates. Key topics are introduced (such as "unprecedented challenges") and enduring topics are updated (such as "psychosocial aspects of cancer") in *OPSW*, which covers all age groups and all populations throughout the continuum of the cancer experience. While focusing on social workers, this book is a superb addition to the personal libraries of all of us in cancer care."

—**Richard J. Gralla**, MD, FACP, Professor of Medicine, Albert Einstein College of Medicine

"Palliative care principles are essential in oncology social work, and this comprehensive text provides an integrated and interdisciplinary approach to these two practice areas. It addresses disparities in health care and is rooted in a framework of social justice, with an antiracist approach that emphasizes cultural humility and sensitivity. It is relevant in the current context of the COVID-19 pandemic and addresses how this has changed the delivery of health care. The text also promotes social activism by providing a guide to social work advocacy of patients at the institutional, community, and government levels. I expect that this book will become a highly valued and much-used reference for social workers in both oncology and palliative care."

—**Cathy Berkman**, PhD, MSW, Professor, Director, Palliative Care Fellowship Director of Continuing Education, Fordham University, Graduate School of Social Service

"Social workers have always been essential members of the oncology multidisciplinary team, and, in many cases are the unsung heroes who tirelessly work to integrate essential services to ease the burdens faced by so many cancer patients and their families. The COVID pandemic clearly underscored the systemic obstacles so many individuals endure during life-threatening and chronic illness, including access to health care, coordination of care, psychosocial support, equity, racism, transportation, and other components of social determinants of health. The editors of the inaugural edition of *Oncology and Palliative Social Work: Psychosocial Care for People Coping With Cancer* have composed an excellent comprehensive text which should be required reading for the entire oncology multidisciplinary team. The book serves to illustrate the need for integrating early palliative care for patients with cancer and the important role social workers embrace in providing psychosocial support services across the cancer trajectory."

—**Al B. Benson III**, MD, FACP, FACCC, FASCO, Professor of Medicine,
Associate Director for Cooperative Groups
Robert H. Lurie Comprehensive Cancer Center, of Northwestern University

"As I sat in my office to write this endorsement, I paused for a moment to scan the many textbooks that I collected over the past 20 years. As I read each title, I again took a moment to think about the focus of each text. After careful thought, the topic of palliative care was missing. As I explored the table of contents for this text, I was amazed to find a significant list of new concepts such as equity, disparities, racism, financial toxicity, spiritual care, pandemics, and many others, including the LGBTQI populations. Now that I have surveyed the entire table of contents for the 28 chapters, the time is here for me to begin to deepen my own perspectives and knowledge on this incredible range of new challenges. Come and join me in using this text to broaden and enhance our approaches to cancer care so that we can truly maximize the benefits of our interventions for cancer patients and their families."

—**James Robert Zabora**, ScD, MSW, Retired,
The Johns Hopkins University School of Medicine

"This comprehensive book will serve as an important resource for oncology and palliative social workers, representing an integrated and interdisciplinary approach to care that embeds principles of palliative care, cultural awareness, and psychosocial skills. The book covers the entire spectrum of cancers from childhood to geriatric cancers. Throughout the book there is a commitment to improving diversity, equity, and inclusion within their workforce to assure more equitable health care access and outcomes for all patients. This is a "must read" textbook that should become an integral part of the education of all students in oncology, palliative care, and social work."

—**Carolyn D. Runowicz**, MD, Professor, Obstetrics & Gynecology, Herbert Wertheim College of Medicine, Florida International University

"*Oncology and Palliative Social Work: Psychosocial Care for People Coping With Cancer* is an essential and valuable book to address the complex needs of people with cancer in our post-COVID world. The book's integration of palliative care into cancer care and emphasis on social determinants and health care disparities addresses the challenges of contemporary oncology social work practice and provides innovative models of care."

—**Diane Blum**, LMSW, FASCO, Former Executive Director, Cancer*Care*

"*Oncology and Palliative Social Work: Psychosocial Care for People Coping With Cancer* provides valuable information that will be an essential source of clinical guidance for both palliative and oncology social workers and examines the important connection between these two social work specialties. This connection is particularly significant since cancer is increasingly a chronic illness with long-standing side effects that is best supported by a comprehensive psychosocial approach inherent in palliative care. In addition, this book is dedicated to examining psychosocial oncology and palliative care within the contexts of racial equity and justice, and cultural humility and ethics (among other topics), providing a much-needed framework that will prove to be an invaluable resource for both experienced clinicians and those newer to the field for many years to come."

—**Penelope Damaskos**, PhD, Editor in Chief, *Journal of Psychosocial Oncology*

"We all pass away, it is as natural a part of life as birth, yet cancer holds a special place in the human existence as an illness that not only steals length of life but also quality of life from those afflicted. The difficult and specific burdens cancer places upon not only cancer patients but on their loved ones and society are unique and complex and range beyond physical pain and symptoms, but include impact on mental health, employment, activities of daily living, interpersonal relationships and finances. In this special book, *Oncology and Palliative Social Work: Psychosocial Care for People Coping With Cancer*, the editors have aimed to provide a guide and framework for addressing all the needs the cancer patient faces and the importance of weaving early into their cancer journey the important support of both palliative care and palliative care social workers. As the director of an NCI Designated Cancer Center (first in San Antonio and now in North Carolina at the Atrium Health Wake Forest Baptist Comprehensive Cancer Center), I have come to strongly endorse from direct observation the crucial role that team-based (social workers, physicians, chaplains, and mental health professionals), holistic, and culturally competent palliative care has on decreasing the burden of cancer. I encourage anyone involved in holistic cancer care to read this book in order to augment the care they provide."

—**Ruben A. Mesa**, MD, FACP, Executive Director of Wake Forest Baptist Comprehensive Cancer Center, President Enterprise Cancer Service Line Atrium Health, Enterprise Senior Vice President Atrium Health, Vice Dean of Cancer Programs and Tenured Professor of Medicine, Wake Forest School of Medicine

"The benefits of early palliative care interventions for patients with advanced cancer have been known for some time, as has the failure of our profession collectively to fully meet these goals and needs. Expansion of the palliative care team to include multiple specialists, including social workers, has numerous advantages. Most importantly, different specialists bring different skills and expertise to the patient and the expanded team can provide more robust and more accessible care. Social workers, in particular, are skilled in providing so much of what patients with advanced cancer and their caregivers need, from counseling services, to strategizing and implementing supportive care services. With this in mind, all palliative care teams should include social workers as key members."

—**Lawrence N. Shulman**, MD, MACP, FASCO, Professor of Medicine, Associate Director, Special Projects, Director, Center for Global Cancer Medicine, Innovation Faculty, Penn Center for Cancer Care Innovation, Abramson Cancer Center, University of Pennsylvania

"Psychosocial aspects of cancer care are essential considerations for patients to experience optimal short- and long-term outcomes. This book provides key insights into a variety of situations that are commonly encountered and provides useful guidance on approaches to use in practice. While primarily intended for social workers, there is valuable information that can benefit all medical providers as they address these issues in their work."

—**John P. Leonard**, M.D. (he/him/his), Senior Associate Dean for Innovation and Initiatives, Chair (Interim), Weill Department of Medicine, Richard T. Silver Distinguished Professor of Hematology and Medical Oncology, Weill Cornell Medicine | New York-Presbyterian

"As we emerge from a pandemic that fully exposed critical health disparities, social inequities, and the essential nature of social work, now is a time to consider new approaches to the care of people affected by cancer. The merging of oncology and palliative social work represents innovation, imagination, creativity, and resilience. Let us use this textbook as a guide to achieve a new normal."

—**Brad Zebrack**, PhD, MSW, MPH, Professor, University of Michigan School of Social Work, Rogel Cancer Center, University of Michigan Health

"The achievements in cancercare over the last decades is a true testament to the strength of common purpose—hundreds of thousands of health care workers and scientists striving to cure cancer. We must now harness that same strength and determination to make these lifesaving discoveries available to all, regardless of gender, ethnicity, race, culture, or economic status. The obstacles are significant, but these medical discoveries belong to all of humanity, and with common purpose, all of humanity can share in the benefit. I recommend this book to all oncology and palliative care disciplines to read."

—**Kate Lathrop**, MD, Associate Professor, Division of Hematology and Oncology, UT Health San Antonio, Breast Medical Oncology, Mays Cancer Center at UT Health San Antonio, Assistant Dean of Undergraduate Research, Long School of Medicine, UT Health San Antonio, Program Director, Medical Oncology and Hematology Fellowship Program, UT Health San Antonio, Program Director, San Antonio Breast Cancer Symposium

"This is an extraordinarily important and timely book. While the medical treatment of cancer is very important, the psychosocial support and palliative care aspects are equally as important. The oncology social worker is an essential part of supporting the patient journey and an increasingly important part of a successful outcome. Palliative care does not mean end-of-life care. It is another critical aspect of supporting the patient during their treatment."

—**Patricia J. Goldsmith**, Chief Executive Officer, Cancer*Care*

"Much praise and thanks are due to the editors and contributors of *Oncology and Palliative Social Work: Psychosocial Care for People Coping With Cancer*, for a timely, clearly written text to improve the care of people with cancer in the ever-changing and blending worlds of oncologic, palliative, and psychosocial oncology. Support of people with cancer must acclimatize to cultural and social trends, especially in a world defined by a once-in-a-lifetime pandemic, as cancer treatments adapt to advances in biology, technology, and pharmacology. This book, with state-of-the-art academic and patient descriptions, helps all those engaged in cancer care appreciate developments in cultural, racial, and sexual diversity, disparities, and bias, providing a unique lens in the wake of the COVID-19 pandemic."

—**Andrew Roth**, MD, FAPOS, Emeritus Member of the Psychiatry Service, Department of Psychiatry & Behavioral Sciences, Memorial Sloan Kettering Cancer Center

"This is the right book at the right time as we hesitantly emerge from the COVID-19 pandemic into a changed and challenging world. The strength of this book is in its integrated and interdisciplinary approach. There is no shrinking from the hard and difficult; as topics include equity, racism, cultural competence, and vulnerable populations amongst others. Readers will find the key concepts at the beginning of each chapter efficient and leave with useful pearls, making this book a useful addition to your library."

—**Michael K. Wong**, MD, PhD, FRCPC, Professor, Division of Cancer Medicine, University of Texas, MD Anderson Cancer Center, Medical Executive—Integration, MD Anderson Cancer Network

"There have been significant advancements in models of early integration of palliative care into oncology practice, yet all communities have not benefited from these advancements equally. This inaugural book, *Oncology and Palliative Social Work: Psychosocial Care for People Coping With Cancer*, is an important contribution to the field of health equity. This book is not only a comprehensive manual addressing the important role that social workers have in providing psychosocial support services across the cancer trajectory but also provides models intended to increase early palliative care in marginalized communities that have historically underutilized these services. As a field, we need to be intentional in our approach towards inclusiveness. I am excited to see the advancements that will be made in culturally congruent and person-centered care because of circulating this important book into practice. This handbook is a great resource for all oncology and palliative social workers regardless of the communities in which they provide care."

—**Lailea Noel**, PhD, MSW, Assistant Professor, Steve Hicks School of Social Work, The University of Texas at Austin, Director of Diversity, Equity, and Inclusion, Association of Oncology Social Work, Health Equity Scholar, American Psychosocial Oncology Society, Board Trustee, Association of Community Cancer Centers

"*Oncology & Palliative Care Social Work: Psychosocial Care for People Coping With Cancer* arrives at a pivotal time in oncology as specialized and complex cancer treatment left less time and effort to care for patients' needs. The book's focus on education, counseling, and advocacy guides both the social worker new to the field and those working with different patient and family populations from diagnosis through survivorship or end-of-life care. It is a must-have desktop reference for all members of the oncology treatment team."

—**Stewart B. Fleishman**, MD, Founding Director of Cancer Supportive Services at Continuum Cancer Centers of New York, now part of the Mt. Sinai Health System; Author, Researcher in Oncology

"The treatment of cancer has become exponentially more complex, in many very good ways (exampled by the rapidly expanding list of targeted, tailored, and personalized therapy options); such progress has necessitated newer, interdisciplinary and adaptive tools and strategies for those interfacing and caring for patients and families. The care team, in taking care of the whole patient and those that care about them, must be attuned to myriad facets—societal, cultural, racial, ethnic, socioeconomic . . . the list goes on—and operate in a pandemic/seemingly unending post-pandemic world where technology continues to morph the human experience. Hats off to the team of authors and the editors assembling *Oncology and Palliative Social Work: Psychosocial Care for People Coping With Cancer* for providing comprehensive, relevant, and timely guidance on how to navigate the delicate and vastly important space of oncology social work and palliative care. So necessary are such skills and knowledge, as palliation should always be an ingredient in the oncology care plan, and the care team is often critically reliant on social work colleagues to truly bring home the care of the whole patient. Never has such a challenge been greater than at present, and no better time than the present for such a collective work as this."

—**Michael J. Mauro**, MD, Leader, Myeloproliferative Neoplasms Program, Member, Memorial Sloan Kettering Cancer Center, Professor, Weill Cornell Medicine

"The need for a comprehensive resource to assist health care professionals caring for persons with cancer and their loved ones has never been greater. In addition to the huge burden the cancer diagnosis and care has always placed, individuals and their families now must face additional health concerns, isolation, and disruption of health care institutions that deliver the care they need brought on by the COVID pandemic. At the same time, all in the health care field have been awakened to inequalities in care and the special needs of the LGBTQI community and other groups and the critical role of all providers and particularly social workers in addressing disparities. This book provides information on and insight into all aspects of the cancer journey. It is a welcome addition."

—**Mark G. Kris**, MD, William and Joy Ruane Chair in Thoracic Oncology, Attending Physician, Thoracic Oncology Service, Department of Medicine, Memorial Sloan Kettering Cancer Center, Professor of Medicine, Weill Cornell Medical College

"Oncology and palliative social workers have shouldered extraordinary changes in their duties to patients during the COVID-19 pandemic. While the toll of cancer has been felt like never before, it may take years to understand how attempts to mitigate this dangerous virus have positively and negatively affected cancer patients and their families. Even as the technology of cancer treatment has improved during the pandemic at a breathtaking pace, those in the oncology field recognize that many cancer patients have not realized the benefits. This important book takes a provocative look at the experience and wisdom oncology and palliative social workers have gained through this difficult time, with a hard look at socioeconomic factors, medical hesitancy and distrust, and other possible causes of health care inequity in oncology during the pandemic. This book is essential and timely reading for all involved in the care of people with cancer."

—**Sarah E. Kerr**, MD, Pathologist, Hospital Pathology Associates, Divisions of Cytopathology, Pulmonary, Gynecologic, and Molecular Pathology, Allina Health Laboratories, Allina Health Cancer Institute

"The editors, Hedlund, Miller, Christ, and Messner, are innovative leaders who were able to bring together a highly respected group of diverse authors to address the strengths and challenges in integrating psychosocial services into cancer care in the current health care climate. The COVID-19 pandemic and social repercussions are causing dramatic changes in health care. These changes have amplified the value of mental-health services, leading to increased demand for services at the same time there are significant staffing shortages. Oncology and palliative care social workers' interventions are vital to successful health care outcomes. Oncology and palliative care social workers reduce patient and family distress and improve quality of life, thereby increasing patient satisfaction, improving efficiencies, and lessening the burden on physicians and health care teams. *Oncology and Palliative Social Work: Psychosocial Care for People Coping With Cancer* will be a significant contribution to the future of the oncology and palliative care social work field and workforce training and development."

—**Courtney Bitz**, LICSW, OSW-C, ACHP-SW, Senior Director, Division of Social Work, Department of Psychosocial Oncology and Palliative Care, Dana-Farber Cancer Institute

"It is worth noting that the proposal for this book was submitted when the world was already amidst a pandemic, and patients and professionals were navigating myriad and rapid changes. The authors and editors, many of whom are nationally recognized, highly skilled practitioners, offer a wonderfully comprehensive and current resource for those working in oncology and palliative social work. In addition to providing clear guidance on clinical practice, the authors identify innovative, empathic approaches to the practical challenges presented by the pandemic as well as essential work still to be done in the realms of health care disparities, provider bias, and systemic racism. This book provides much-needed wisdom and perspective, squarely located in the context of the current times. I enthusiastically recommend *Oncology & Palliative Care Social Work: Psychosocial Care for People Coping With Cancer* as a standard addition to the library of oncology and palliative care social workers and those working alongside them."

—**Leora Lowenthal**, LICSW, OSW-C, MPA, FAOSW (she/her), Sr. Clinical Social Worker, Department of Psychosocial Oncology and Palliative Care, Dana-Farber Cancer Institute, President, Association of Oncology Social Work (2023)

Oncology and Palliative Social Work

Psychosocial Care for People Coping With Cancer

Edited by

Susan Hedlund, Bryan Miller, Grace Christ, and Carolyn Messner

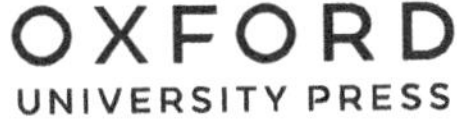

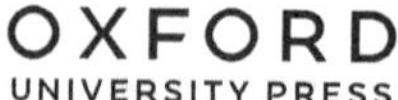

Oxford University Press is a department of the University of Oxford. It furthers the University's objective of excellence in research, scholarship, and education by publishing worldwide. Oxford is a registered trademark of Oxford University Press in the UK and certain other countries.

Published in the United States of America by Oxford University Press, 198 Madison Avenue, New York, NY 10016, United States of America.

Library of Congress Cataloging-in-Publication Data
Names: Hedlund, Susan, editor. | Miller, Bryan (Social worker), editor. | Christ, Grace, editor. | Messner, Carolyn, editor.
Title: Oncology and palliative social work : psychosocial care for people coping with cancer / Susan Hedlund, Bryan Miller, Grace Christ, Carolyn Messner.
Description: New York, NY : Oxford University Press, [2024] | Includes bibliographical references and index.
Identifiers: LCCN 2023032610 (print) | LCCN 2023032611 (ebook) | ISBN 9780197607299 (hardback) | ISBN 9780197607312 (epub) | ISBN 9780197607329
Subjects: LCSH: Medical social work. | Cancer—Patients—Services for. | Cancer—Psychosomatic aspects. | Cancer—Palliative treatment.
Classification: LCC HV687 .O47 2024 (print) | LCC HV687 (ebook) | DDC 362.19699/4—dc23/eng/20230814
LC record available at https://lccn.loc.gov/2023032610
LC ebook record available at https://lccn.loc.gov/2023032611

DOI: 10.1093/oso/9780197607299.001.0001

Printed by Integrated Books International, United States of America

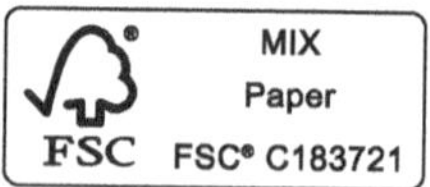

Oncology and Palliative Social Work: Psychosocial Care for People Coping With Cancer *has been written to capture the voices of oncology and palliative social workers and of people coping with cancer, their caregivers, cancer survivors, and the bereaved with whom we have the great privilege to work. Their lived experiences have informed this book immensely. Oncology and palliative social workers share a common bond to make a difference in the lives of people coping with cancer. And it is people coping with cancer to whom this book is dedicated. As you read the chapters, listen to their voices.*

Oncology and Palliative Social Work: Psychosocial Care for People Coping With Cancer, *is a repository of this era and written as a reference for each of you. These have not been easy times for our profession with a global pandemic, health care disparities, systemic racism, disparate access to health care, trauma, and so many people without safe harbor. As the scientific breakthroughs in oncology and palliative care grow, there are many patients who lack access to these breakthroughs. As oncology and palliative social workers, we are often referred those patients and caregivers for whose needs there are no easy solutions. We hope that in this book, you will find solace, novel approaches to your work, and reflective time to discover innovative solutions and renewed resilience to take on the challenges that lie ahead for all of us.*

Contents

List of Illustrations xix
Preface: Pairing Oncology and Palliative Social Work: Why Now? xxi
Acknowledgments xxiii
List of Contributors xxv

SECTION I PERSPECTIVES IN ONCOLOGY AND PALLIATIVE SOCIAL WORK
Susan Hedlund

1. **Overview of Diagnosing and Treating Cancer** 3
Susan Hedlund and Ana Maria Lopez

2. **The Changing Landscape of Cancer Treatment** 17
Heidi Ko, Eric Chang, Marcela Mazo Canola, Zoe Tao, Daniel Hughes, Krista Nelson, and Timothy Siegel

3. **Equity, Racism, Cultural Competence, and Cultural Humility in Oncology Social Work Practice** 32
Eucharia Borden and Jennifer M. Dunn

4. **Social Determinants of Health: Cancer-Related Health Disparities and Financial Toxicity** 45
Iris Cohen Fineberg and Jessica Savara

5. **Unprecedented Challenges: Cancer Care Amid Pandemics, Disasters, and Other Traumatic Events** 57
Karen Bullock

6. **Beyond Survival: Survivorship, Integrative Programs, Lifestyle, and Rehabilitation** 69
Randi Lyn Hornyak, Yvette Colón, and Mary Lou Galantino

7. **Innovative Models in Palliative Care in Oncology** 81
Jennifer J. Halpern and Eunju Lee

SECTION II CLINICAL ISSUES AND INTERVENTIONS

Cecilia L. W. Chan

8. **Beyond Distress Screening: The Future of Psychosocial Oncology and Palliative Care** 97
   Brad Zebrack, Meredith Doherty, and Katrina R. Ellis

9. **Psychosocial Aspects of Cancer** 110
   Angelique Caba, Maria Chi, and Stewart B. Fleishman

10. **Finding Comfort: Pain, Symptom, and Treatment-Related Toxicity Management** 123
    Sara Taub, Kamel Abou Hussein, Victoria Puzo, and Jason A. Webb

11. **A Novel Collaborative Care Model for People With Cancer and Serious Mental Illness** 141
    Amy Corveleyn, Vilmarie Rodriguez, and Kelly Irwin

12. **Interprofessional Spiritual Care Along the Cancer Care Trajectory** 154
    Debra Mattison, Sandra Blackburn, and Christopher Brady

13. **The Burdens and Rewards of Informal Cancer Caregivers: Issues and Interventions** 167
    Kelly R. Tan, Tamryn F. Gray, Alyson Erardy, and Erin E. Kent

14. **Palliative and Hospice Care at the End of Life: Walking Alongside Patients and Families** 181
    Jamie Newell and Stephanie B. Broussard

15. **Grief, Loss, and Bereavement in Oncology and Palliative Care** 195
    Kimarie Knowles, Abigail Nathanson, Danetta Hendricks Sloan, and Grace Christ

SECTION III POPULATION HIGHLIGHTS: UNDERREPRESENTED, UNDERSERVED, AND VULNERABLE POPULATIONS

Guadalupe Palos

16. **The Older Person With Cancer** 215
    Danielle Saff, Sarah Kelly, and Lisa Petgrave-Nelson

17. **Cancer in Middle Age** 227
Meredith Cammarata, Samantha Fortune, and Carissa Hodgson

18. **Children, Adolescents, and Young Adults With Cancer** 240
Nancy Cincotta, Sarah Paul, and Arika Patneaude

19. **Palliative Care for Lesbian, Gay, Bisexual, Transgender, Queer, and Intersex (LGBTQI) Persons Coping With Cancer** 261
Mandi L. Pratt-Chapman, Gary Stein, Cathy Berkman, and Andre Pruitt

20. **America's Growing Multicultural and Diverse Populations: Implications for Oncology and Palliative Care** 275
Guadalupe Palos, Mi (Emma) Zhou, and Yanette Tactuk

SECTION IV PROFESSIONAL ISSUES
Eucharia Borden

21. **Ethical and Legal Issues in Oncology and Palliative Care Social Work** 295
Lori Eckel, Phylicia L. Woods, and Kathryn M. Smolinski

22. **Living and Working Through Pandemics, Disasters, and Other Traumatic Events: Impact on Professionals** 309
Susan Hedlund, Bryan Miller, and Leena Nehru

23. **Professional Social Work Development and Sustainability** 322
Alison Snow and Heather Honoré Goltz

24. **The Increasing Role of Credentialing, Certification, and Continuing Education** 340
Brittany Nwachuku, Jennifer Bires, and Vickie Leff

25. **How Technology Is Transforming Oncology and Palliative Care: Opportunities and Challenges** 352
Michael Wong, A. J. Cincotta-Eichenfield, Carolyn Messner, and Sunita Jadhav

26. **Leadership Development in Oncology and Palliative Care Social Work** 369
Penelope Damaskos, Linda Mathew, and LaKeisha Jackson

27. **Creating Partnerships: Fostering Collaboration and Managing Conflict** 384
Stephanie Fooks-Parker, Barbara Jones, and Tara Schapmire

28. **Capturing the Contribution of International Oncology and Palliative Social Work** 397
Geok Ling Lee and Cecilia Lai Wan Chan

Epilogue: Oncology Social Work Leadership: Innovators in a Changing World 409
Susan Hedlund, Bryan Miller, Grace Christ, and Carolyn Messner

Index *413*

Illustrations

Figures

3.1 The system of racism causes racial inequities in the key areas of the social determinants of health. 38

11.1 Bridge: Person-centered collaborative care for serious mental illness and cancer. 144

20.1 Determinants of disparities in cancer and palliative care. 280

20.2 Example of social work intervention for an undocumented immigrant needing palliative care services. 285

20.3 Future priorities in oncology and palliative care social work with multicultural groups. 288

21.1 Ethical issues influence and action. 296

27.1 IPEC interprofessional collaboration competency domain (2016). 392

27.2 IPEC core competencies for interprofessional collaborative practice (2016). 393

Tables

13.1 Examples of Conceptual Frameworks Related to Caregiving 172

13.2 Selected Exemplar Interventions 176

15.1 Common/Typical Grief Symptoms 199

15.2 Bereavement Intervention: Three Levels of Care 207

18.1 Development, Disruption, and Coping During the Cancer Journey for Children, Adolescents, and Young Adults 242

18.2 Questions According to Age 251

19.1 Basic Terminology 265

19.2 Resources for LGBTQI Elders 272

20.1 Matrix of Social Work Practice Interventions and Models for At-Risk Multicultural Groups 282

23.1 Opportunities for Developing OSW Competencies: Professional Organizations that Offer National Conferences/Continuing Education and Mentorship 328

23.2 Opportunities for Developing OSW Competencies: Fellowships/Internships/Mentoring 328

Preface

Pairing Oncology and Palliative Social Work: Why Now?

When the editors first submitted the proposal for this book, we were in the midst of the COVID-19 pandemic. The United States had recently reached and exceeded the ominous number of 100,000 deaths. We felt we would be remiss if we failed to acknowledge this and what it was like to practice during that time. In the early days, vaccines and adequate testing were unavailable, and we lacked the ability to conceive of a return to "normal" in the foreseeable future. The financial fallout and impact of the pandemic worldwide continue to be experienced. The delivery of cancer care and psychosocial support services have been affected in intense and dynamic ways.

To live with cancer during a pandemic added complexity to treatment and treatment decisions and reinforced the need for palliative care principles to be well integrated into care. Additionally, the approach to diagnosing and treating cancer continues to evolve in novel ways. Well-integrated palliative care offered concurrently with standard oncology treatment is highly beneficial, regardless of the stage of disease or expected prognosis. The current shortage of palliative care specialists has created an opportunity for all oncology practitioners to adapt methods used by palliative care teams. We have attempted to integrate these principles throughout the book.

Additionally, health care disparities, provider bias, and systemic racism are significant problems that all oncology social workers should work to eliminate. The pandemic further underscored these disparities and the disproportionate burden of illness and access to care on vulnerable populations. Using our voices to advocate for individual clients while also pushing for policy changes within our institutions, communities, and government are important aspects of oncology social work practice. We have actively sought to have diverse voices represented in this book.

Now, three years later, we have all personally worked our way through the different iterations of the pandemic and attempted to adapt our practices accordingly while still serving our oncology patients. We have witnessed innovation, creativity, and resilience. It is said that the worst of times bring out the best and the worst in people. We choose to focus on the best.

What we have attempted to create is a book that will be a resource to oncology and palliative social workers, representing an integrated and interdisciplinary approach to care that embeds principles of palliative care, cultural awareness, and psychosocial skills throughout. We hope you will find these chapters helpful in your practice.

With gratitude,

Susan Hedlund, LCSW, FAOSW
Director, Patient & Family Services
Knight Cancer Institute
Oregon Health & Sciences University

Bryan Miller, LCSW, OSW-C
Director of Psychosocial Support Services
Atlanta Cancer Care
affiliated with Northside Hospital Cancer Institute

Grace Christ, PhD, DSW, FAOSW
Professor Emerita, Research Scientist
Columbia University School of Social Work

Carolyn Messner, DSW, BCD, FNAP, FAPOS, FAOSW, LCSW-R
Senior Director of Education and Training
Cancer*Care*

Acknowledgments

We could not have edited this inaugural book, *Oncology and Palliative Social Work: Psychosocial Care for People Coping With Cancer*, without all our section heads and authors. We are very grateful to each of them for their tireless work, wonderful energy and enthusiasm that made the publication of this book possible during the pandemic. We especially wish to thank our colleague, Stuart Fleishman, MD, for his invaluable assistance, consultation, and support to us. We also wish to thank Heather Lee Miller, PhD, for her copyediting assistance. We are indebted to our Oxford team for their unwavering encouragement and support of this inaugural book. Bryan would like to personally thank Hiba Tamim, MD, for her enduring leadership, philanthropic efforts, support of oncology social work, and sportsmanship—the numerous triathlons and trail run races have been genuinely treasured—over the span of more than 17 years of working together.

Contributors

Cathy Berkman, PhD, MSW, Fordham University

Jennifer Bires, MSW, LCSW, OSW-C, CST, Inova Schar Cancer Institute

Sandra Blackburn, MSW, LSW, Abramson Cancer Center Penn Medicine

Eucharia Borden, MSW, LCSW, OSW-C, Cancer Support Community

Christopher Brady, MDiv, THM, MSSW, North Carolina Conference of the United Methodist Church

Stephanie B. Broussard, MSSW, LCSW-S, APHSW-C, Texas Oncology

Karen Bullock, PhD, LICSW, FGSA, APHSW-C, Boston College

Angelique Caba, LCSW, Cancer*Care*

Ann M. Callahan, PhD, LCSW, Eastern Kentucky University

Meredith Cammarata, LCSW-R, Memorial Sloan Kettering Cancer Center

Marcela Mazo Canola, MD, UT Health San Antonio Mays Cancer Center

Cecilia Lai Wan Chan, BSocSc, MSocSc, PhD, RSW, JP, The University of Hong Kong

Eric Chang, MD, Oregon Health & Science University Knight Cancer Institute

Maria Chi, DSW, LCSW-R, Perlmutter Cancer Center—NYU Langone Health

Grace Christ (Editor), PhD, DSW, FAOSW, Columbia University

Nancy Cincotta, M.Phil, LCSW, CPA, Columbia University

A. J. Cincotta-Eichenfield, LMSW, OSW-C, Cancer*Care*

Yvette Colón, PhD, BCD, FAOSW, LMSW-C, Eastern Michigan University

Amy Corveleyn, MSW, LICSW, Massachusetts General Hospital

Penelope Damaskos, PhD, LCSW, OSW-C, FAOSW, *Journal of Psychosocial Oncology*

Meredith Doherty, PhD, LCSW, University of Pennsylvania

Jennifer M. Dunn, MSW, LCSW, OSW-C, Washington University School of Medicine in St. Louis

Lori Eckel, LCSW, APHSW-C, Legacy Medical Group

Katrina R. Ellis, PhD, MPH, MSW, University of Michigan

Alyson Erardy, LCSW, Westchester Medical Center

Iris Cohen Fineberg, PhD, MSW, OSW-C, FNAP, FAOSW, Stony Brook University

Stewart B. Fleishman, MD, American College of Surgeons, Commission on Cancer

Stephanie Fooks-Parker, MSW, LSW, OSW-C, Children's Hospital of Philadelphia

Samantha Fortune, LCSW, Cancer*Care*

Mary Lou Galantino, PT, PhD, MSCE, FAPTA, Stockton University

Heather Honoré Goltz, PhD, LCSW, MEd, MPH, University of Houston-Downtown

Tamryn F. Gray, PhD, RN, MPH, Dana-Farber Cancer Institute and Harvard Medical School

Jennifer J. Halpern, PhD, LMSW, APHSW-C, Fordham University

Susan Hedlund (Editor), LCSW, FAOSW, Oregon Health & Sciences University Knight Cancer Institute

Carissa Hodgson, LCSW, OSW-C, Bright Spot Network

Randi Lyn Hornyak, PT, DPT, Gaspar Doctors of Physical Therapy

Daniel Hughes, PhD, MEd, University of Texas Health – San Antonio

Kamel Abou Hussein, MD, MD Anderson Cancer Center at Cooper

Kelly Irwin, MD, MPH, Harvard Medical School, Massachusetts General Hospital Cancer Center

LaKeisha Jackson, MSW, LCSW, LICSW, Anne Arundel Medical Center

Sunita Jadhav, PhD, MSW, Tata Memorial Hospital

Barbara Jones, PhD, MSW, Boston University

Sarah Kelly, MSW, LCSW-R, Cancer*Care*

Erin E. Kent, PhD, MS, University of North Carolina at Chapel Hill

Kimarie Knowles, LCSW-R, Memorial Sloan Kettering Cancer Center

Heidi Ko, DO, UT Health San Antonio-Mays Cancer Center

Eunju Lee, MSW, MSOD, APHSW-C, LCSW, Memorial Sloan Kettering Cancer Center,

Geok Ling Lee, PhD, FT, RSW, National University of Singapore

Vickie Leff, MSW, LCSW, BCD, APHSW-C, Advanced Palliative Care & Hospice Social Work Certification Program

Ana Maria Lopez, MD, MPH, MACP, FRCP, Sidney Kimmel Medical College and Sidney Kimmel Cancer Center—Jefferson Health—New Jersey

Linda Mathew, DSW, MSW, LCSW-R, Memorial Sloan Kettering Cancer Center

Debra Mattison, LMSW, OSW-C, ACSW, BCD, University of Michigan

Carolyn Messner (Editor), DSW, BCD, FNAP, FAPOS, FAOSW, LCSW-R, Cancer*Care*

Bryan Miller (Editor), LCSW, OSW-C, Atlanta Cancer Care affiliated with Northside Hospital Cancer Institute

Abigail Nathanson, DSW, LCSW, APHSW-C, ACS, New York University

Leena Nehru, MSW, LCSW, OSW-C, Wellstar Kennestone Cancer Center

Krista Nelson, LCSW, OSW-C, FAOSW, FAPOS, Providence Cancer Institute

Jamie Newell, MSW, LCSW, Providence Portland Medical Center

Brittany Nwachuku, EdD, LCSW, LISW, OSW-C, Alliant International University

Guadalupe Palos, DrPH, LMSW, RN, The University of Texas MD Anderson Cancer Center (Retired)

Arika Patneaude, MSW, LICSW, APHSW-C, Seattle Children's Hospital

Sarah Paul, LCSW, OSW-C, Cancer*Care*

Lisa Petgrave-Nelson, LMSW, OSW-C, The Cancer Institute at St. Francis Hospital

Mandi L. Pratt-Chapman, MA, PhD, Hon-OPN-CG, The George Washington University School of Medicine and Health Sciences

Andre Pruitt, PhD, LCSW, Rustic Sage LLC

Victoria Puzo, LCSW, Cancer*Care*

Vilmarie Rodriguez, LCSW, Cancer*Care*

Danielle Saff, MSW, LCSW, Cancer*Care*

Jessica Savara, LCSW, CADC II, Oregon Health & Science University Knight Cancer Institute

Tara Schapmire, PhD, MSSW, OSW-C, FAOSW, University of Louisville

Timothy Siegel, MD, FACS, Oregon Health & Science University Knight Cancer Institute

Danetta Hendricks Sloan, PhD, MSW, MA, John Hopkins Bloomberg of Public Health

Kathryn M. Smolinski, JD, MSW, Wayne State University

Alison Snow, PhD, LCSW-R, OSW-C, Mount Sinai Downtown Cancer Centers

Gary Stein, PhD, Yeshiva University

Yanette Tactuk, LCSW-R, Memorial Sloan Kettering Cancer Center

Kelly R. Tan, PhD, RN, University of North Carolina at Chapel Hill Lineberger Comprehensive Cancer Center

Zoe Tao, MD, Oregon Health & Science University Knight Cancer Institute

Sara Taub, MD, MBE, FAAP, Oregon Health & Science University Knight Cancer Institute

Jason A. Webb, MD, DFAPA, FAAHPM, Oregon Health & Science University Knight Cancer Institute

Michael K. Wong, MD, PhD, FRCPC, The University of Texas MD Anderson Cancer Center

Phylicia L. Woods, JD, MSW, GRAIL, Inc.

Brad Zebrack, PhD, MSW, MPH, University of Michigan

Mi (Emma) Zhou, MSW, LCSW, The Blavatnik Family Chelsea Medical Center at Mount Sinai

SECTION I

PERSPECTIVES IN ONCOLOGY AND PALLIATIVE SOCIAL WORK

Susan Hedlund

In this first section of the book, the authors lay a foundation to reflect on the history of cancer treatment and where we are today in considering both novel and evolving therapies, as well as the rationale for integrating palliative care throughout the treatment trajectory. While many people are living longer after the diagnosis of and treatment for cancer, other issues have evolved that include the need to address long-term or late effects, survivorship issues, and financial toxicity. One chapter focuses specifically on survivorship issues, lifestyle, and rehabilitation. Also reviewed in this section are issues of long-standing systemic racism in health care, as well as challenges of access and equity that are essential for oncology and palliative care social workers to understand and address. Developing cultural competence and understanding cultural humility are foundational skills to deal with these challenges. Relatedly, recognizing the connection between social determinants of health and cancer-related health disparities are critical components to address and understand. Living through and practicing during the COVID-19 pandemic has been an unprecedented challenge. Finally, new and innovative models for the provision of palliative care are offered for consideration.

1

Overview of Diagnosing and Treating Cancer

Susan Hedlund and Ana Maria Lopez

Key Concepts

- Accurately diagnosing the type, stage, and molecular profile of cancer is essential in guiding treatment decisions.
- Numerous approaches to treatment exist and continue to evolve.
- The type, stage, prognosis, and treatment approaches will have an impact on and guide psychosocial care.
- Attention to the psychosocial impact of cancer is important.
- Oncology social workers work with anxiety, depression, and quality-of-life issues for patients and families.

Keywords: cancer, chemotherapy, diagnosis, immunotherapies, oncology social work, psychosocial impact, radiation therapy, surgery

Cancer is a group of diseases involving abnormal cell growth with the potential to invade or spread to other parts of the body. These contrast with benign tumors, which do not spread.

The development of the modern microscope in the nineteenth century led to a greater ability to study diseased tissues and fostered the rise of scientific oncology. This technology not only allowed for a better understanding of the damage cancer can do but also aided in the development of cancer surgery (Mukherjee, 2010). The field has continued to grow and led to change as better understanding of cell biology and the mechanisms of cancer growth has evolved.

Cancer affects one in three people in the United States. The human body is made up of trillions of cells that over a lifetime grow and divide as needed. When cells are abnormal or get old, they usually die. Cancer starts when something goes wrong in this process. Cells continue to grow—making new

Susan Hedlund and Ana Maria Lopez, *Overview of Diagnosing and Treating Cancer* In: *Oncology and Palliative Social Work.* Edited by: Susan Hedlund, Bryan Miller, Grace Christ, and Carolyn Messner, Oxford University Press.
 DOI: 10.1093/oso/9780197607299.003.0001

cells while the old or abnormal cells do not die as they should. For growing numbers of people, cancer can be treated successfully or have its growth limited. This in turn has increased the number of cancer survivors living well after treatment (Siegel et al., 2020).

Cancer is not one disease. Cancer is a conglomerate of disease processes where the normal controls of cell birth, growth, and death have gone awry, and this loss of normal signaling (coordination between the cells among the cells themselves) can occur in any tissue. Broadly speaking, malignant disease may be divided into hematologic cancers and solid tumor cancers. Hematologic cancers originate in the blood, marrow, or lymph fluid, and include leukemia, lymphomas, multiple myeloma, and myeloproliferative neoplasms. Solid tumors originate in the various body organs and include breast, prostate, lung, and colorectal, among many other cancers.

Cancer treatment has traditionally consisted of the triumvirate of surgical therapy, radiation therapy, and systemic therapy. Treatment options vary based on the cancer type, stage, and a patient's general health. Most recently, oncologists have used genomic testing to help inform and tailor treatment choices. Options may be used concurrently, sequentially, or not at all. Treatment goals must be aligned with a careful understanding of the natural history of the disease, the treatment options available, and the patient's other health conditions and functional status. Treatment goals may also change over the course of the illness depending on the type of cancer and stage of disease. Early in the disease process, the goal of treatment could be cure. Later in the disease process, the goal of treatment may be containing the growth of the cancer to prolong survival or improve symptom control (palliate). Treatment goals may also overlap and coexist in various sequences as a patient's need changes.

Diagnosing Cancer

The diagnosis of cancer requires understanding the size, location, type, and most recently, "molecular portrait" of the disease. Screening, lab tests, biopsies, imaging, and other tests contribute to understanding the type of cancer and its stage of disease as well as determining what treatments may be most effective. Cancer staging refers to the extent of the disease and typically takes into account the tumor's location and size, the cell type, and whether the cancerous cells have spread to nearby lymph nodes or elsewhere in the body. Tumor grade refers to how abnormal the cells look and how likely the tumor is to grow and spread.

Solid tumors refer to a mass of cancer cells that grow in organ systems and can occur anywhere in the body (e.g., breast, colon, lung). Surgery, chemotherapy, and/or radiation may all be used to treat solid tumors. Many hematologic cancers are diagnosed by a bone marrow aspiration, in which a small piece of marrow is removed and examined by a pathologist. Others are diagnosed by an excisional biopsy of a lymph node. These hematological cancers occur in the blood, bone marrow, or lymph nodes and include types of leukemia, lymphoma, multiple myeloma, and myeloproliferative disorders.

Hematological cancers are treated systemically and/or with a combination of chemotherapy and stem cell transplant (previously referred to as bone marrow transplant). A stem cell transplant replaces diseased bone marrow with healthy cells. The replacement cells can either come from one's own body or from a donor. A stem cell transplant, also known as a hematopoietic stem cell transplant, can be used to treat leukemia, myeloma, lymphoma, and other blood and immune system diseases that affect bone marrow.

Treating Cancer

Surgical Therapy

Oncologists use several types of surgical methods to diagnose, stage, and treat cancer and precancerous conditions, as well as to manage functional problems or appearance changes caused by cancer and/or its treatment. Surgery may involve a full or partial removal of solid malignant tumors and be used alone or in combination with other anticancer therapies. In certain situations, anticancer therapies like chemotherapy or radiation therapy, may be given to shrink larger cancers before surgery. Surgical techniques have been refined over time and are more precise, promote easier recovery, and are less disfiguring, in general. Similarly, assessment of local cancer spread is also more precise. Side effects may be related to other health conditions or surgical complications with potential impact subsequent physical function. Longer-term effects such as lymphedema may also occur (Morita et al., 2018).

Radiation Therapy

The concept of using radiation to treat cancer emerged in the early twentieth century. The primary goal of radiation therapy is to minimize spread to adjacent tissues. Radiation therapy is most commonly delivered through an external beam. The radiation dose and the frequency of delivery, once or twice daily, depends on the type and location of the cancer and its stage. Radiation may also be delivered directly into the tumor as brachytherapy. Brachytherapy is not an option for all cancers. These developments in radiation oncology have resulted in more precise and directed therapy. Common side effects are local skin changes and fatigue. Occasionally, nearby organs may be adversely affected (Gunderson & Tepper, 2015). For advanced solid tumors, radiation therapy is used to treat bone metastases and symptoms.

Systemic Therapy

The chemicals used in cytotoxic (cell destroying) treatments were initially developed for warfare in World War I. The observation that mustard gas destroyed lymphatic tissue led to experiments by Louis Goodman and Alfred Gilman at Yale. In 1946, they published an article in the *Journal of the American Medical Association* and reported that systemic therapy or chemotherapy had caused cancer regression in their studies.

Scientists' understanding of the molecular and genetic biology of cancer has grown dramatically in the twenty-first century. Therapeutic options for systemic control may include hormonal blockade for tumors sensitive to hormonal manipulation, immunotherapies, and targeted therapies. Immunotherapies may include treatments that restore the patient's own immune response—monoclonal antibodies. These monoclonal antibodies block cancer cell growth by attaching to its intended "antigen" target. Some drugs are combination cytotoxic chemotherapy and monoclonal antibody. Targeted therapies block specific proteins critical to cancer cell growth, may be used to inhibit cancer cell growth in hereditary cancers, and are often used in combination with other cancer drug therapies. Immunotherapies in development include cancer vaccines.

Systemic therapies are intended to enter the bloodstream to reach their intended target after being delivered intravenously, subcutaneously, orally, or directly into an area affected by the cancer, such as intravesical chemotherapy into the bladder, chemoembolization into the tumor itself, or intrathecal chemotherapy into the spinal column. Single drug or combination drug therapies may be utilized depending on the type of cancer and its stage. All dividing cells are thought to be susceptible to chemotherapy. Although an array of side effects is possible, the individual patient's experience is not clearly predictable. Side effects are generally attributed to the disruption and destruction of rapidly growing normal cells such as hair and cells in the reproductive system or gastrointestinal tract. Additionally, side effects may affect the brain and emotions directly or indirectly. The impact of a cancer diagnosis on the person's emotional and spiritual being can be significant (Kerr & Baumann, 2016).

Clinical Trials

Clinical trials provide the foundation on which clinical progress is built. Carefully designed and undertaken in all aspects of cancer therapy—surgical, radiation, and systemic, clinical trials help oncologists understand which treatments best improve outcomes and teach all members of the care team about the disease process and treatment effects. The incredible vision, trust, and compassion of the clinical research teams and the patients and families who have participated in these studies over time have changed the course of cancer.

Emerging Therapies

As noted, oncologists are increasingly considering emerging treatment approaches such as immunotherapy. A dramatic shift in how we treat cancer, immunotherapy is a type of biological therapy that uses substances made from living organisms to treat cancer by reinforcing the body's defenses. As part of its normal function, the immune system detects and destroys abnormal cells and likely prevents or curbs the growth of many cancers. Even though the immune system can prevent or slow cancer growth, cancer cells can sometimes evade destruction by the immune system.

Two leading forms of approved immunotherapies are immune checkpoint inhibitors and cellular immunotherapy. Immune checkpoint inhibitors work by teaching immune cells to attack the pathways where cancer grows. Tumor cells can camouflage themselves by sending false signals to immune cell "checkpoints" so they look harmless. Checkpoint inhibitor drugs block these false signals, so the immune system is not tricked into ignoring tumors. Chimeric antigen receptor therapy (CAR-T) is a form of cellular immunotherapy that uses modified white blood cells—T cells—to attack cancer cells. A sample of T cells is taken from the patient's body and reengineered in a lab setting to produce chimeric antigen receptors (CARs). When they are reinfused into the patients' body as CAR-T cells, they can recognize cancer cells and prevent their growth. Although not yet as widely used as surgery, chemotherapy, or radiation therapy, immunotherapy is emerging as the future of treatment for many cancers, particularly blood cancers.

History of Oncology Social Work

Oncology social work has enjoyed a rich and evolving history over the past 50 years. The practice has mirrored the evolution of cancer treatment and the need to support the "whole person" versus simply treating the disease. Unsurprisingly, the clinical interventions that oncology social workers bring to the field have evolved accordingly to match the changing needs of cancer survivors and cancer treatment.

Social workers have contributed to the care of the medically ill since the early twentieth century. In the early 1970s, oncology social work emerged as a subspecialty of medical social work that provided direct psychosocial care to people with cancer and their loved ones. Oncology social workers help patients by providing emotional, practical, and social supports for the challenges cancer brings, including coping with the diagnosis itself, communicating with family and friends, employment concerns, access to health care coverage, and other practical concerns. The psychological impact of cancer can include distress, anxiety, depression, grief, and bereavement. Oncology social workers are often the primary providers of mental health for patients on the oncology team (Fleishman & Messner, 2015).

As the field of oncology social work has evolved, social workers have established themselves as integral members of interdisciplinary cancer care teams. Oncology social workers provide education and support programs not only to patients but often also to staff. As advocates for patients affected by cancer and who may have limited access to care, oncology social workers are also increasingly involved with psychosocial research and in policymaking.

Another significant shift that has occurred in the field of cancer treatment is that most care is now provided in the outpatient or ambulatory setting. Much of the supportive care that a patient once received in a hospital setting they now receive in the outpatient arena or from family, friends, and other loved ones of the patient. Because cancer affects not just the patient but all those who care for and about them, social workers tailor psychosocial services in a manner that considers the needs of the patient and their extended community.

One of the first books published about social work practice in oncology was Ruth Abrams's 1974 *Not Alone With Cancer*. Abrams reflected on the fears, anxieties, and suffering that cancer generated and the "wall of silence" that existed around cancer when she was writing. Not knowing the etiologies of the disease or the ways to eradicate it created a widespread fear of contagion that resulted in stigmatization and isolation of cancer patients (Hedlund, 2015).

During the 1990s, as a result of progress in understanding and treating cancer, society's thinking about the disease began to shift from always seeing cancer as an acute, life-threatening illness to addressing it more like a chronic disease. With this shift came a greater emphasis on quality of life and how to cope with chronic illness. At the same time, researchers worked to develop cancer treatments that were effective in curing or treating the disease but with fewer side effects.

Cancer-related psychosocial care has become a firmly established field with its own journals, scientific meetings, and professional societies. Support groups have emerged as a resource for information and support and a place for people to share experiences. Groups and other psychosocial services are most often provided by oncology social workers, which has increased professional and patient and family confidence in the therapeutic value of psychosocial support and strengthened the social work role.

Current Trends in Psychosocial Care

As cancer treatments have become more complex, so has psychosocial care. With the shift to outpatient care as the norm for treatment, families are needing to access services that provide support during the experience. While less toxic treatments create fewer side effects, receiving care at home or in an outpatient facility has presented different challenges to patients and families. Some people report experiencing isolation in the cancer journey, a phenomenon that seems to be occurring more often than when there was frequent contact with an inpatient cancer team.

The 2008 Institute of Medicine report, *Cancer Care for the Whole Person: Meeting Psychosocial Health Needs*, brought important attention to the need for greater support for patients and families than what we have been providing. The report presented substantial evidence for the effectiveness of a range of psychosocial services, including counseling and psychotherapy, self-management and self-care programs, family and caregiver education, and health promotion interventions. The study also reported that despite the evidence that these interventions were successful, many individuals who could benefit from these services did not receive them.

The National Comprehensive Cancer Network was among the first organizations to propose interdisciplinary guidelines related to psychosocial care.

These guidelines, first issued in 1999, focus on the recognition and management of distress in patients with cancer, which led to the inclusion of distress screening as a routine part of care. In 2012, the American College of Surgeons' Commission on Cancer (COC) initiated new standards for all accredited cancer programs that has affected the role of psychosocial support services. By 2015, all accredited cancer centers had to implement three components of psychosocial care: patient navigation, which attempts to assess, identify, and eliminate barriers to access to cancer treatment; implementation of distress screening for all newly diagnosed patients being treated at the cancer center; and implementation of survivorship care planning (COC, 2022). Each of these standards has evolved over time, and oncology social workers (who also are represented on the COC) have given input to strengthen and fine-tune these important initiatives.

A range of models of psychosocial support exist nationally. In smaller, community-based health care systems, oncology social workers in hospitals may assist patients with discharge planning and coordinate care with community-based agencies, such as the American Cancer Society, Cancer*Care*, or the Leukemia and Lymphoma Society. They also facilitate support or psychoeducation groups. Technology has made some of these services available over the telephone or via the Internet, increasing patient access.

In larger settings, including academic medical settings, oncology social workers may provide psychosocial screening and assessment of at-risk patients, offer short- and/or long-term counseling regarding adjustment to illness, engage in patient and colleague advocacy, and participate in program development and research. All oncology social workers, however, help patients and families better understand treatments and services and cope with the emotions surrounding cancer and its treatment; assist with managing treatment-related side effects; suggest behavioral changes to minimize disease impact; manage disruptions in work, school, and family life; and locate and secure financial assistance.

Psychosocial Needs of Oncology Patients

Numerous studies have demonstrated the association of psychosocial morbidity with maladaptive coping, reduction of quality of life, impairment in social relationships, risk of suicide, longer rehabilitation time, poorer treatment compliance, and family distress. The most frequently reported psychological challenges for people with cancer are adjustment disorders (20%–25%).

Depressive disorders have also received much attention in oncology, with 25%–75% of oncology patients reporting symptoms (Caruso et al., 2017). The prevalence of depression varies depending on the studies, the contexts, and the stage of cancer. Approximately 30% of oncology patients report having anxiety and stress-related disorders. Increasingly, post-traumatic stress disorder is being identified in oncology patients, with 7%–15% prevalence (Cordova et al., 2017). Cancer diagnosis and treatment can be traumatic stressors; additionally, many patients may have preexisting experiences of trauma. Oncology social workers, as the primary mental health providers in oncology settings, can and should be well trained to identify, assess, and either treat or refer for care.

Additionally, as cancer survivorship is now recognized as a distinct phase along the cancer continuum, and as the COC now evaluates programs on their survivorship initiatives, oncology social workers are often involved in developing services and programs to serve the diverse needs of cancer survivors. As is woven throughout this book, palliative care is increasingly offered concurrently with cancer treatment; in many settings, it is embedded within the oncology service line and clinics. Ideally, this serves to enhance patients' quality of life regardless of the stage of disease.

Challenges of New Treatment Approaches

The emergence both of new therapies such as CAR-T and other immunotherapies and genetic testing as a form of cancer prevention is both exciting and challenging, as they present new issues for patients to consider. Decisions about treatment, clinical trials, and genetic risk are all complex issues to navigate both practically and psychologically. Oncology social workers can help patients navigate many of these concerns.

Additionally, treatment—including new treatments—can be expensive. Studies have revealed how the financial toxicity of cancer has had serious effects on cancer patients and their families (Carrera et al., 2018). While pharmaceutical drug manufacturers are often willing to provide some therapies to patients at no charge, minimizing the costs, for other patients, the out-of-pocket expenses are extreme. Medical expenses can devastate a patient's finances; in some cases, patients and families are forced to declare medical bankruptcy. Social workers can and should continue to advocate for change that provides better and more equitable access to care and medication. All these emerging therapies will create new needs in the realm of cancer survivorship and needed support services (Box 1.1).

Box 1.1

Peter is a 20-year-old male who presented to his college's health center with concerns for increasing fatigue and sense of general malaise. These symptoms had worsened over the last two weeks. When he began to feel feverish on the morning of presentation, he thought he had developed the flu, and sought care. Clinical evaluation resulted in the diagnosis of acute lymphoblastic leukemia, Ph chromosome positive. The medical team met with the patient and outlined a treatment approach that included standard chemotherapy plus a targeted therapy to address the finding of Philadelphia chromosome positivity. They explained that the addition of targeted therapy in this setting will increase his chance for remission. The clinical team also discussed the impact of the diagnosis and the treatment on a patient's life. They introduced the multidisciplinary approach to cancer care and, specifically, offered fertility preservation interventions and a meeting with the medical social worker to address potential financial toxicity risks and psychosocial stressors.

The medical social worker subsequently met with the patient and his parents to discuss the treatment course, disruption of his normal life (interruption of school, need to move back home with parents, and insurance issues). They also discussed the possibility of "normal" psychological reactions to the diagnosis, including fear, grief, sadness, and existential distress. Resources were offered that included patient and family counseling, referral to a young adult cancer support group, and financial assistance. Additional proactive referrals included referrals to nutritional care, pre-habilitative care, and integrative care with the goal of normalizing "need" and maintaining well-being.

The field of cancer treatment has changed in important and profound ways in the past 50 years. Greater attention to care of the "whole person" including managing physical side-effects, quality of life, attending to the psychosocial aspects of care, and working as an interdisciplinary team will remain important as the field continues to grow and change. As always, the patient should be at the center of all we do.

Guiding Best Practices for the Future

Cancer Disparities and Access to Care

Recent attention to access to care and the deep disparities that exist for patients of color and other marginalized and underserved communities has sounded an alarm in cancer programs across the nation (Zavala et al., 2021). America's long history of systemic structural racism, discrimination, and distrust and decreased access to health care results in late diagnoses and worsened health outcomes. Compounded by comorbidities, disparate exposures to carcinogens and psychosocial stress, genetics, and differences in the individual's microbiome, disparities in outcomes are the product of multiple factors (Tsion et al., 2021). Improvements in health equity will require a multifaceted, multidisciplinary, whole-system, team-based approach. Understanding and addressing these disparities has become a priority for many national cancer-related organizations as well as for individual health systems. New laws, such as the Affordable Care Act, and associated policies have increased equitable access to care; however, much work has yet to be done. Social workers are trained to understand the important influence of social determinants of health. Oncology social workers can also partner with communities and agencies that represent vulnerable populations to enhance awareness, build trusting relationships, and address barriers to care through social interventions and advocacy.

The Impact of COVID-19 on Cancer Care

Significant disruptions in breast, colorectal, and cervical cancer screenings during COVID-19 have been noted in cancer programs across the United States. Of particular concern is the considerable number of postponed screenings in the federally qualified health systems that typically serve the most vulnerable (Fisher-Borne et al., 2021). Delays in screening may result in later diagnosis and poorer treatment outcomes. Without purposeful intervention, pandemic-related disruptions in preventive services may widen cancer disparities.

The ultimate impact of COVID-19 pandemic on cancer care has yet to be determined. Researchers are concerned about the risks of "long COVID" symptoms and syndromes to cancer patients. Additionally, the impact of delays in treatment due to COVID-19 will result in cancer progression and mortality. Fortunately, state and national agencies have created COVID-19 databases with cancer registries to study the impacts. The medical community has come together in unprecedented ways to investigate, collaborate, and innovate with technology. The longitudinal data regarding the consequences of COVID-19 on patient care and outcomes will be important to study (Desai et al., 2021).

Patient/Family Advisory Councils

Increasingly, medical practitioners are seeking the patient voice in cancer program development. Patient/family advisory councils (PFACs) have existed for a while in some National Cancer Institute–designated cancer programs, and the "triple aim," which focuses on better outcomes, reduced costs, and patient satisfaction has elevated the focus on having the patient voice at the table (Berwick et al., 2008; Institute for Patient- and Family-Centered Care, n.d.). The benefits include having an effective mechanism for receiving and responding to patient input. PFACs can also lead to increased understanding and respectful and effective partnerships among patients, families, and professionals.

The Need for Team-Based Care

As the complexities of cancer treatment continue to emerge as well as the focus on treating the "whole person," the need for team-based care is more evident than ever. In addition to the physician specialists in various oncology treatments, the value of skilled nurses, rehabilitation specialists, dieticians, pharmacists, chaplains, social workers, and other mental health providers are paramount. Patients and their loved ones can benefit from having access to these specialists. Additionally, these professionals can support one another in treating patients, developing programs, and sharing the "journey" of caring for seriously ill patients together. The expression "it takes a village" is well-applied to the cancer experience.

Pearls

- Cancer treatment is tailored to cancer biology.
- Cancer treatment impacts the whole person.
- Cancer clinical trials advance knowledge.
- Psychosocial support services should be offered proactively.

Pitfalls

- Cancers are many diseases, so no "one approach" will fit all.
- Cancer survivors are a varied and diverse group, and further study is needed to tailor care to individuals.
- Health equity remains a challenge in access to care and treatment. This will not be quickly or easily resolved.
- Financial toxicity is an essential topic yet to be resolved.

Additional Resources

American Society of Clinical Oncology (ASCO) Cancer Basics: www.cancer.net/navigating-cancer-care/cancer-basics
Cancer*Care*: www.cancercare.org
ASCO, Current Initiatives: https://www.asco.org/news-initiatives/current-initiatives/cancer-care-initiatives/team-based-care-oncology
National Cancer Institute (NCI): www.cancer.gov
NCI Center to Reduce Cancer Health Disparities: www.cancer.gov/about-nci/organization/crchd
American College of Surgeons Commission on Cancer, Standards and Resources: https://www.facs.org/quality-programs/cancer/coc/standards
Yale School of Medicine, Clinical Trials: https://medicine.yale.edu/ycci/clinicaltrials/learnmore/tradition/chemotherapy/

References

Abrams, R. (1974). *Not alone with cancer: A guide for those who care, what to expect, what to do.* Charles C. Thomas.
Berwick, D. M., Nolan, T. W., & Whittington, J. (2008). The triple aim: Care, health, and cost. *Health Affairs*, *27*(3), 759–769. https://doi.org/10.1377/hlthaff.27.3.759
Carrera, P. M., Kantarjian, H. M., & Binder, V. S. (2018). The financial burden and distress of patients with cancer: Understanding and stepping-up action on the financial toxicity of cancer treatment. *CA: A Cancer Journal for Clinicians*, *68*(2), 153–165. https://doi.org/10.3322/caac.21443
Caruso, R., Nanni, M. G., Riba, M. B., Sabato, S., & Grassi, I. (2017). The burden of psychosocial morbidity related to cancer: Patient and family issues. *International Review of Psychiatry*, *29*, 389–402. https://doi.org/10.1080/09540261.2017.1288090
Commission on Cancer. (2022). *Optimal resources for cancer care.* Retrieved July 28, 2023, from https://www.facs.org/quality-programs/cancer-programs/commission-on-cancer/standards-and-resources/2020/
Cordova, M. J., Riba, M. B., & Speigel, D. (2017). Post-traumatic stress disorder and cancer. *Lancet Psychiatry*, *4*, 330–338. https://doi.org/10.1016/S2215-0366(17)30014-7
Desai, A., Mohammed, T. J., & Duma, N. (2021, September 2). COVID-19 and cancer: A review of registry-based pandemic response. *JAMA Oncology*, *7*(12), 1882–1890. https://doi.org/10.1001/jamaoncol.2021.4083
Fisher-Borne, M., Isher-Witt, J., Comstock, S., & Perkins, R. B. (2021). Understanding COVID-19 impact on cervical, breast, and colorectal cancer screening among federally qualified healthcare centers participating in "Back on track with screening" quality improvement projects. *Preventive Medicine*, *151*, 106681. https://doi.org/10.1016/j.ypmed.2021.106681
Fleishman, S. B., & Messner, C. (2015). Cancer in contemporary society: Grounding in oncology and psychosocial care. In C. Christ, C. Messner, & L. Behar (Eds.), *Handbook of Oncology Social Work* (pp. 3–8). Oxford University Press.
Gunderson, L. L., & Tepper, J. E. (2015). *Clinical radiation oncology*. Elsevier Health Sciences.
Hedlund, S. (2015). Oncology social work: Past, present, and future. In G. Christ, C. Messner, & L. Behar (Eds.), *Handbook of Oncology Social Work* (pp. 9–14). Oxford University Press.

Institute for Patient- and Family-Centered Care. (n.d.). *Effective patient and family advisory councils*. Retrieved June 19, 2022, from https://www.ipfcc.org/bestpractices/sustainable-partnerships/engaging/effective-pfacs.html

Institute of Medicine. (2008). *Cancer care for the whole patient: Meeting psychosocial health needs*. National Academies Press. https://doi.org/10.17226/11993.

Kerr, D. J., & Baumann, M. (Eds.). (2016). *Oxford textbook of oncology*. Oxford University Press.

Morita, S. Y., Balch, C. R., Klimberg, V. S., Pawlik, T. M., Posner, M. C., & Tanabe, K. K. (2018). *Textbook of complex general surgical oncology*. McGraw Hill.

Mukherjee, S. (2010). *The emperor of all maladies: A biography of cancer*. Scribner.

Siegel, R. L., Miller, K. D., & Jemal, A. (2020). Cancer statistics, 2020. *CA: A Cancer Journal for Clinicians, 70*(1), 7–30. https://doi.org/10.3322/caac.21590

Tsion, Z. M., Kiely, M., Aja, A., & Ambs, S. (2021). An overview of cancer health disparities: New approaches and insights and why they matter. *Carcinogenesis, 42*(1), 2–13. https://doi.org/10.1093/carcin/bgaa121

Zavala, V. A., Bracci, P. M., Carethers, J. M., Carvajal-Carmona, L., Coggins, M. B., Curz-Correa, M. R., Davis, M., deSmith, A. J., Dutil, J., Figueiredo, J. C., Fox, R., Graves, K. D., Gomez, S. L., Llera, A., Neuhausen, S. L., Newman, L., Nguyen, T., Palmer, J. R., Palmer, N. R., . . . Fejerman, L. (2021). Cancer health disparities in racial/ethnic minorities in the United States. *British Journal of Cancer, 124*(2), 315–332. https://doi.org/10.1038%2Fs41416-020-01038-6

2

The Changing Landscape of Cancer Treatment

Heidi Ko, Eric Chang, Marcela Mazo Canola, Zoe Tao, Daniel Hughes, Krista Nelson, and Timothy Siegel

Key Concepts

- As the understanding of the mechanisms of cancer grows, so do treatment approaches that also integrate palliative care along the continuum.
- Great disparities exist in screening, access, and treatment affecting diverse populations and the vulnerable poor.
- The costs of cancer care and resulting financial toxicities are essential issues for oncology social workers to address.
- As cancer survivors live longer, support services should be developed that are tailored to their unique needs.

Keywords: chemotherapy, financial toxicity, immunotherapy, novel treatments, palliative care, radiation therapy, surgery, survivorship

Cancer as a Chronic Disease

In the war against cancer, strategic battles have been won. Although cancer incidence rates continue in a seemingly inevitable, upward trend, advances in early detection and treatments have improved survival rates for nearly all cancers. Indeed, individuals with advanced "incurable" solid tumors and hematologic malignancies are now celebrating more birthdays due to these key advancements. As a result, cancer has shifted from being a disease characterized as always and rapidly fatal to more of a chronic condition that patients may deal with for an extended period of their lives (American Cancer Society, 2019). The effect of this elongated disease trajectory on the psychosocial well-being of patients is just now starting to become apparent. With long-term

Heidi Ko, Eric Chang, Marcela Mazo Canola, Zoe Tao, Daniel Hughes, Krista Nelson, and Timothy Siegel, *The Changing Landscape of Cancer Treatment* In: *Oncology and Palliative Social Work*. Edited by: Susan Hedlund, Bryan Miller, Grace Christ, and Carolyn Messner, Oxford University Press. © Oxford University Press 2024. DOI: 10.1093/oso/9780197607299.003.0002 cancer survivorship comes a need for allied health care professionals to better understand and help patients, caregivers, and the larger community and help them meet previously invisible and misunderstood needs.

Another change in the landscape of cancer treatment is the emergence of precision medicine in oncology. Precision medicine takes into account individual differences in genetic composition, environment, and lifestyle as well as tumor variability in molecular phenotypes to prevent, diagnose, and treat cancer (Lancet, 2021). Understanding the inter- and intratumor variability in genes and tumor microenvironment has led to development of immunotherapy that modulates the tumor microenvironment and therapies targeted toward the specific oncogenic drivers of the tumor. This inter- and intravariability approach should also be applied when assessing the biopsychosocial impact of these treatments on the individual, their primary caregivers, and the communities to which they belong. Little is known of the long-term psychosocial implications of precision medicine on the cancer patient's life, which means individualized precision management of the psychosocial aspects of their survivorship will be equally as important as treating the biological cancer. This chapter discusses advances in medical, radiation, and surgical oncology; how practitioners in these fields have recalibrated their approach; and the importance of social workers in integrating a meaningful psychosocial support as part of the overall treatment strategy.

Targeted Therapy Toward Molecular and Genetic Alterations

One of the earliest targeted therapies was applied in cases of breast cancer after George Thomas Beatson made the critical observation that surgical removal of the ovaries and subsequent reduction in a patient's circulating estrogens led to regression of breast cancer growth and clinical improvements (Marth, 2008; Meisel et al., 2018). Formulated in the late 1960s, a selective estrogen receptor modulator, tamoxifen, became the first clinically usable antiestrogen drug that was an alternative to surgical removal or radiotherapeutic ablation of endocrine glands. Tamoxifen blocks the effects of estrogen in the breast tissue by binding to estrogen receptors on cell surfaces in a competitive manner; it has become the mainstay of endocrine intervention in breast cancer. The discovery of tamoxifen marked the beginning of the era of precision oncology (Meisel et al., 2018). Other early targeted therapies emerged from scientific advances related to understanding the amplification of the gene that encodes human epidermal growth factor receptor 2 (HER2) cell surface protein (1980s) and understanding kinase structure variations (2000s).

In the early 1990s, a humanized monoclonal antibody directed at the extracellular domain of the transmembrane receptor HER2, trastuzumab, was developed and found to be safe and effective in HER2+ breast cancer. In 1989, trastuzumab became the first HER2-targeted therapy approved by the U.S. Food and Drug Administration (FDA) for treatment of HER2-overexpressing metastatic breast cancer (Nahta & Esteva, 2007). Similarly, in chronic myelogenous leukemia, breakthroughs in research around the molecular significance of chromosomal translocation between chromosomes 9 and 22 led to development of effective treatment strategy with small molecule tyrosine kinase inhibitor called imatinib or Gleevec in the early 2000s (Capdeville et al., 2002).

More recently, increasing knowledge of molecular pathways has led to exponential growth of technologies for detecting actionable genetic alterations and availability of targeted agents. For example, related to treatments for non-small-cell lung cancer (NSCLC), researchers have identified such actionable molecular alterations as epidermal growth factor receptor (EGFR), anaplastic lymphoma kinase gene rearrangement, RAS mitogen-activated protein kinase (RAS-MAPK), and NTRK/ROS1. Several drugs targeting these molecular alterations have emerged as first-line treatments and effective therapies in NSCLC. In colorectal cancer, drugs targeted at molecular pathways such as vascular endothelial growth factor, EGFR, and BRAF/MEK/MAP kinase have increasingly emerged as important treatment strategies.

The discovery of novel targeted therapies has led to increased tumor testing and sequencing. A recent National Cancer Institute Molecular Analysis for Therapy Choice (NCI-MATCH) study reported that in this era of precision oncology, clinicians can perform large-scale, pan-cancer tumor testing to identify clinically actionable molecular alterations (Flaherty et al., 2020). Similarly, genetic testing for cancer susceptibility genes has also expanded. The most common mutations are among homologous recombination (HR) pathway genes and Lynch syndrome, a heritable colon cancer. Germline mutations in HR pathway genes, such as BRCA 1/2 mutations, account for 5%–10% of all breast cancers and are associated with an elevated lifetime risk of breast, ovarian, pancreatic, and prostate cancer. Poly (ADP-ribose) polymerases (PARP) inhibitors (PARPi) are a class of anticancer drugs that use a principle called "synthetic lethality" in which simultaneous occurrence of two defects results in cell death. These drugs target PARP enzymes, which are responsible for repairing single-strand breaks (SSBs) in DNA; when this process is interrupted, SSBs progress into double-strand breaks (DSBs) in DNA. In normal cells, HR pathway genes can repair DSBs; however, HR-deficient cells, such as in BRCA 1/2-mutant tumors, cannot repair the damage from PARP inhibitors, which causes subsequent cell death. PARP inhibitors such as olaparib, talazoparib, and rucaparib have shown clinical benefits in many germline HR-deficient tumors (breast, ovarian, prostate, and pancreatic) (Bernstein-Molho et al., 2021; Owens et al., 2019).

In this changing landscape of oncology, all allied health care professionals including oncology and palliative care social workers must ensure that all patients have access to advanced types of testing and treatment and address social determinants of health (SDOH), such as inadequate insurance coverage or financial instability, in the practice setting so that SDOH in no way interfere with equitable access to these advances.

Immunotherapy: Immune Checkpoint Inhibitors, CAR-T Cell, and Cancer Vaccines

Many people think of immunotherapy as a recent medical achievement; however, it originated in the third century with the use of inoculation with variola minor virus to prevent smallpox. Considered the "father of immunotherapy," around 1891 William Bradley Coley directly observed several cases of patients that went into spontaneous remission after developing erysipelas. His observation led him to inoculate tumors with different mixtures of inactive *Streptococcus pyogenes* and *Serratia marcescens*, the first immune-based treatment for cancer. Coley's clinical results were described in 1893 with durable and complete responses in several tumor types. Despite this success, few oncologists used the "Coley Toxins" due to their lack of knowledge about how the action mechanism worked (Dobosz & Dzieciatkowski, 2019).

Interest in immunotherapy resurfaced in the 1960s with the discovery of T cells and understanding of their crucial role in immunity, which paved the way for later physicians and scientists to pioneer bone-marrow transplant as a treatment for hematological malignancies (Pavletic & Armitage, 1996). With further understanding of the basics of cancer immunotherapy, Schreiber et al. (2011) proved that T cells were able to provide antitumor responses—this led to the discovery of antibody-based therapies.

Undoubtedly the most promising medications in cancer research are immune checkpoint inhibitors (ICIs). Brunet et al. discovered the first ICI molecule in 1987 and named it cytotoxic T lymphocyte antigen 4 (CTLA-4). Later, CTLA-4 was tested in animals, which led to the development of ipilimumab in 2011 for the treatment of advanced melanoma. Since then, other ICIs such as nivolumab, atezolizumab, and pembrolizumab have helped multiple patients around the world.

Vaccines have had a significant, positive impact on medicine and global health. Just as the immune system protects humans from harmful bacteria and parasites, it also plays a vital role in cancer prevention. Research that led to the development of the human papillomavirus (HPV) and hepatitis B vaccine (HBV), for example, highlighted how viral carcinogenesis works, and widespread vaccination for these viruses has prevented infection and effectively lowered incidences of the cancers that they once caused. To date, there are two main types of cancer vaccines under development. Whereas autologous vaccines use the patient's own cells, which are extracted and multiplied in a laboratory setting and then reinjected into the circulatory system, allogenic vaccines are made from laboratory-cultivated cells from external individuals of the same species. Both work by triggering the immune system, which in turn attacks cancer cells. Although these new vaccines are in the initial stages of research and development, multiple approaches are under investigation combining emerging technologies with conventional treatments.

Another revolutionary therapy is the use of chimeric antigen receptor T cells (CAR-T cells), which are T cells genetically modified to target cancer cells. First described in the 1990s, CAR-T cell therapy was FDA approved (after years of research) in 2017 for the treatment of hematologic malignancies. CAR-T cell therapy has been successful in reducing the presence of cancer cells. However, the treatment is expensive and has also been associated with a potential serious side effect called cytokine release syndrome (CRS) that can lead to hyperinflammatory syndrome and ultimately, organ damage. Although treatment with CAR-T cells has produced remarkable clinical responses, many challenges persist (Sterner & Sterner, 2021).

The impact of the increased availability of innovative therapies on the psychosocial well-being on patients with cancer and their care partners is still being realized. With the increased availability and use of self-administered oral cancer therapies, cancer treatment has transitioned increasingly into the home setting. As a result, social workers are seeing both the burden of care delivery and associated financial costs falling on individual patients and their support team (if they have one). For example, patients are only eligible for CAR-T cell therapy if they have a 24-hour caregiver, due to potential side effects such as neurotoxicity and cognitive changes. This requirement disproportionately impacts lower socioeconomic populations as well as younger patients who may not have access to a caregiver who is available to provide constant care because they need to work or have no paid leave benefits.

Social workers have been addressing SDOH—"the conditions in which people are born, grow, work, live, age, and the wider set of forces and systems shaping the conditions of daily life" (World Health Organization, n.d.)—for over a hundred years. All health care professionals, however, should pay special attention to how they can effectively address the negative impacts SDOH have on many patients and ensure that all people have equitable access to individualized treatments and high-quality care.

Radiation Oncology and Palliative Care

Radiation oncology, medical oncology, and surgical oncology are the three main branches of oncology care. Paralleling innovations in medical oncology, radiation therapy has also seen significant technological advancements in its delivery, which have improved accuracy and efficacy while also sparing more normal tissues and reducing toxicity. Radiation therapy remains a mainstay of treatment for many types of cancer, with approximately 50% of all cancer patients receiving radiation therapy over the course of their illness, both in the curative and palliative settings (Baskar et al., 2012). As prognoses continue to improve across multiple disease sites, understanding the long-term effects of radiation therapy and how it may be best employed to minimize those effects have become increasingly important. Health care practitioners and oncology social workers have increasingly recognized the importance of involving allied professionals both in the treatment and survivorship of patients treated with radiation therapy in effort to minimize its potential adverse effects on patient's daily functioning and quality of life.

Over the past few decades, radiation oncology has made significant technological advances with the advent of intensity-modulated radiation therapy (IMRT). First introduced in the 1990s, IMRT utilizes complex computer algorithms to design and deliver highly conformal dose distributions, which allows for improved "shaping" of radiation dose around the tumor while sparing adjacent normal tissues (Hong et al., 2005). This technology permits dose escalation, which has increased tumor control and decreased acute and chronic toxicities and morbidity across multiple disease sites (Hong et al., 2005). IMRT rapidly became a fundamental part of radiation therapy, and its use has led to the increase of definitive treatment from 22% in 2004 to 58% in 2017 (Hutten et al., 2022). IMRT also increases the feasibility of organ preservation for patients who may not otherwise tolerate or who may have substantial morbidity from surgical resection.

In particular, IMRT has played a significant role in the treatment of cancers of the head and neck, disease sites in which the effects of radiation therapy can be particularly negatively life-altering (Bhide et al., 2012). Definitive radiotherapy to the head and neck is intensive and often requires the support of social workers, registered dieticians, speech pathologists, physical/occupational therapists, and dentists to effectively manage acute and chronic adverse effects both during and after the completion of treatment. New radiation therapy processes coupled with improvements in prognosis for many subsites. In part, this is driven by increasing prevalence of HPV-mediated oropharynx cancers, which have significantly improved survival rates compared to HPV-negative tumors (Ang et al., 2010). The positive result of patients living longer has raised a corollary need for greater support managing such long-term complications as dry mouth, chronic pain, fatigue, and dysphagia. Studies suggest 60%–65% of patients have at least one unmet survivorship need. Beyond physical symptoms, treatment can have psychological affects due to changes in functionality or appearance, challenges to interpersonal or sexual relationships, and difficulty returning to work (head and neck cancer patients often returning to work less often than patients with other cancers); patients dealing with these "side effects" of survivorship will likely benefit from involvement of mental health services (Miller, 2020; Nguyen & Ringash, 2018). Advances in radiation technology such as IMRT thus must be met with greater research in survivorship care to more effectively support patients with complex disease.

More recently, the development of stereotactic radiosurgery (SRS) and stereotactic body radiation therapy (SBRT) have dramatically altered the approach to and need for traditional radiation therapy. These techniques utilize strict patient immobilization, organ motion management techniques, and stereotactic planning systems to deliver extremely precise, high-dose radiation in either a single dose or small number of treatments with subcentimeter accuracy (Tipton et al., 2011). Across disease sites, these ablative techniques offer a noninvasive outpatient alternative to surgical interventions—for example, in the treatment of brain metastases or early-stage lung cancers—often with minimal morbidity. Particularly significant has been the use of SRS/SBRT in advanced-stage cancer patients, for whom locally aggressive treatments were previously often viewed as futile in the setting of progressing metastatic disease. Improvements in early detection have allowed more diagnoses of patients with single or limited organ metastases, and using SRS/SBRT has led to improved survival rates among these patients (Alongi et al., 2012). Growing evidence exists that using SRS/SBRT for all metastatic sites in patients with limited metastatic burden may improve overall survival in comparison with the current standard of care; this in turn indicates that there may be a role for locally aggressive treatments even in the setting of metastatic disease (Palma et al., 2020). Due to improvements in systemic therapies for metastatic cancer at certain disease sites, health care professionals, patients, and caregivers can now more easily conceptualize cancer as a chronic disease. This is a positive outcome that nonetheless further reinforces the importance of multidisciplinary involvement throughout the entire cancer trajectory since patients who can live with their cancer as a chronic disease are also at risk for developing cumulative toxicities from multiple treatments.

Radiation oncologists play a significant role in managing patients with advanced cancer, with roughly 40% of radiation therapy delivered purely with the palliative intent of relieving morbidity associated with progressing disease (Lam & Tseng, 2019). As such, not all recent developments in the field of radiation oncology have been technological in nature. For example, while not typically considered traditional members of the palliative care team, it has become clear that in addition to delivering palliative radiation therapy, radiation oncologists may also contribute to the multidisciplinary, psychosocial care of patients with advanced cancer by participating in engaging in primary palliative care assessments, goals of care conversations, and discussions of prognosis (Lam & Tseng, 2019). The ability to contribute to a larger care team has coupled with greater recognition of palliative radiation therapy as a unique discipline in which treatment priorities differ from those being treated with curative intent with greater focus on improving patient tolerability, shortening treatment duration, maximizing patient convenience, and reducing financial toxicity. Multiple cancer centers have created dedicated palliative radiation therapy programs that have demonstrated wide-ranging improvements, including increased timeliness of and access to radiation therapy; shorter courses of treatment; improved communication among providers, patients, and caregivers; and more referrals to specialized service providers who can help manage palliative care needs (Johnstone, 2019). Many of these programs directly integrate the support of social work services, which has led to multiple benefits to patients, such as increased completion of advance directives (Cammy, 2017).

Surgical Oncology and Palliative Care

In recent years, palliative care has become increasingly integrated into surgical oncology practice and medical philosophy. While surgery's role in alleviating or worsening suffering is well established, oncology surgeons are interested in developing standards of care and patient education regarding how surgeries can have either or both curative and palliative intent as well as cultivating palliative care competencies among surgical trainees (Fahy, 2013; Miner et al., 2004).

Primary palliative care refers to the ability of nonsubspecialty providers to practice aspects of palliative care such as complex decision-making and pain and symptom management (Ernecoff et al., 2020). Surgeons frequently encounter patients with an abundance of pain, nausea, and functional limitations and must therefore guide both medical and surgical management. Whereas some these patients are near end of life, many may live a number of years more than they might have before technological advancements in cancer treatments but face debilitating acute or chronic conditions.

Starting in 2003, the American College of Surgeons formalized several core competencies of palliative care in surgical training that included communication, pain management, and end-of-life care, underscoring the growing value and emphasis of the alleviation of suffering among surgical patients (Fahy, 2013). Subsequently, many training programs have developed curricula to cultivate primary palliative care skills among surgical trainees (Bradley et al., 2010; Klaristenfeld et al., 2007).

Surgeons also encounter patient scenarios where cure of a primary disease process is unlikely but alleviation of symptoms such as nausea from an obstructing tumor is possible. Surgical procedures performed with palliative intent aim to reduce pain and symptom burden while carefully weighing the risks of morbidity and mortality associated with a given procedure. Examples of procedures with palliative intent are diverse; Shinall (2021) gives the noncancer example of a lower extremity vascular bypass, which does not reverse a patient's underlying peripheral vascular disease but can improve pain and function. Miner et al. (2004) studied over a thousand cancer surgeries performed with palliative intent at a major urban cancer center and found that symptom improvement or resolution was attained within 30 days of the procedure for 80% of the prospective cohort. Notable outcomes related to palliative surgeries are quality-of-life centered, and their success is difficult to quantify by traditional surgical outcome measures such as mortality or length of hospital length. Additionally, disease-specific decision-making regarding palliative surgery can be complex. For patients with poor preoperative functional and nutritional status, palliative procedures may have an unacceptable level of associated morbidity (Miner et al., 2004).

Enhanced recovery pathways for individual procedures, which protocolize preoperative and postoperative treatments such as thromboembolic prophylaxis and advancement of diet following surgery, can decrease length of hospital stays and readmission rates (Li et al., 2022). Preoperative frailty assessments have also gained popularity in determining potentially adverse postoperative outcomes for patients discharged to a rehabilitation or skilled nursing facility (Feng et al., 2015). Additionally, routine implementation of multidisciplinary cancer care for many diseases has allowed extensive lymph node and multivisceral resections to fall out of favor in lieu of sequential cancer treatment involving combinations of chemotherapy, radiation, surgery, and other treatments. For example, as research has demonstrated that extensive resections do not necessarily contribute to survival and can actually lead to worsened morbidity, surgeons have turned to less invasive gastric resection procedures in the 21st century (Terashima, 2021). Subsequently, timely initiation of multiple diagnostic and therapeutic modalities where indicated is considered standard of care and may not always benefit from surgery (Di et al., 2017; Ju et al., 2020).

The surgical community is working to develop an improved evidence base for optimizing patient selection for palliative surgeries, emphasizing quality-of-life measures in curative-intended procedures and teaching and fostering primary palliative care skills in future practicing surgeons. Enthusiasm for palliative care within the surgical community has increased along with a deep desire to become adept in the psychosocial aspects of illness; indeed, these skills have become essential components of good perioperative care.

Integrating the Components of Interdisciplinary Care

Changes in the landscape of medical, radiation, and surgical oncology and palliative care, as previously described, have created a wide array of correlated psychosocial implications that need illumination, understanding, and proper management. For example, many new anticancer medications can now be administered orally, which offers the convenience of avoiding infusion visits. However, this process can leave patients with varying levels of personal health literacy responsible for managing the dose of their medication, enduring potential financial toxicity, and suffering potentially serious physical side effects in a somewhat unsupervised home setting.

Unfortunately, the same cancer treatments that extend the years a patient can live with cancer often do collateral damage to other organs or systems of the body; the results of those damages can manifest themselves immediately or even many years after treatment therapies are completed (Cohen & Jefferies,

2018; Galvão et al., 2018; Sturgeon et al., 2019). Cancer survivorship as a chronic condition will continually challenge survivors' health-related quality of life (HR-QOL) from diagnosis through the end of life (Cohen & Jefferies, 2018; Schmitz et al., 2019). Thus all professional health care providers need to consider the psychosocial constructs of patients living with cancer being managed as a chronic disease, including sometimes less visible factors such as individual health literacy, financial toxicity, time constraints, and concerns about lost productivity or employment for not only the patients but also those who care for them.

The onslaught of the chronic stressors the cancer experience often causes can lead to a long-term downward spiral for a cancer patient's HR-QOL. HR-QOL is multidimensional, consisting of not only physical but also mental and spiritual domains of the human experience. To optimize long-term survivorship and HR-QOL for patients with cancer, a shift is needed that focuses on the "whole" person (body, mind, and spirit). Each survivor is on an individual cancer journey with different starting points and long-term potential trajectories. For many patients with cancer, the cancer experience often constrains their HR-QOL by reducing their functional capacities and social connectedness and increasing the financial toxicity they face and their perceived level of stress.

Guiding Best Practices for the Future

Innovations in both communication and science have helped social workers better understand the mechanisms of cancer and advanced the development of novel therapies and approaches to cancer treatment. Not only has the presence of "silos" among medical, surgical, and radiation therapies diminished but a stronger focus on palliative care has also seen wider integration throughout the subspecialties. As cancer survivors live longer, the entire care team—especially social workers—must pay greater attention to the long-term impacts of survival on both patients and their loved ones from a "whole person" perspective. Additionally, social workers must be aware how disparities persist that limit screening, access to treatment, and approaches to care for people of color and/or the vulnerable poor. More research is needed to understand the barriers that exist to equitable access to quality cancer care and find ways to overcome those barriers (e.g., optimal and equitable use of telehealth) in order to increase access to care for those most affected. Finally, attention must be paid to the negative financial impacts and resulting financial toxicity of cancer treatment, especially in light of ever-increasing health care costs. The ideal approach to "whole person" cancer care should be both transdisciplinary and trans-specialty.

Pearls

- As treatment approaches for cancer evolve, so must the understanding of needed support for "whole person" care.
- Cancer survivors are diverse. Support services should be tailored accordingly.
- A transdisciplinary, trans-specialty approach to cancer care is ideal.

Pitfalls

- While much progress in cancer treatment has been made, disparities in screening and access to high-quality and innovative treatments continue to exist.
- The financial burden and resulting financial toxicity of care is increasing as novel treatments develop.
- More research is needed to understand the impact of cancer on diverse populations.

Additional Resources

- National Cancer Institute: www.cancer.gov/about-cancer
- Center to Advance Palliative Care: www.capc.org
- Cancer Support Community, *Get Educated and Inspired*: www.cancersupportcommunity.org/get-educated-inspired

References

Alongi, F., Arcangeli, S., Filippi, A. R., Ricardi, U., & Scorsetti, M. (2012). Review and uses of stereotactic body radiation therapy for oligometastases. *Oncologist*, *17*(8), 1100–1107. https://doi.org/10.1634/theoncologist.2012-0092

American Cancer Society. (n.d.). *Managing cancer as a chronic illness*. Retrieved from https://www.cancer.org/treatment/survivorship-during-and-after-treatment/long-term-health-concerns/cancer-as-a-chronic-illness.html

Ang, K. K., Harris, J., Wheeler, R., Weber, R., Rosenthal, D. I., Nguyen-Tân, P. F., Westra, W. H., Chung, C. H., Jordan, R. C., Lu, C., Kim, H., Axelrod, R., Silverman, C. C., Redmond, K. P., &

Gillison, M. L. (2010). Human papillomavirus and survival of patients with oropharyngeal cancer. *New England Journal of Medicine*, *363*(1), 24–35. https://doi.org/10.1056/NEJMoa0912217

Baskar, R., Lee, K. A., Yeo, R., & Yeoh, K. W. (2012). Cancer and radiation therapy: Current advances and future directions. *International Journal of Medical Sciences*, *9*(3), 193–199. https://doi.org/10.7150/ijms.3635

Bernstein-Molho, R., Evron, E., Yerushalmi, R., & Paluch-Shimon, S. (2021). Genetic testing in patients with triple-negative or hereditary breast cancer. *Current Opinion in Oncology*, *33*(6), 584–590. https://doi.org/10.1097/CCO.0000000000000784

Bhide, S. A., Newbold, K. L., Harrington, K. J., & Nutting, C. M. (2012). Clinical evaluation of intensity-modulated radiotherapy for head and neck cancers. *British Journal of Radiology*, *85*(1013), 487–494. https://doi.org/10.1259/bjr/85942136

Bradley, C. T., Webb, T. P., Schmitz, C. C., Chipman, J. G., & Brasel, K. J. (2010). Structured teaching versus experiential learning of palliative care for surgical residents. *American Journal of Surgery*, *200*(4), 542–547.

Brunet, J. F., Denizot, F., Luciani, M. F., Roux-Dosseto, M., Suzan, M., Mattei, M. G., & Golstein, P. (1987). A new member of the immunoglobulin superfamily—CTLA-4. *Nature*, *328*(6127), 267–270. https://doi.org/10.1038/328267a0

Cammy, R. (2017). Developing a palliative radiation oncology service line: The integration of advance care planning in subspecialty oncologic care. *Journal of Social Work in End-of-Life & Palliative Care*, *13*(4), 251–265. https://doi.org/10.1080/15524256.2017.1400494

Capdeville, R., Buchdunger, E., Zimmermann, J., & Matter, A. (2002). Glivec (STI571, imatinib), a rationally developed, targeted anticancer drug. *Nature Reviews: Drug Discovery*, *1*(7), 493–502. https://doi.org/10.1038/nrd839

Cohen, L., & Jefferies, A. (2018). *Anticancer living: Transform your life and health with the mix of six*. Viking.

Di, L., Wu, H., Zhu, R., Li, Y., Wu, X., Xie, R., Li, H., Wang, H., Zhang, H., Chen, H., Zhen, H., Zhao, K., Yang, X., & Tuo, B. (2017). Multi-disciplinary team for early gastric cancer diagnosis improves the detection rate of early gastric cancer. *BMC Gastroenterology*, *17*(1), 1–9. https://doi.org/10.1186/s12876-017-0711-9

Dobosz, P., & Dzieciątkowski, T. (2019). The intriguing history of cancer immunotherapy. *Frontiers in Immunology*, *10*, 2965. https://doi.org/10.3389/fimmu.2019.02965

Ernecoff, N. C., Check, D., Bannon, M., Hanson, L. C., Dionne-Odom, J. N., Corbelli, J., Klein-Fedyshin, M., Schenker, Y., Zimmermann, C., Arnold, R. M., & Kavalieratos, D. (2020). Comparing specialty and primary palliative care interventions: Analysis of a systematic review. *Journal of Palliative Medicine*, *23*(3), 389–396. https://doi.org/10.1089/jpm.2019.0349

Fahy, B. N. (2013). Palliative care for the surgical oncologist: Embracing the palliativist within. *Surgery*, *153*(1), 1–3. https://doi.org/10.1016/j.surg.2012.06.002

Feng, M. A., McMillan, D. T., Crowell, K., Muss, H., Nielsen, M. E., & Smith, A. B. (2015). Geriatric assessment in surgical oncology: A systematic review. *Journal of Surgical Research*, *193*(1), 265–272. https://doi.org/10.1016/j.jss.2014.07.004

Flaherty, K. T., Gray, R. J., Chen, A. P., Li, S., McShane, L. M., Patton, D., Hamilton, S. R., Williams, P. M., Iafrate, A. J., Sklar, J., Mitchell, E. P., Harris, L. N., Takebe, N., Sims, D. J., Coffey, B., Fu, T., Routbort, M., Zwiebel, J. A., Rubinstein, L. V., . . . NCI-MATCH Team. (2020). Molecular landscape and actionable alterations in a genomically guided cancer clinical trial: National Cancer Institute Molecular Analysis for Therapy Choice (NCI-MATCH). *Journal of Clinical Oncology*, *38*(33), 3883–3894. https://doi.org/10.1200/JCO.19.03010

Galvão, D. A., Taaffe, D. R., Spry, N., Cormie, P., Joseph, D., Chambers, S. K., Chee, R., Peddle-McIntyre, C. J., Hart, N. H., Baumann, F. T., Denham, J., Baker, M., & Newton, R. U. (2018). Exercise preserves physical function in prostate cancer patients with bone metastases. *Medicine & Science in Sports & Exercise*, *50*(3), 393–399. https://doi.org/10.1249/MSS.0000000000001454

Hong, T. S., Ritter, M. A., Tomé, W. A., & Harari, P. M. (2005). Intensity-modulated radiation therapy: Emerging cancer treatment technology. *British Journal of Cancer, 92*(10), 1819–1824. https://doi.org/10.1038/sj.bjc.6602577

Hutten, R. J., Weil, C. R., Gaffney, D. K., Kokeny, K., Lloyd, S., Rogers, C. R., & Suneja, G. (2022). Worsening racial disparities in utilization of intensity modulated radiation therapy. *Advances in Radiation Oncology, 7*(3), 100887. https://doi.org/10.1016/j.adro.2021.100887

Johnstone, C. (2019). Palliative radiation oncology programs: Design, build, succeed! *Annals of Palliative Medicine, 8*(3), 264–273. https://doi.org/10.21037/apm.2018.12.09

Ju, M., Wang, S. C., Syed, S., Agrawal, D., & Porembka, M. R. (2020). Multidisciplinary teams improve gastric cancer treatment efficiency at a large safety net hospital. *Annals of Surgical Oncology, 27*(3), 645–650. https://doi.org/10.1245/s10434-019-08037-9.

Klaristenfeld, D. D., Harrington, D. T., & Miner, T. J. (2007). Teaching palliative care and end-of-life issues: A core curriculum for surgical residents. *Annals of Surgical Oncology, 14*(6), 1801–1806. https://doi.org/10.1245/s10434-006-9324-1

Lam, T. C., & Tseng, Y. (2019). Defining the radiation oncologist's role in palliative care and radiotherapy. *Annals of Palliative Medicine, 8*(3), 246–263. https://doi.org/10.21037/apm.2018.10.02

Lancet. (2021, May 15). *20 years of precision medicine in oncology* [Editorial]. *Lancet, 397*(10287), 1781. https://doi.org/10.1016/S0140-6736(21)01099-0

Li, N., Liu, Y., Chen, H., & Sun, Y. (2022). Efficacy and safety of enhanced recovery after surgery pathway in minimally invasive colorectal cancer surgery: A systemic review and meta-analysis. *Journal of Laparoendoscopic & Advanced Surgical Techniques*. Part A, advance online publication. https://doi.org/10.1089/lap.2022.0349

Marth, C. (2008). Endocrine therapy—What else? *Breast Care 3*(5), 301–302. https://doi.org/10.1159/000160910

Meisel, J. L., Venur, V. A., Gnant, M., & Carey, L. (2018). Evolution of targeted therapy in breast cancer: Where precision medicine began. *American Society of Clinical Oncology Educational Book, 38*, 78–86. https://doi.org/10.1200/EDBK_201037

Miller, A. (2020). Returning to work after head and neck cancer. *Current Opinion in Otolaryngology & Head & Neck Surgery, 28*(3), 155–160. https://doi.org/10.1097/MOO.0000000000000628

Miner, T. J., Brennan, M. F., & Jaques, D. P. (2004). A prospective, symptom related, outcomes analysis of 1,022 palliative procedures for advanced cancer. *Annals of Surgery, 240*(4), 719–727. https://doi.org/10.1097/01.sla.0000141707.09312.dd

Nahta, R., & Esteva, F. J. (2007). Trastuzumab: Triumphs and tribulations. *Oncogene, 26*(25), 3637–3643. https://doi.org/10.1038/sj.onc.1210379

Nguyen, N. A., & Ringash, J. (2018). Head and neck cancer survivorship care: A review of the current guidelines and remaining unmet needs. *Current Treatment Options in Oncology, 19*(8), 44. https://doi.org/10.1007/s11864-018-0554-9

Owens, K., Schlager, L., & Welcsh, P. L. (2019). The impact of germline testing for hereditary cancer postdiagnosis. *American Journal of Managed Care* [Special issue], *25*(9), SP285–SP287.

Palma, D. A., Olson, R., Harrow, S., Gaede, S., Louie, A. V., Haasbeek, C., Mulroy, L., Lock, M., Rodrigues, G. B., Yaremko, B. P., Schellenberg, D., Ahmad, B., Senthi, S., Swaminath, A., Kopek, N., Liu, M., Moore, K., Currie, S., Schlijper, R., . . . Senan, S. (2020). Stereotactic ablative radiotherapy for the comprehensive treatment of oligometastatic cancers: Long-term results of the SABR-COMET Phase II randomized trial. *Journal of Clinical Oncology, 38*(25), 2830–2838. https://doi.org/10.1200/JCO.20.00818

Pavletic, Z. S., & Armitage, J. O. (1996). Bone marrow transplantation for cancer—An update. *Oncologist, 1*(3), 159–168. https://doi.org/10.1634/theoncologist.1-3-159

Schmitz, K. H., Campbell, A. M., Stuiver, M. M., Pinto, B. M., Schwartz, A. L., Morris, G. S., Ligibel, J. A., Cheville, A., Galvão, D. A., Alfano, C. M., Patel, A. V., Hue, T., Gerber, L. H., Sallis, R., Gusani, N. J., Stout, N. L., Chan, L., Flowers, F., Doyle, C., . . . Matthews, C. E. (2019). Exercise is medicine in oncology: Engaging clinicians to help patients move through cancer. *CA: A Cancer Journal for Clinicians*, *69*(6), 468–484. https://doi.org/10.3322/caac.21579

Schreiber, R. D., Old, L. J., & Smyth, M. J. (2011). Cancer immunoediting: Integrating immunity's roles in cancer suppression and promotion. *Science, 331*(6024), 1565–1570. https://doi.org/10.1126/science.1203486

Shinall, M. C., Jr. (2021). "Aren't surgery and palliative care kind of opposites?" *AMA Journal of Ethics*, *23*(10), E823–E825. https://doi.org/10.1001/amajethics.2021.823.

Sterner, R. C., & Sterner, R. M. (2021). CAR-T cell therapy: Current limitations and potential strategies. *Blood Cancer Journal*, *11*(4), 69. https://doi.org/10.1038/s41408-021-00459-7

Sturgeon, K. M., Mathis, K. M., Rogers, C. J., Schmitz, K. H., & Waning, D. L. (2019). Cancer- and chemotherapy-induced musculoskeletal degradation. *JBMR Plus*, *3*(3), e10187. https://doi.org/10.1002/jbm4.10187

Terashima, M. (2021). The 140 years' journey of gastric cancer surgery: From the two hands of Billroth to the multiple hands of the robot. *Annals of Gastroenterological Surgery*, *5*(3), 270–277. https://doi.org/10.1002/ags3.12442

Tipton, K. N., Sullivan, N., Bruening, W., Inamdar, R., Launders, J., Uhl, S., & Schoelles, K. M. (2011). *Stereotactic body radiation therapy*. Rockville, MD: Agency for Healthcare Research and Quality.

World Health Organization. (n.d.). *Social determinants of health*. Retrieved November 28, 2022, from https://www.who.int/health-topics/social-determinants-of-health#tab=tab_1

3

Equity, Racism, Cultural Competence, and Cultural Humility in Oncology Social Work Practice

Eucharia Borden and Jennifer M. Dunn

Key Concepts

- Health inequities in cancer outcomes persist despite significant advancements in research, prevention, and treatment.
- Racism is a public health crisis and a root cause of health inequity.
- Eliminating racism in cancer care requires cultural humility and ethical consideration from social workers.

Keywords: equity, ethics, health care, oncology, palliative care, power imbalance, racism

Cancer Health Disparities in the United States

Despite significant advancements in research and treatment, cancer continues to be a challenging public health crisis in the United States. According to the National Cancer Institute's (NCI), National Institute of Health, cancer incidence and mortality rates are declining in all segments of the U.S. population, however some segments of the population remain at greater risk of developing and dying from certain diagnoses, perpetuating a history of inequities in cancer care. According to the NCI, cancer health disparities occur when there are higher rates of new diagnoses and cancer-related deaths among racial and ethnic groups (NCI, 2022). Despite efforts to equalize outcomes, variations are associated with factors such as race/ethnicity, sexual orientation and gender identity, age, geography, socioeconomic status, and health literacy. Research indicates that Black men and women, people living in rural

Eucharia Borden and Jennifer M. Dunn, *Equity, Racism, Cultural Competence, and Cultural Humility in Oncology Social Work Practice* In: *Oncology and Palliative Social Work*. Edited by: Susan Hedlund, Bryan Miller, Grace Christ, and Carolyn Messner, Oxford University Press. © Oxford University Press 2024. DOI: 10.1093/oso/9780197607299.003.0003 areas, and populations with lower income and education levels continue to experience worse outcomes for any cancer regardless of stage at diagnosis (American Association for Cancer Research [AACR], 2021).

The NCI's Surveillance, Epidemiology, and End Results (SEER) program continues to monitor inequities in cancer incidence specific to race, ethnicity, and demographics. Despite making up only 13% of the U.S. population, Black Americans continue to carry the burden of cancer disparities with rates of prostate, breast, lung, and colorectal cancers greater than any other racial or ethnic group. Regardless of similarities in diagnosis rates, the risk of Black women dying from breast cancer is 39% higher than that of White women. The rate of prostate cancer incidence is one and a half times greater for Black American men, and the death rate is two times greater than any other racial/ethnic group. The incidence rates of Black Americans with multiple myeloma and stomach cancer are significantly higher, with a death rate at least double that of their White counterparts (AACR, 2021).

Although Black Americans carry the greatest burden of cancer health disparities, adverse differences in cancer prevalence are documented among multiple racial and ethnic groups. According to the 2020 AACR Cancer Disparities Progress Report, Asian American/Pacific Islander adults are twice as likely to die from stomach cancer as White adults, while American Indian/Alaska Native adults are twice as likely to develop liver and bile duct cancer as their White counterparts. Due to significantly lower rates of cervical cancer screening, incidence and death rates have been higher for Latina women compared to White women for more than two decades (AACR, 2021).

The etiologies of cancer health disparities are multifactorial and a reflection of the intersection of several factors, including social determinants of health (SDOH). According to the NCI, SDOH are the conditions in which people are born, grow, live, work, and age and are linked with those who are economically, socially, and environmentally disadvantaged creating greater obstacles to health care (NCI, 2022). Structural and institutional racism experienced by communities that are historically marginalized remains an ongoing obstacle to equitable health care. Eliminating disparities in cancer outcomes requires increased attention to racial and ethnic populations and commitment to increasing equity in health care so all persons have a fair and just opportunity to be as healthy as possible.

Health Equality Versus Health Equity

Reducing and eliminating health disparities requires ongoing efforts and long-term commitment to addressing imbalanced social systems that perpetuate inequities in access to health care. According to the Centers for Disease Control and Prevention (CDC), equity in health care is achieved when every person can attain their full health potential, and no one is at a disadvantage because of their socially determined circumstances (NCI, 2022). Per the Race Matters Institute, assuring equity in health care will not be achieved by treating everyone equally. The Equality and Human Rights Commission defines equality as the distribution of the same resources and opportunities to every individual across a population, however, distributing resources equally does not assure fair and nondiscriminatory delivery of services. As defined by the World Health Organization, equity is customized distribution of resources and opportunities to assure no groups are at a particular disadvantage in achieving maximum wellness (Kurapati, 2020). Solely focusing on equal distribution of resources does not account for disparities or SDOH. Health equity redirects resources toward those at greatest risk of poor health outcomes due to their social circumstances while guaranteeing no person is denied access or services for belonging to a population that is historically marginalized. As a result, health disparities are the outcomes used to measure progress toward health equity. Reduction in health disparities indicates movement toward greater health equity and is achieved by commitment to improving the health of those who experience marginalization, both socially and economically (Braveman, 2014).

In 2009, the American Society of Clinical Oncology (ASCO) published the Policy Statement on Cancer Care Disparities affirming the commitment of oncology physicians and health care providers to address disparities that have plagued cancer outcomes and later established a Health Disparities Committee. In 2018, the committee was renamed the Health Equity Committee to reflect the changing focus of improving health equity across the continuum of cancer care and laid out a comprehensive set of strategic goals to achieve cancer health equity. These goals include improving equitable access to cancer care, ensuring equity in clinical research, addressing structural barriers in health care that perpetuate disparities, and increasing awareness of health inequities that result in measurable actions toward achieving cancer health equity for all (Patel et al., 2020). In addition to ASCO's policy statement, many other professional organizations are committed to combating health disparities and inequities. The National Association of Social Workers (NASW), Social Work Hospice and Palliative Care Network, National Hospice and Palliative Care Organization, and Association of Oncology Social Work are all examples of organizations with policies and/or statements about their commitment to improving diversity, equity, and inclusion within their workforce to assure more equitable health care access and outcomes.

Emergence of Racism as a Public Health Crisis

It is important not only to describe the inequalities that plague communities that are historically marginalized but also to identify the root causes of ill health and premature death that persist in these populations. Following the public murder of George Floyd Jr. on May 25, 2020, more than 200 declarations of racism as a public health crisis were passed in 37 states across the country (American Public Health Association [APHA], 2021). At the end of 2020, the American Medical Association declared racism an urgent public health threat that contributes to health inequities among communities that have been historically marginalized (Elk, 2021). APHA declared racism a public health crisis and was joined by other health care organizations and professional medical societies searching to find the means by which to eliminate the various systems that perpetuate health inequities in our society (APHA, 2021). Racism in the United States can be traced back to the enslavement of African men and women over 400 years ago and remains deeply ingrained in American culture. Racism is a social system in which one racial group has the power to create a hierarchy within which other racial groups are deemed inferior (Yearby et al., 2020). Racism assigns value based on how one looks (presumed to be associated with race) that unfairly disadvantages some individuals while benefiting those in power (Diop et al., 2021). Declaring racism a public health crisis acknowledges that racism exists in our society and that systemic oppression and unequal access to resources and opportunities negatively affects the health of those who experience racial discrimination in their daily lives.

Racism and discrimination have a multitude of negative effects on the overall health of communities that are underserved, particularly for Black Americans. Discrimination is a form of stress that contributes to a person's allostatic load or "wear and tear" on the body because of repeated exposure to chronic stressors. Chronic stress is highly prevalent among Black communities and contributes to unequal outcomes in health care. Communities that have been socially and economically marginalized have greater exposure to chronic stress because of several disadvantages, including unstable employment opportunities, lack of adequate housing, and increased community violence, while having greater access to high-fat foods, alcohol, and illicit drugs. Exposure to chronic stress can impact both physical and mental well-being and have long-term effects on overall health. People who experience chronic stress throughout their lifetime experience dysregulation on the cellular level resulting in accelerated aging, as well as shortened telomere length and increased levels of inflammation. Chronic stress can contribute to impaired cardiovascular functioning, metabolic dysregulation, and a weakened immune system, leaving individuals more susceptible to infection and disease, such as cancer (Hudson, 2019). Discrimination is also associated with mental well-being and can contribute to low self-esteem as well as increased levels of depression and anxiety (Diop et al., 2021). To combat the effects of racism on the health of historically underserved communities, practitioners must identify the many systems within health care that perpetuate these outcomes.

Racism as a System in Health Care

Understanding how racism within the health care system continues to shape the experience of these populations is essential to improving health care access and the quality of care provided to groups that are historically marginalized. As previously discussed, racism in the United States is a hierarchy where the racial group in power deems all other racial groups as inferior. In the health care system, this hierarchy is supported by social norms and institutional practices that result in disparities in health outcomes. In 2020, the Institute of Healing Justice & Equity at Saint Louis University, Data for Progress and the Justice Collaborative Institute published *Racism Is a Public Health Crisis. Here's How to Respond.* The report describes four types of racism that support these social norms and institutional practices within the health care system: structural, institutional, interpersonal, and intrapersonal.

Structural racism is the way in which health care is structured to benefit the group in power while depriving historically disadvantaged populations (p. 3). Access to health care in the United States remains more based on one's ability to pay than one's medical needs. Ethnic and racial minorities in this country are disproportionately poorer than their White counterparts, have decreased access to affordable health care or health insurance, and are more likely to forgo necessary treatment due to inability to pay for care, resulting in disparities in health outcomes and mortality (p. 5).

Institutional racism is the process in which an institution's seemingly "neutral" practices and policies create barriers for racial and ethnic groups, reinforcing the hierarchy that these populations are inferior to their White counterparts (p. 4). In health care facilities, this manifests in policies that restrict the admission of certain individuals. Closure, relocation, or privatization of health care facilities can also affect racially underserved communities. Institutional racism can also look like the "dumping" or transferring of unwanted patients to public facilities that are often underfunded and overburdened, often resulting in substandard care. These practices tend to disproportionately affect people of color and ethnic minorities and prioritize the lives of White individuals (p. 6).

Interpersonal racism in health care is defined by how a provider's conscious (explicit) and/or unconscious (implicit) bias or prejudice comes into play during individual interactions with patients and families and negatively affects a patient's access to equal care (p. 4). Research in this area indicates that physicians provide less than the recommended care to Black patients. As a result, Black patients are less likely to be referred to specialists for further exploration of their needs and are less likely to be referred to higher quality institutions for care (p. 6).

Intrapersonal racism or internalized racism is the process by which ethnic and racial groups accept stereotypes about themselves and believe that members of other racial groups are superior to their own (p. 4). The belief in their own inferiority can result in harm, both physically and mentally. Research indicates that Black men with internalized experiences of racism have shorter telomeres than their White counterparts, which can result in accelerated aging and predisposition to disease (p. 6).

Lack of trust in the health care system among underrepresented racial and ethnic groups is a result of unequal treatment that is a consequence of racism, unconscious bias, and discrimination experienced over generations of time. To create a system free of racism that provides equitable care, all providers, including social workers, must recognize that racism exists in health care and work together to dismantle the systems that lead to disparities in health outcomes (Figure 3.1).

The Emergence of Cultural Humility

Social work literature first mentioned "cultural competence" in the early 1980s, and the term has been widely used since in medical education and in health care settings. Cultural competence can be defined as a set of attitudes, skills, behaviors, and policies that enable individuals and organizations to establish effective interpersonal working relationships that supersede cultural differences. A decade later, the term "culturally competent practice" was introduced and became foundational to social work practice for counseling with people of color (Danso, 2018; Foronda et al., 2016).

Melanie Tervalon and Jann Murray-García (1998) recognized that quantitative assessments in medical education required mastery of knowledge and endpoints for learning, which was narrow in the scope of clinical practice with people from diverse backgrounds. What they mean is that medical

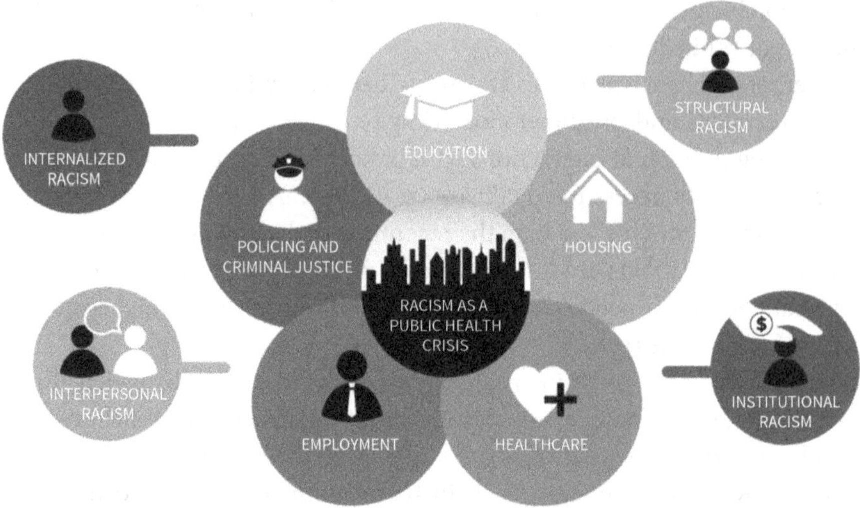

Figure 3.1 The system of racism causes racial inequities in the key areas of the social determinants of health (education, employment, health care, housing, and law enforcement), which are associated with racial health disparities (Yearby et al., 2020).

education relies heavily on assessments of knowledge that are quantitative in nature (e.g., exams and tests). Learning endpoints refers to the "mastery of" a subject area. With cultural competency, this approach is troublesome because one cannot truly "master" the culture of another. It also means that one's behavior and/or biases may remain the same. Thus, they coined the term "cultural humility" as an alternative to cultural competence. Tervalon and Murray-García highlighted that while learning about community practices is important, medical trainees had increased their knowledge without necessarily altering their own implicit biases and behaviors.

Cultural competence models emphasize knowledge acquisition while cultural humility emphasizes the need for accountability, on not only an individual but also an institutional level (Fisher-Borne et al., 2015). Tervalon and Murray-García (1998) highlighted that in introducing a new framework, they were not discounting the value of learning about health care practices of communities one serves; rather, cultural humility incorporates three dimensions: lifelong learning and a commitment to self-reflection and self-evaluation; redressing power imbalances; and institutional accountability.

Through lifelong learning and self-reflection, cultural humility emphasizes self-awareness on the part of providers and acknowledges the ways in which cultural values and structural forces shape experiences of the people we serve (Fisher-Borne et al., 2015). Focusing on being flexible and humble enough to approach each interaction with the attitude of "not knowing," lifelong learning allows for the patient or client to remain the expert on their own experiences. Criticism in the literature asserts that one cannot measure their own sense of being "humble"; however, being humble implies "reflecting, expressing, or offering in a spirit of deference, or submission" (Merriam-Webster, n.d.), which is "immeasurable in the care of the patient as well as their future clinical practice" (Tervalon & Murray-García, 1998, p. 119).

Cultural humility acknowledges power imbalances within interactions that clients or patients have in health care where patterns of racism, classism, and homophobia are reinforced, often unintentionally (Tervalon & Murray-García, 1998). If a Black patient seeks care at a health care institution where upon arrival, the only people who look like them are performing service roles and most of the physicians and nurses are White, an imbalance has immediately been observed and internalized, even prior to meeting with a member of any health care team. As highlighted already in this chapter, structural racism exists in health care and is "perpetuated inadvertently by well-meaning, but unaware, institutional representatives" (Ford et al., 2019, p. 286). Social workers must acknowledge their positions of power and the ways in which the language they use to describe behaviors (e.g., "noncompliant") and the labels they assign to patients in treatment team meetings or in medical record documentation reinforce biases. Practicing with cultural humility requires shifting power imbalances.

In recent years, discussions about institutional accountability have increased as organizations and/or institutions have been more intentional about publicly stating the ways in which they plan to actively address factors such as racism, disparities, and inequalities. Just as self-reflection is addressed at an individual level, institutions must do the same in an approach that embodies cultural humility. How your institution engages with the surrounding community, responds to systemic and structural barriers, promotes inclusivity, or addresses known gaps in service delivery to certain populations are examples of what cultural humility looks like on a macro level. Cultural humility emphasizes the development of mutually beneficial community partnerships and mitigating the direct impact of institutional practices on the health of people in underrepresented communities (Ford et al., 2019).

While literature often discusses cultural humility as an alternative to cultural competency, some writers also highlight that one does not have to choose either cultural humility or cultural competence (Greene-Moton & Minkler, 2020); rather, social workers can effectively incorporate valuable aspects of both into their interactions with diverse populations along a continuum with other cross-cultural practice concepts (Danso, 2018; Greene-Moton & Minkler, 2020). Imperative is a commitment to ongoing interpersonal, intrapersonal, and institutional evaluation versus a compartmentalized understanding or approach that leads to the persistence of health disparities.

Integrating Cultural Humility: Guiding Best Practices for the Future

Social work education teaches us to meet people where they are; however, recognizing the extent to which we meet people where *we* think they are is a challenge that reflects our own biases and assumptions. Cultural humility seeks to cultivate self-awareness on the part of providers and acknowledges the ways in which (our) cultural values and structural forces shape client/patient experiences.

Integrating cultural humility into social work practice begins with asking essential questions at both individual and institutional levels to assess cultural humility. According to Fisher-Borne et al. (2015, p. 176, Table 2), questions should address power imbalances (e.g., "How do we 'actively' address inequalities?" and "What social and economic barriers affect a client's ability to receive effective care?") and critical self-reflection (for example, "What do I learn about myself through listening to clients who are different than me?" and "Is our leadership reflective of the populations/communities we serve?").

Acknowledging that we are each accountable is also an important part of implementation. Our accountabilities exist on every level of practice to truly dismantle the systems in place that perpetuate racism in health care. Accountability includes building our own resourcefulness. In 2015, the NASW published the *Standards and Indicators for Cultural Competence in Social Work Practice* (2015), which provides guidance on implementation across 10 standards (ethics and values; self-awareness, cross-cultural knowledge; cross-cultural skills; service delivery; empowerment and advocacy; diverse workforce; professional education; language and communication; and leadership to advance cultural competence). Achieving health equity through implementing cultural humility also means building a culture that centers equity. Equity in the Center's Awake to Woke to Work model provides "insights, tactics, and best practices to shift organizational culture and operationalize equity" (Equity in the Center, 2020).

The Role of Social Work in Eliminating Health Inequities

Social workers have played an integral role in health care since the early 20th century and remain present in a variety of settings, including oncology and palliative care. According to the 2005 NASW *Standards for Social Work Practice in Health Care Settings*, a hallmark of social work's commitment to health and wellness is the profession's ongoing attention to health inequality in the United States. Social workers have a unique understanding of how SDOH, such as poverty, discrimination, and lack of health insurance, have a disproportionate impact on rates of acute illness and chronic disease for groups that have been socially and economically marginalized. The NASW established that social work's primary mission is to enhance the well-being of all people, with special attention placed on the needs of communities most vulnerable, oppressed, or living in poverty. Social workers practicing in health care settings have an ethical obligation to address the needs of people most affected by SDOH and to advocate for change to assure equitable access to care (NASW, 2005).

Improving outcomes in cancer disparities is a continuous process that begins by acknowledging the existence of racism in the health care system and its impact on health inequities among racial and ethnic communities. Social workers in oncology have an obligation to conduct themselves in an ethical manner and maintain an understanding of equity as it relates to health outcomes, especially in cancer care. The NASW *Code of Ethics* (2021) directs health care social workers to advocate for social, economic, and political justice efforts that promote equitable care for everyone. Social workers recognize high-quality health care as a basic human right and understand that barriers to such care are a result of power imbalances and social policies. Social workers understand how the health care system may oppress communities that are historically marginalized and are empowered to advocate for policies within their institutions that eliminate barriers to quality health services. The NASW endorses lifelong learning, self-exploration, and self-awareness that encourages social workers to manage their personal bias and allow professional values to guide ethical decision-making. Supervision in social work is employed to explore one's own bias and exercise cultural humility in daily practice. Social workers are encouraged to remain competent in culturally sensitive research, draw from evidence-based approaches, and evaluate their own practice to practice ethically and from a social justice perspective (Williams et al., 2013). Oncology social workers draw on these strengths and professional values to support equitable access to high-quality cancer care across the continuum, from prevention and early detection to survivorship and end-of-life care.

Pearls

- It is important to acknowledge that racism does exist in health care and work together to dismantle the systems that lead to disparities in health outcomes.
- Achieving health equity is everyone's responsibility.
- Incorporating dimensions of cultural humility into social work practice enriches provider–patient interactions.
- Oncology social workers have an ethical obligation to challenge social injustice.

Pitfalls

- Minimizing the harmful impact of racism in health care perpetuates disparities in cancer health outcomes.
- Placing blame (intentionally or unintentionally) on members of communities with disparate health outcomes undermines the impact of SDOH.
- Assuming that competency is derived from being "educated" about another person's culture can reinforce harmful stereotypes.
- Social workers contribute to power imbalances by prioritizing their own comfort (e.g., choosing not to interrupt racist remarks) over professional ethics, which explicitly call us to take meaningful action against injustice.

Additional Resources

Articles

Ford, C., Griffith, D., Bruce, M., & Gilbert, K. (2019, November). Racism: Science and tools for the public health professional. In *APHA's 2019 Annual Meeting and Expo (Nov. 2–6)*. APHA. https://ajph.aphapublications.org/doi/book/10.2105/9780875533049

Greene-Moton, E., & Minkler, M. (2020). Cultural competence or cultural humility? Moving beyond the debate. *Health Promotion Practice, 21*(1), 142–145. https://journals.sagepub.com/doi/full/10.1177/1524839919884912

Winkfield, K. M., Regnante, J. M., Miller-Sonet, E., González, E. T., Freund, K. M., & Doykos, P. M. (2021). Development of an actionable framework to address cancer care disparities in medically underserved populations in the United States: Expert roundtable recommendations. *JCO Oncology Practice, 17*(3), e278–e293. https://ascopubs.org/doi/10.1200/OP.20.00630

Websites

Association of American Medical Colleges (AAMC) Center for Health Justice: https://www.aamchealthjustice.org/

Centers for Disease Control and Prevention, Racism and Health: https://www.cdc.gov/minorityhealth/racism-disparities/

Kaiser Family Foundation, Racial Equity and Health Policy: https://www.kff.org/racial-equity-and-health-policy/

Racial Equity Tools: https://www.racialequitytools.org/

The Winters Group, Inc.: https://www.wintersgroup.com/resources/

References

American Association for Cancer Research. (2021, October 26). *Cancer disparities progress report 2020*. https://cancerprogressreport.aacr.org/disparities/

American Public Health Association. (2021). *Analysis: Declarations of racism as a public health crisis*. https://apha.org/topics-and-issues/health-equity/racism-and-health/racism-declarations

Braveman, P. (2014). What are health disparities and health equity? We need to be clear. *Public Health Reports, 129*(Suppl 2), 5–8. https://doi.org/10.1177%2F00333549141291S203

Danso, R. (2018). Cultural competence and cultural humility: A critical reflection on key cultural diversity concepts. *Journal of Social Work, 18*(4), 410–430. https://doi.org/10.1177%2F1468017316654341

Diop, M. S., Taylor, C. N., Murillo, S. N., Zeidman, J. A., James, A. K., & Burnett-Bowie, S. A. M. (2021). This is our lane: Talking with patients about racism. *Women's Midlife Health, 7*(1), 1–8. https://doi.org/10.1186/s40695-021-00066-3

Elk, R. (2021). The intersection of racism, discrimination, bias, and homophobia toward African American sexual minority patients with cancer within the health care system. *Cancer, 127*(19), 3500–3504. https://doi.org/10.1002/cncr.33627

Equity in the Center. (2020). *Awake to woke to work: Building a race equity culture*. https://equityinthecenter.org/aww/.

Fisher-Borne, M., Cain, J. M., & Martin, S. L. (2015). From mastery to accountability: Cultural humility as an alternative to cultural competence. *Social Work Education, 34*(2), 165–181. https://doi.org/10.1080/02615479.2014.977244

Ford, C., Griffith, D., Bruce, M., & Gilbert, K. (2019, November). Racism: Science and tools for the public health professional. In *APHA's 2019 Annual Meeting and Expo (Nov. 2–6)*. APHA. https://ajph.aphapublications.org/doi/book/10.2105/9780875533049.

Foronda, C., Baptiste, D. L., Reinholdt, M. M., & Ousman, K. (2016). Cultural humility: A concept analysis. *Journal of Transcultural Nursing, 27*(3), 210–217.

Greene-Moton, E., & Minkler, M. (2020). Cultural competence or cultural humility? Moving beyond the debate. *Health Promotion Practice, 21*(1), 142–145. https://doi.org/10.1177%2F1524839919884912

Hudson, D. L. (2019). How racism has shaped the health of Black Americans and what to do about it. In C. L. Ford, D. M. Griffith, M. A. Bruce, & K. L. Gilbert (Eds.), *Racism: Science and tools for the public health professional* (pp. 429–444). American Public Health Association.

Kurapati, S. (2020, March 9). Health equality vs. health equity. American Medical Women's Association. *Premed Division Blog*. https://www.amwa-doc.org/health-equality-vs-health-equity/

Merriam-Webster. (n.d.). *Merriam-Webster.com dictionary*. https://www.merriam-webster.com

National Association of Social Workers. (2005). *NASW standards for social work practice in health care settings*. NASW Press.

National Association of Social Workers. (2015). *Standards and indicators for cultural competence in social work practice*. NASW Press. https://www.socialworkers.org/LinkClick.aspx?fileticket=PonPTDEBrn4%3D

National Association of Social Workers. (2021). *Code of ethics of the National Association of Social Workers*. NASW Press.

National Cancer Institute, National Institutes of Health. (2022). *Cancer disparities*. https://cancer.gov/about-cancer/understanding/disparities

Patel, M. I., Lopez, A. M., Blackstock, W., Reeder-Hayes, K., Moushey, E. A., Phillips, J., & Tap, W. (2020). Cancer disparities and health equity: A policy statement from the American Society of Clinical Oncology. *Journal of Clinical Oncology*, *38*(29), 3439–3448. https://doi.org/10.1200/jco.20.00642

Tervalon, M., & Murray-García, J. (1998). Cultural humility versus cultural competence: A critical distinction in defining physician training outcomes in multicultural education. *Journal of Health Care for the Poor and Underserved*, *9*(2), 117–125. https://doi.org/10.1353/hpu.2010.0233

Williams, J. H., Brunet, T. C., Des Marais, E. A., & National Association of Deans and Directors of Schools of Social Work (United States). (2013). *Advanced social work practice behaviors to address behavioral health disparities*. National Association of Deans and Directors of Schools of Social Work.

Yearby, R., Lewis, C., Gilbert, K., & Banks, K. (2020). *Racism is a public health crisis: Here's how to respond*. Institute for Healing Justice and Equity at Saint Louis University, Data for Progress and Justice Collaborative Institute.

4

Social Determinants of Health

Cancer-Related Health Disparities and Financial Toxicity

Iris Cohen Fineberg and Jessica Savara

Key Concepts

- Social determinants of health (SDOH) are structural elements that can affect certain population groups' health and health experiences.
- Some SDOH lead to systematic health disparities that reflect discrimination and stigmatization.
- Cancer prevention, detection, treatment, and experience of care, including palliative care, can be affected by SDOH.
- Financial toxicity is a particular and noteworthy consequence of some SDOH.
- The field of social work, which is fundamentally oriented to social justice, advocacy, and the impact of the environment on people's experiences, has much to contribute to addressing SDOH and health disparities.

Keywords: financial toxicity, health disparities, oncology, oncology social work, palliative care, palliative social work, social determinants of health, social work

The concept of social determinants of health (SDOH) and how they create health disparities that privilege some groups' overall health and access to health care while negatively affecting other groups have become central to discussions of the public's health and intensified attention to social inequities. The social work profession has long paid attention to the components that make up the social determinants that can lead to negative (and positive) health outcomes among certain groups of people; however, social work has not used that specific terminology and has approached these topics from an ecological perspective that centers on the patient, family, group, or community. Understanding the definitions, relationships, and significance of

Iris Cohen Fineberg and Jessica Savara, *Social Determinants of Health* In: *Oncology and Palliative Social Work*. Edited by: Susan Hedlund, Bryan Miller, Grace Christ, and Carolyn Messner, Oxford University Press.
 DOI: 10.1093/oso/9780197607299.003.0004

different SDOH and how they create health disparities is important for social workers as interprofessional colleagues, advocates, clinicians, educators, and policymakers. This chapter addresses topics and offers insight into their connection with cancer prevention, diagnosis, treatment, and palliative care experiences. We use the example of breast cancer to illustrate the numerous intersections of social determinants, health disparities, cancer, and palliative care. In addition, we pay specific attention to the concept of financial toxicity.

Introduction to Social Determinants of Health and Health Disparities

Social work is fundamentally oriented toward the relationship between people and their environment, a concept that encompasses multiple ecological elements: social, economic, political, cultural, and physical forces (Cederbaum et al., 2019; Pardeck, 1988). Since its origin, social work has recognized the critical and transactional relationship between the environment and people's life experiences, reinforcing the long-standing history of social work with direct application of the ecological perspective (Pardeck, 1988). The profession is grounded in the person-in-environment perspective and social workers thus understand the human experience as bound to the environment in which it occurs (Bullock et al., 2021).

Social Determinants of Health

The terminology of SDOH is used in the fields of medicine and public health, and public health and social work have shared dedication to the ecological factors that constitute SDOH (Bachman, 2017). Awareness of SDOH has been growing since 1998, when the World Health Organization (WHO) published a brief but important report on SDOH (Wilkinson et al., 1998); 10 years later, WHO commissioned a more extensive report on social determinants of health (WHO, 2008), thereby signaling WHO's recognition of social determinants' critical nature. Today, WHO (n.d.) defines SDOH as, "the non-medical factors that influence health outcomes. They are the conditions in which people are born, grow, work, live, and age, and the wider set of forces and systems shaping the conditions of daily life. These forces and systems include economic policies and systems, development agendas, social norms, social policies, and political systems."

The U.S. Department of Health and Human Services Healthy People 2030 program (n.d.) divides SDOH into the five areas of economic stability, education access and quality, health care access and quality, neighborhood and built environment, and social and community context. The variations in these factors influence health outcomes among social groups in ways that lead to a number of different health disparities. Of key significance is that social determinants are systematic and structural in society—in other words, they operate on the grand scale of population health. Social determinants of health particularly contribute to health disparities through discrimination (e.g., racism or homophobia) and stigmatization (Alcaraz et al., 2020; Cogburn, 2019). People with cancer and their families experience these disparities directly.

Health Disparities

Health disparities are the differences in health status and experiences based on group affiliation. These disparities are understood as a consequence or outcome of the social determinants of health. People in socially disadvantaged groups often bear the negative version of these differences. "Health disparities are systematic, plausibly avoidable health differences according to race/ethnicity, skin color, religion, or nationality; socioeconomic resources or position (reflected by, e.g., income, wealth, education, or occupation); gender, sexual orientation, gender identity; age, geography, disability, illness, political or other affiliation; or other characteristics associated with discrimination or marginalization" (Braveman et al., 2011, p. S151). Thus, for example, the SDOH "access to health care" can lead to disparities in health status through variations in disease detection, quality of care, and treatment outcomes between people who have good access and those who have little or no access.

Relationships Among SDOH, Health Disparities, and Social Work

Social work is fundamentally rooted in viewing the human experience in the context of the social environment. The profession works on the levels of both SDOH and health disparities, aiming to affect both the causes and consequences of health inequities. In that sense, social work has long specialized in SDOH (Zerden et al., 2020). The profession is dedicated to advancing social equity and assisting people who are socially marginalized and disenfranchised. With health disparities understood as measures of health equity (Braveman et al., 2011) and social work's dedication to equity and social justice, it is evident that social work would have strong interests in SDOH and health disparities (Braveman et al., 2011; Moniz, 2010). Social work's acute attention to culture and understanding of issues of power and power dynamics in society, communities, and health care, make the profession well suited for leading advocacy and social change in the social determinants that impact health.

SDOH and Cancer-Related Health Disparities

The intersection of SDOH and cancer-related health disparities is apparent in all phases of the cancer experience: cancer prevention and etiology, screening, detection, treatment, and survivorship. According to the National Cancer Institute, disparities are visible across groups through such measures as cancer screening rates, stage at diagnosis, and the numbers of new cases and deaths (cited in American Association for Cancer Research, n.d.). Similarly, the intersection is evident in disparities in knowledge about, access to, and experience of palliative care in the context of cancer care (Griggs, 2020).

Connecting SDOH to Cancer Prevention and Detection

Social determinants of health like education level, employment status, geography, race, and socioeconomic status (SES) connect with knowledge about, engagement with, and lived conditions related to cancer prevention and detection. For example, SES influences the neighborhoods in which people live, with lower SES neighborhoods often having higher proportions of people of color. Lower SES neighborhoods tend to have fewer fresh-food markets and more fast-food restaurants. Consequently, these communities have poor access to healthy foods known to support cancer prevention while consuming higher proportions of cheaper, processed food known to be less healthy (Alcaraz et al., 2020). People living in lower-SES communities also face increased cancer risks through higher rates of exposure to causes of cancer such as industrial pollution. Disparities in cancer detection also result from social determinants such as race, sexual and gender minority status (Matthews et al., 2018), SES, and geography—people of color or a sexual/gender identity minority who perceive or have experienced discrimination in health care settings, for example, may not feel safe pursuing cancer screenings. Other SDOH, such as living in a rural area or experiencing homelessness, serve as barriers to cancer screening and early detection because of distance to appropriate medical clinics and a lack of affordable transportation to those services.

SDOH, Cancer, and Palliative Care Experiences

Social determinants of health have a direct bearing on cancer and palliative treatment and care. Low education levels or poor health literacy may affect a person's understanding of the importance of maintaining consistent adherence to medication schedules, which can lead to negative cancer treatment outcomes or higher pain levels. Low education also may affect a person's type of employment, which in turn may limit access to health insurance, paid leave, work-schedule flexibility, or job security. Each one of these elements would affect a person's decisions about if, where, and when to seek and engage with cancer care. Patterns resulting from SDOH are notable in not only oncology care but also palliative care. For example, Mayeda and Ward (2019) found that people in minority groups face three types of barriers to palliative care: lower health literacy, poorer access to health care resources, and lack of effective communication caused by differences in language or culture. Cancer patients from racial and ethnic minorities also face disparities in symptom palliation (Griggs, 2020). People in primarily minority neighborhoods may face difficulties accessing pain medications due to supply limitations in neighborhood pharmacies (Johnson, 2013). People experiencing homelessness are often unable to access palliative care until late in their illness (Henry et al., 2017). The scenarios above reflect just a few examples of how SDOH and associated systematic health disparities affect the experiences of people needing oncology and palliative care.

Breast Cancer

People's experience of breast cancer provides an example of the impact of SDOH across the trajectory of illness. Consider the SDOH of a Black woman living in a low-income neighborhood, working in a restaurant that offers no health insurance. People in the neighborhood have poor access to nutritious foods, few safe places to exercise, and limited medical care facilities, all of which disadvantage the woman's access to breast cancer prevention and early detection, such as mammography. Several other SDOH affect her potential cancer trajectory. Experiences of racism contribute to breast cancer disparities through greater risks of chronic stress and maladaptive health behaviors such as smoking and increased alcohol use. Unsurprisingly, women living in disadvantaged neighborhoods often are in later stages of breast cancer at diagnosis (Coughlin 2019; Gehlert et al, 2021). Lack of health insurance is also associated with diagnoses at later stages. Once diagnosed with breast cancer, the woman's ability to attend chemotherapy or radiation treatment appointments may be compromised by the cost or schedule of transportation. Not having paid sick time and a fear of missing work or losing a job may affect treatment decisions more than consideration of what is the most effective breast cancer treatment. Ultimately, the consequences of the various social determinants are disparities in breast cancer mortality (Gehlert et al., 2021).

Financial Toxicity in the Context of Oncology and Palliative Care

Social determinants of health affect people's ability to bear the financial impact of cancer. Cancer care costs have increased exponentially and are projected to continue with advancements in diagnostics, treatment, and supportive services. Health care providers and patients alike are experiencing increasing concern about the financial harms—often described as financial toxicity—associated with oncology and palliative care.

The term "financial toxicity" has come into use in the last decade to describe the negative economic effects and resulting stressors from cancer and its treatment on a person and their household. The term borrows from the concept of physical toxicities associated with cancer treatment and reframes the harms associated with cancer care to include the financial burdens it imposes on patients and their families (Abrams et al., 2021). De Souza et al. (2017, p. 476) define financial toxicity as "the objective financial consequences of cancer, as well the subjective financial concerns." The extent of financial adversity and distress from treatment varies among patients and is dependent on patients' unique medical and psychosocial circumstances—cancer diagnosis and associated standard of care, SES, insurance coverage, and other SDOH. While research exists to support the use of some tools for the screening and assessment of financial toxicity among cancer patients and survivors, little research exists that supports specific methods for prevention and interventions.

Causes of Financial Toxicity for Those Experiencing Cancer

The economic burden of care to a cancer patient and their household includes direct and indirect costs. Direct costs include medical costs like cancer medications, health insurance, and out-of-pocket expenses. As treatment costs have soared, health insurance plan providers have shifted the costs of care to the patient (Zafar et al., 2013). Indirect costs can include childcare, transportation, parking fees, and lodging (Abrams et al., 2021; Iragorri et al., 2021). Costs of care can result in material losses like reduced income due to sick days and credit card debt and associated interest and fees; in extreme cases, patients have lost their jobs or homes or had to declare bankruptcy. Financial toxicity can lead to patients spending less on food, paying for and taking only some medications, and not completing care or forgoing treatment altogether. Some studies point to severe financial toxicity as a risk factor for early mortality among cancer patients (Ramsey et al., 2016). Many of these negative impacts and outcomes extend to caregivers.

Social Work Roles in Addressing SDOH and Health Disparities in Oncology and Palliative Care

Social workers have the imperative, knowledge, and skills to understand the sources and mitigate the consequences of SDOH. While SDOH and health disparities work at a population level, social workers' roles are to provide knowledge about and assistance with SDOH not only to individual patients and their families but also within organizations, larger communities, and society as a whole. In the setting of oncology and palliative care, social workers conduct comprehensive biopsychosocial-spiritual assessments that can identify the sources of SDOH that are affecting and may affect the patient and family experience. The social work role in the setting of interprofessional and team care includes communicating with the team about specific SDOH and health disparities that should be considered in planning, delivering, and communicating about care with patients and families. With individuals and families, social workers help mitigate the impact of SDOH and health disparities by connecting people to resources, advocating and supporting self-advocacy, and finding mechanisms to minimize future disparities.

Social work's core connection to social justice and advocacy also translates to action in the larger community, illuminating social work's commitment to and leadership in addressing SDOH (Moniz, 2010; Zerden et al., 2020). In 2013, the American Academy of Social Work and Social Welfare created the Grand Challenges for Social Work (GCSW) that reflect social work's application of concepts shared with the public health perspective underlying the SDOH (Cederbaum et al., 2019). Social work advocacy for structural and procedural changes on the organizational and societal level, including legislative transformations, aims to reduce and eliminate health disparities. In the context of palliative care, Bullock et al. (2021) offer three strategies for social workers to address health inequities: having the social worker on the team identify the greatest burdens and unmet needs in the population served; leading with purpose to reduce health inequity by developing and adhering to an equity strategic plan; and listening to patients and families about their greatest worries and what matters to them most.

While social work is dedicated to identifying and addressing the environmental factors that impact patients' and families' lives (Moniz, 2010), social workers must remember they are part of, not external to, this environment. It is important to acknowledge the social worker's identity, including their social and professional positioning, when working with oncology and palliative care patients. Social workers are themselves affected by SDOH. At times, they may share social identities with patients and families. In other situations, a social worker's possible social affiliations, such as being of a dominant racial group or SES, may contrast with their patient's affiliation. Both similarities and differences in positioning impact the relationship dynamic. As a profession dedicated to self-reflection and self-awareness, social work emphasizes the responsibility of its members to notice and attend to such social identities and dynamics in service to providing high-quality patient and family care.

Social determinants of health and health disparities are variations (at the societal level) among social groups that influence the many phases of cancer and palliative care. Social workers must recognize that people's identities, cultures, and social groups are fundamentally connected with health disparities that affect their illness experience. Financial toxicity reflects how systemic economic stressors can burden cancer patients and their families. While the terminology of SDOH and health disparities is conceptual and not necessarily the language social workers would use in direct clinical care, it is important to ask about the socioenvironmental forces that affect cancer patients and their families. Future research is needed to guide oncology and palliative care professionals on how to best assist patients and families with the consequences of SDOH.

Guiding Best Practices for the Future

As professionals oriented to the person-in-environment approach to patient and family care, social workers have the responsibility to explore and address the SDOH and resulting health disparities that are most relevant to their clients' oncology and palliative care. Strategies for this work begin with thorough and thoughtful biopsychosocial-spiritual assessments that explore SDOH that might be influencing, or could influence, the illness experience. Particular attention should be paid to the experiences of minority populations who have been subject to systemic discrimination and social exclusion. Social workers can build relationships with patients/families and create inviting and supportive care settings that mitigate the negative consequences of SDOH and health disparities. Social workers have important roles to play in educating their interprofessional colleagues and team members (through personal conversations and professional presentations) on the impacts of SDOH on high-quality oncology and palliative care. Furthermore, social workers must be key advocates in their organizations and communities for helping identify and change policies that perpetuate health disparities, especially those related to cancer prevention, screening, treatment, survivorship, and palliative care.

Pearls

- Social workers fundamentally have expertise in identifying and understanding SDOH that impact patients and families.
- SDOH and the resulting health disparities reflect structural, systemic issues that affect population groups.
- The effects of the intersection of SDOH and cancer-related health disparities reveal themselves in all phases of the cancer experience and palliative care.
- Financial toxicity illustrates how SDOH affect the lives of oncology patients and families, differentially burdening portions of the populations.
- Social work's provision of assessment, intervention, resource identification, patient/family and interprofessional colleague education, and multilevel advocacy represent some of the profession's critical roles in mitigating and eliminating health disparities.

Pitfalls

- SDOH include not only race, ethnicity, and SES but also numerous social elements such as geography, age, and sexual and gender identities.
- While social workers often assist individuals and families with the impact of SDOH and health disparities, it is important to remember that these exist on the larger, population group level of society.

- Financial toxicity reflects economic consequences of cancer that are caused by systemic and structural forces, such as history and policies, rather than individual failings.
- Social work advocacy addressing health disparities happens not only on the clinical level of oncology and palliative care but through the settings and vehicles of systemic change such as organizations, communities, policies, and governmental legislation.

Additional Resources

Readings

Koroukian, S. M., Schiltz, N. K., Warner, D. F., Given, C. W., Schluchter, M., Owusu, C., & Berger, N. A. (2017). Social determinants, multimorbidity, and patterns of end-of-life care in older adults dying from cancer. *Journal of Geriatric Oncology*, *8*, 117–124. https://doi.org/10.1016/j.jgo.2016.10.001

Singh, G. K., Daus, G. P., Allender, M., Ramey, C. T., Martin, E. K., Perry, C., De Los Reyes, A. A., & Vedamuthu, I. P. (2017). Social determinants of health in the United States: Addressing major health inequality trends for the nation, 1935–2016. *International Journal of MCH and AIDS*, *6*(2), 139–164. https://doi.org/10.21106/ijma.236

Websites

American Cancer Society, Advancing Health Equity—Addressing Cancer Disparities: https://www.cancer.org/about-us/what-we-do/health-equity.html

American Society of Clinical Oncology: https://www.cancer.net/research-and-advocacy/health-disparities-and-cancer/resources-cancer-disparities-and-health-equity

National Cancer Institute, Cancer Health Disparities Research: https://www.cancer.gov/research/areas/disparities

U.S. Department of Health and Human Services, Office of Disease Prevention and Health Promotion, Healthy People 2030: https://health.gov/healthypeople/objectives-and-data/social-determinants-health

References

Abrams, H. R., Durbin, S., Huang, C. X., Johnson, S. F., Nayak, R. K., Zahner, G. J., & Peppercorn, J. (2021). Financial toxicity in cancer care: Origins, impact, and solutions. *Translational Behavioral Medicine*, *11*(11), 2043–2054. https://doi.org/10.1093/tbm/ibab091

Alcaraz, K. I., Wiedt, T. L., Daniels, E. C., Yabroff, K. R., Guerra, C. E., & Wender, R. C. (2020). Understanding and addressing social determinants to advance cancer health equity in the United States: A blueprint for practice, research, and policy. *CA: A Cancer Journal for Clinicians*, *70*, 31–46. https://doi.org/10.3322/caac.21586

American Association for Cancer Research. (n.d.). *Cancer health disparities*. Retrieved August 20, 2023, from https://www.aacr.org/patients-caregivers/about-cancer/cancer-health-disparities/

Bachman, S. S. (2017). Social work and public health: Charting the course for innovation. *American Journal of Public Health*, *107*(53), S220. https://doi.org/10.2105/AJPH.2017.304209

Braveman, P. A., Kumanyika, S., Fielding, J., LaVeist, T., Borrell, L. N., Manderscheid, R., & Troutman, A. (2011). Health disparities and health equity: The issue is justice. *American Journal of Public Health*, *101*(S1), S149–S155. https://doi.org/10.2105/AJPH.2010.300062

Bullock, K., Damiano, S., & Sinclair, S. (2021, April 24). *Social workers can lead the way in addressing health inequities*. Retrieved from https://www.capc.org/blog/social-workers-can-lead-the-way-in-addressing-health-inequities/

Cederbaum, J. A., Ross, A. M., Ruth, B. J., & Keefe, R. H. (2019). Public health social work as a unifying framework for social work's grand challenges. *Social Work*, *64*(1), 9–17. https://doi.org/10.1093/sw/swy045

Cogburn, C. D. (2019). Culture, race, and health: Implications for racial inequities and population health. *Milbank Quarterly*, *97*(3), 736–761. https://doi.org/10.1111/1468-0009.12411

Coughlin, S. S. (2019). Social determinants of breast cancer risk, stage, and survival. *Breast Cancer Research and Treatment*, *177*, 537–548. https://doi.org/10.1007/s10549-019-05340-7

de Souza, J. A., Yap, B. J., Wroblewski, K., Blinder, V., Araújo, F. S., Hlubocky, F. J., Nicholas, L. H., O'Connor, J. M., Brockstein, B., Ratain, M. J., Daugherty, C. K., & Cella, D. (2017). Measuring financial toxicity as a clinically relevant patient-reported outcome: The validation of the Comprehensive Score for financial Toxicity (COST). *Cancer*, *123*(3), 476–484. https://doi.org/10.1002/cncr.30369

Gehlert, S., Hudson, D., & Sacks, T. (2021). A critical theoretical approach to cancer disparities: Breast cancer and the social determinants of health. *Frontiers in Public Health*, *9*, 674736. https://doi.org/10.3389/fpubh.2021.674736

Griggs, J. J. (2020). Disparities in palliative care in patients with cancer. *Journal of Clinical Oncology*, *38*(9), 974–979. https://doi.org/10.1200/JCO.19.02108

Henry, B., Dosani, N., Huynh, L., & Amirault, N. (2017). Palliative care as a public health issue: Understanding disparities in access to palliative care for the homeless population living in Toronto, based on a policy analysis. *Current Oncology*, *24*(3), 187–191. https://doi.org/10.3747/co.24.3129

Iragorri, N., de Oliveira, C., Fitzgerald, N., & Essue, B. (2021). The out-of-pocket cost burden of cancer care: A systematic literature review. *Current Oncology*, *28*(2), 1216–1248. https://doi.org/10.3390/curroncol28020117

Johnson, K. S. (2013). Racial and ethnic disparities in palliative care [Special report: NIA white paper]. *Journal of Palliative Medicine*, *16*(11), 1329–1334. https://doi.org/10.1089/jpm.2013.9468

Matthews, A. K., Breen, E., & Kittiteerasack, P. (2018). Social determinants of LGBT cancer health inequities. *Seminars in Oncology Nursing*, *34*(1), 12–20. https://doi.org/10.1016/j.soncn.2017.11.001

Mayeda, D. P., & Ward, K. T. (2019) Methods for overcoming barriers in palliative care for ethnic/racial minorities: A systematic review. *Palliative and Supportive Care*, *17*, 697–706. https://doi.org/10.1017/S1478951519000403

Moniz, C. (2010). Social work and the social determinants of health perspective: A good fit. *Health and Social Work*, *35*(4), 310–313. https://doi.org/10.1093/hsw/35.4.310

Pardeck, J. T. (1988). An ecological approach for social work practice. *Journal of Sociology and Social Welfare*, *15*(2), 133–142. https://https://doi.org/10.15453/0191-5096.1855

Ramsey, S. D., Bansal, A., Fedorenko, C. R., Blough, D. K., Overstreet, K. A., Shankaran, V., & Newcomb, P. (2016). Financial insolvency as a risk factor for early mortality among patients with cancer. *Journal of Clinical Oncology*, *34*(9), 980–986. https://doi.org/10.1200/JCO.2015.64.6620

U.S. Department of Health and Human Services, Office of Disease Prevention and Health Promotion, Healthy People 2030. (n.d.). *Social determinants of health*. Retrieved July 30, 2023, from https://health.gov/healthypeople/objectives-and-data/social-determinants-health

Wilkinson, R. G., Marmot, M., & World Health Organization. (1998) . *The solid facts: Social determinants of health*. World Health Organization Regional Office for Europe. https://apps.who.int/iris/handle/10665/108082

World Health Organization. (n.d.). *Social determinants of health*. Retrieved June 11, 2022, from https://www.who.int/health-topics/social-determinants-of-health#tab=tab_1

World Health Organization, Commission on Social Determinants of Health. (2008). *Closing the gap in a generation: Health equity through action on the social determinants of health*. https://www.who.int/publications/i/item/WHO-IER-CSDH-08.1

Zafar, S. Y., Peppercorn, J. M., Schrag, D., Taylor, D. H., Goetzinger, A. M., Zhong, X., & Abernethy, A. P. (2013). The financial toxicity of cancer treatment: A pilot study assessing out-of-pocket expenses and the insured cancer patient's experience. *Oncologist*, *18*(4), 381–390. https://doi.org/10.1634/theoncologist.2012-0279

Zerden, L. D., Cadet, T. J., Galambos, C., & Jones, B. (2020). Social work's commitment and leadership to address social determinants of health and integrate social care into health care. *Journal of Health and Human Services Administration*, *43*(3), 309–323. https://doi.org/10.37808/jhhsa.43.3.5

5

Unprecedented Challenges

Cancer Care Amid Pandemics, Disasters, and Other Traumatic Events

Karen Bullock

> I'm sick and tired of being sick and tired.
>
> —**Fannie Lou Hamer (1964)**

Key Concepts

- A cancer diagnosis exacerbates the effects of the unprecedented challenges—pandemics, natural disasters, and other traumatic events—that are ravaging communities locally, regionally, nationally, and globally.
- Decreased screening and cancer treatments during the COVID-19 pandemic exacerbated already extant disparities in cancer care.
- Oncology social work best practices for addressing challenges demand particular attention to patterns of inequality rooted in historical racism.
- It behooves oncology social workers to align our clinical practice approaches with theoretical models, awareness, skills, and knowledge to cultivate cultural competence as a tool for addressing systemic and structural racism in cancer care.
- Oncology clinicians are uniquely prepared to provide leadership that is social-justice focused, aligned with the National Association of Social Work's Code of Ethics, values, and cultural competence to support diverse patients and families.

Keywords: COVID-19, disaster, disparities, health equity, traumatic events

A cancer diagnosis exacerbates the effects of the unprecedented challenges—pandemics, natural disasters, and other traumatic events—that are ravaging

Karen Bullock, *Unprecedented Challenges* In: *Oncology and Palliative Social Work.* Edited by: Susan Hedlund, Bryan Miller, Grace Christ, and Carolyn Messner, Oxford University Press. © Oxford University Press 2024.
DOI: 10.1093/oso/9780197607299.003.0005

communities locally, regionally, nationally, and globally. Specifically, the COVID-19 pandemic highlighted the disproportionate impacts of traumatic events on persons living with cancer (Siker et al., 2020). The reality of being immunosuppressed by the disease and its treatments compounded by exposure to predisposing factors for cancer, including but not limited to smoking and obesity, introduced adverse outcomes for patient infected by COVID-19 during the pandemic. In addition, persons diagnosed with cancer already have a higher risk of mortality and twice the morbidity rate from COVID-19 than the general population (Venkatesulu et al., 2021; Wang & Li, 2020).

Cancer was the second leading cause of death in the United States prior to the COVID-19 pandemic. Furthermore, racial disparities in cancer incidence and mortality, risk factors, screening, and treatment outcomes have existed as long as cancer research and interventions (American Cancer Society, 2022; Centers for Disease Control and Prevention, n.d.; Siker et al., 2020). Cancer disparities were already impossible to ignore not only in health care systems and access to medical treatment but also in the allocation of resources toward research across racial groups (Bullock & Allison, 2015; Ejem et al., 2019; Kamal et al., 2017; Sanders et al., 2016), pre-COVID-19.

Black, Indigenous, Hispanic/Latino, Asian, and Pacific Islander patients and families have been front and center of COVID-19—arguably, the worst public health crisis of the century. The pandemic led to unanticipated, pronounced challenges around how to care for populations of people for whom structural and systemic racism were already social determinants of health, leaving them disproportionately at risk for preexisting health conditions that the coronavirus exacerbated (American Cancer Society Cancer Action Network [ACSCAN], n.d.). Moreover, as a historically marginalized group, Black people were already experiencing barriers to equitable serious illness care including but not limited to hospice and palliative care. The pandemic illuminated the racial disparities in access to care and culturally bound decision-making factors influenced by historical and contemporary sociocultural values and lived experiences (Crawley et al., 2000). Research has focused on documenting the disparities among patients and families of racially marginalized groups in terms of identifying and addressing the psychosocial needs of culturally diverse and underserved patients living and dying of serious illness and disease (Ejem et al., 2019; Sanders et al., 2016). What has become abundantly clear is that social workers have an important role to play in cancer care amid pandemics, disasters, and other traumatic events.

During a pandemic or other natural disasters, responding to care needs by delivering patient-centered symptom management requires timely, complex decisions in the face of uncertainty and in many instances, the delay of diagnosis and treatment (Patt et al., 2020). For many oncology social workers this means adapting standards of care such as advance care planning conversations, family members at the bedside of the patient while their loved one is receiving care, extended time to develop trusting relationships with clinicians and the engagement of pastoral care and spiritual support. Yet, for Black patients who were already facing barriers to equitable care, including cancer care, receiving worse care than White patients (Sanders et al., 2016) and mistrusting of health care systems (Crawley et al., 2000), the natural disaster of a pandemic further alienated them from cancer care options.

Oncology social workers should continuously challenge each other to reflect on contemporary issues in the larger society that impact the lives of our patients, prior to their illness encounter and quest for the best possible health outcomes. At the core of ethical social work practice is a commitment to and value for diversity, equity, and culturally competent care (National Association of Social Workers [NASW], 2017). An examination of cancer care amid pandemics, disasters, and/or other traumatic events requires particular attention to the patient populations that have been disproportionately impacted by the COVID-19 pandemic and historically experienced barriers to equitable health care (ACSCAN, n.d.; Cadet et al., 2021). Everyone has experienced the unprecedented challenges of the COVID-19 public health emergency as a disaster fraught with traumatic events, but the pandemic has disproportionately affected Black and Brown people and communities. In light of this, it behooves oncology social workers to consider the implications of systemic injustices for patients in need of cancer care. Given the long history of racial disparities in cancer care (ACSCAN, 2022) and now the undeniable inequities and impacts of COVID-19 on communities of color (Elbaum, 2020), there is no better time to prioritize the alignment of the basic values, ethical principles, and ethical standards of the social work profession (NASW, 2017) and the practice of oncology social work.

For nearly two decades, health services research has considered history and heritage as explanatory factors in addressing barriers to care for racial and ethnic populations (Aaron et al., 2021; Crawley et al., 2000). It is time that social workers now do the same for patients receiving cancer care and their families, especially those populations that have experienced substantial inequities over their life course (Siker et al., 2020). While disparate standards of and limited access to care associated with the COVID-19 pandemic have been felt globally and universally, the full range of gaps in oncology and palliative care for racially and culturally diverse patients is not yet well understood or well documented in the health care literature. We must begin to consider racism as a social determinant of cancer outcomes in order to address historical inequities, and the context of unprecedented challenges amid a pandemic, disasters, and other times of traumatic events may reveal areas for improvement in health care systems where individuals of Black, Indigenous, Hispanic/Latino/a/x, and Asian and Pacific Island backgrounds were already experiencing barriers such as distrust (Crawley et al., 2000) and delayed diagnosis and slower time for cancer care screening and treatment (Siker et al., 2020). A cancer diagnosis is not a protective factor from the disparate racial inequities.

Even prior to the COVID-19 pandemic, the unequal burden of cancer on racially diverse populations was well documented through reports of far worse health outcomes than their White counterparts (Acquati et al., 2021; ACSCAN, 2022; Elbaum, 2020; Hooper et al., 2020). In particular, Black patients have faced long-standing disparities in cancer risk factors, cancer incidence, treatment, survivorship, and mortality. Moreover, research suggests that the causes of these disparities and barriers to health equity are multifactorial inside and outside of cancer care delivery systems. Furthermore, racism has been spotlighted as a driver of health outcomes (Elbaum, 2020).

Times of disaster and traumatic events, including the COVID-19 pandemic, propel grave consequences for cancer care, including disrupted treatment protocols, more stringent allocation of scarce resources, disrupted service delivery, and devasting patient outcomes, including accelerated death. The momentum to attend to the traumatic events experienced across racial lines (Wang et al., 2020) was spawned by the evidence that White communities, while certainly affected, were not experiencing the escalated death rates and lack of restorative health outcomes in proportion to Black and Brown communities (Hooper et al., 2020).

Access to medical treatment has always been less readily available to some populations than others (Bullock & Allison, 2015; Washington, 2006). For example, persons experiencing homelessness while living with a cancer diagnosis during the COVID-19 pandemic were at greater risk of inequitable access than White persons (Bullock-Johnson & Bullock, 2020). Moreover, people who were marginalized, with limited access to resources prior to the COVID19, often found that they were not able to wear personal protective equipment to minimize exposure to hazards that cause workplace injuries and illnesses, layoffs, or housing security (Bullock-Johnson & Bullock, 2020). Coupled with traumatic, life-threating events, the parallel process of increased exposure to racialized violence and systemic racism in health care systems created unprecedented challenges during COVID-19.

The future trajectory of this pandemic, disasters, and other traumatic events are uncertain, and social workers must continue to prepare for such public health unpredictability in cancer care. As the health care crisis surrounding COVID-19 continues to evolve, social workers' overarching goals are to provide compassionate, equitable care for patients with cancer. We must aim for culturally competent care, consistent with our social work *Code of Ethics* (2017), as this pandemic continues to affect patients in need of oncology care. In so doing, social workers must take into account racial equity when also dealing with disasters and traumatic events.

Racial Inequity, Disasters, and Traumatic Events

Structural racism is an identifiable and preventable barrier to access to health care. Historically, White people have had greater access to insurance and user-pay systems than Black and Brown people (Wang et al., 2020; Washington, 2006), which has disadvantaged these racial groups. People who have not had the privilege of access to preventive care over their lifetime has brought these disparities into stark relief, especially in light of a cancer diagnosis (Acquati et al., 2021). Consequently, groups that have been historically marginalized and denied equal access to education, health care, and other basic necessities of life are devasted by the coronavirus with a greater likelihood of reduced life expectancies three to four times larger than their White counterparts during the COVID-19 pandemic (Wang et al., 2020). In summary, the disproportionate impacts of COVID-19 have been felt through incidence risk and mortality that should be taken into consideration through a contextual lens of multiple factors that affect palliative care outcomes, such as lack of racial concordance between patients and care providers, historical distrust and mistrust (Crawley et al., 2000), and chronic fatigue that may be linked to racism (Brooks & Houck, 2013; Bullock-Johnson & Bullock, 2020; Washington, 2006).

Racism Fatigue

Oncology researchers have debated the impacts and implications of vicarious trauma and resilience (e.g., Mattison, 2015). Studies that explore stress as a clinical and research concept have resulted in widespread acknowledgment of the personal toll cancer patients face in the form of unrest and a longing to escape the cumulative impact of and exposure to emotional and psychological pain, trauma, and loss. To date, however, the research into and discourse around stress have ignored the concept of racism fatigue. Disparities in how people experience the world around us create significant differences in how people experience each other on a personal and professional level.

Many people in the United States witnessed traumatic events during the COVID-19 pandemic; however, Black individuals and communities, in particular, experienced firsthand the devastating results of how the toxic legacy of racialized trauma that they have long endured served to exacerbate the COVID-19 pandemic among them. Preexisting racial and health inequities result in poor cancer care and palliative care outcomes. A study that examined the impact of the COVID-19 pandemic on cancer care and health-related quality of life for non-Hispanic Black or African American, Hispanic/Latina, and non-Hispanic White women diagnosed with breast cancer in the United States, revealed evidence that pandemic conditions, public health crises, and global traumatic events do not serve as a protective factor against racial disparities in serious illness care (Acquati et al., 2021; Ejem et al., 2019). The study belies the assumption that during a crisis or pandemic circumstances, all patients would receive the same care, compassion, and access to resources for recovery—research clearly shows otherwise. Preexisting racial and health inequalities associated with social determinants of health did not result in a shift that prioritized patients with a higher risk of morbidity and mortality in the COVID-19 pandemic. Instead, Black and Brown people were less likely to receive scarce medical resources and endured longer delays in access to screening, diagnosis, and treatment (Hooper et al., 2020)—in other words, they continued to face structural racism in palliative care (Bullock et al., 2022). These stark differences require social workers (indeed all medical professionals) to acknowledge racism as a social determinant of cancer care in order to move toward health equity.

Acknowledging Racism as a Social Determinant of Health Outcomes in Cancer Care

Cancer is the second leading cause of death in the United States, and Blacks suffer the highest rates of cancer morbidity and mortality of any racial group (ACSCAN, 2022). Furthermore, for centuries, Black Americans have not only experienced specific instances of traumatic and racist medical research but also endured the dreadful results of racial inequity in U.S. health care systems (Washington, 2006). In cancer care and other medical treatments for health and disease, Black or African American people have been deemed expendable. Historically, such medical atrocities have taken a toll on Black patients, families, and clinicians, which has yet to be fully addressed in the serious illness care literature. In light of this dark past, exploring antiracist approaches to improving care is essential for all oncology social work and medical practitioners. To understand the depth and extent of racist, inequitable treatment for patients and families, social workers must gain cross-cultural knowledge that goes beyond idle curiosity or an academic exercise that claims to help clinicians recognize unconscious bias in the care encounter (Bullock et al., 2022; Curseen & Bullock, 2022). The NASW *Code of Ethics* (2017) clearly sets forth cultural competence as a standard of practice for social workers. In order to reduce inequitable health practice behaviors, social workers should demonstrate awareness of cultural differences (including their own implicit biases), acquire knowledge of how these differences manifest as disparities in a health care setting, and learn and implement specific antiracist skills that are transferrable across care settings. Social workers should obtain education and training that increases their capacity to function effectively across cultural groups with the aim to detect and tear down barriers that perpetuate oppression, racism, discrimination, and racial inequities.

Addressing Systemic Racism in Cancer Care

Racism in U.S. health care systems has been both historically legal and lethal (Elbaum, 2020). This chapter has emphasized a plethora of sources, including scholarly research, social and news media, Grand Rounds presentations, webinars, workshops, and classroom lectures and seminars is that the lifelong learning that the NASW espouses in the *Code of Ethics* is only as good or effective as those doing the teaching and those engaged in the learning. In other words, one cannot teach what they do not know. If social workers are to address racism in serious illness care, they must commit individually and as a profession to education that is action oriented and inclusive of theories and frameworks that decenter Whiteness. Racism is a social determinant of health, especially through the lack of preventive cancer care that historically marginalized populations experience due to unequal access to education, employment, housing opportunities, and many other social factors (Elbaum, 2020; Washington, 2006). Black people, in particular, are exhausted by structural racism and the legacy of unfair treatment they have experienced in health care settings. Social workers and other practitioners need a clear roadmap that outlines the specific steps needed to innovate and create alternative ways to ensure access to cancer care, even in the face of a pandemic, disaster, or traumatic event.

Moving into postpandemic times, oncology social workers must unify against racism. The guiding principles offered in the next section can help us provide equitable care to patients and families that have experienced (and continue to experience) both past racism and unprecedented challenges as a result of negative and traumatic events. We should recognize first, though, that racially and ethnically diverse patients and families should not bear the burden of convincing oncology clinicians, government officials (elected or paid), health care executives, higher education administrators, business owners, educators, clergy, physicians, nurses, social workers, or other health care providers that their cultural preferences and values should be honored and respected. Basic steps that any/all individuals can take on micro, mezzo, or macro levels are to *lean in*, *speak up*, and *speak out* loudly and often about disparities and the need for racial equity in cancer care in our daily practice of providing person-centered, goal-concordant, culturally competent holistic cancer care.

Guiding Best Practices for the Future

Oncology social workers are members of professional teams with specialized knowledge, skills and training required to support patients, families, and colleagues facing and managing serious illness under some of the most stressful circumstances and crisis conditions. Providing person-centered care is a best practice in social work practice (NASW, 2017). In order to optimize quality of life and mitigate suffering among people with serious, complex illnesses, social workers should aim for cultural competence in alignment with the NASW *Code of Ethics* (2017). Whether the focus is on managing a cancer diagnosis, on the crisis points that ebb and flow when dealing with cancer over the care continuum, on instilling hope in coping, or on galvanizing resources and concrete services, social workers lead with standards for and indicators of cultural competence. It is important in cancer care to address issues of racial inequity experienced by historically marginalized populations that have been victimized by structural and systemic racism.

Serious illness care clinicians working in interdisciplinary teams that include social workers are promoting cultural competence as a tool for educating team members about how best to engage effectively with racially and ethnically diverse patients (Boucher & Johnson, 2021). In offering person-centered cancer care and seeking to understand the importance of equity in cancer care during or after a pandemic, natural disaster, of other traumatic event, oncology social workers must seek to address structural and systemic racism through an antiracist cancer care approach. The five essentials steps on the journey to becoming more cultural competent are (1) awareness of and (2) acknowledgment that the problem of racism exists as a barrier to health equity, (3) considering antiracist practices, (4) contemplating what kinds of professional development oncology social workers can engage in to move along the continuum from a lack of awareness of one's implicit bias to awareness of racial disparities and the cultivation of humility, and finally, (5) initiating specific actions in support of individual patients, families, communities, and oncology colleagues that feel ignored, oppressed, silenced, and marginalized in our struggle for equity and justice. Working toward cultural competence will build a bridge to action-oriented practice that moves beyond cultural humility to more individualized, goal-concordant care (Bullock et al., 2022; Curseen & Bullock, 2022).

Pearls

- Identifying psychosocial distress and trauma associated with racial inequities in cancer care and understanding the historical lack of access to culturally competent clinicians and the distrust of health care systems these things have caused among historically excluded and marginalized populations must become a priority in oncology social work education, training, and practice.
- Developing a workforce of culturally competent oncology social workers prepared to provide restorative practices and services for patients and families that have experienced historical racism is essential.
- Incorporating social work values, ethical practice standards, and a commitment to social justice and racial equity to increase the likelihood historically marginalized populations will receive person-centered cancer care is critically important to their health outcomes.

Pitfalls

- Placing the burden on patient and families to educate clinicians to move beyond cultural humility to cultural competence amounts to blaming the victim and perpetuates entrenched inequities in access to quality cancer care.
- Failing to identify the impacts of structural and systemic racism during pandemics, disasters, and other traumatic events can perpetuate

justifiable fears among patients and families that they will also face racial inequity in the cancer care setting.
- Failing to recognize how Black and Brown patients and families have been and still are marginalized and systematically excluded from equitable health care perpetuates their exclusion from culturally congruent cancer care.

Additional Resources

Books

Matthew, D. B. (2022). *Just health: Treating structural racism to heal America*. NYU Press.
Barr, D. A. (2019). *Health disparities in the United States: Social class, race, ethnicity, and the social determinants of health* (3rd ed.). Johns Hopkins University Press.
Skloot, R. (2010). *The immortal life of Henrietta Lacks*. Random House.

Websites

Bullock, K., Samiano, S., & Sinclair, S. (2021, April 24). *Health equity: Social workers can lead the way in addressing health inequities*. Center for Advancing Palliative Care: https://www.capc.org/blog/social-workers-can-lead-the-way-in-addressing-health-inequities/
Three practical steps that palliative care leaders can take to empower their social work colleagues and help bridge gaps in health equity.
Morehouse School of Medicine. *Cancer Health Equity Institute (CHEI)*: https://www.msm.edu/cancerhealthequityinstitute/index.php
Established in 2015, CHEI brings together people using their energy, talents, and skills to provide the best care for patients and discover new ways to prevent and combat cancer.
American Cancer Society. Cancer disparities in the Black community: https://www.cancer.org/about-us/what-we-do/health-equity/cancer-disparities-in-the-black-community.html
A resource for evidence-based information about racial/ethnic health disparities.

References

Aaron, S. P., Gazaway, S. B., Harrell, E. R., & Elk, R. (2021). Disparities and racism experienced among older African Americans nearing end of life. *Current Geriatrics Reports*, *10*(4), 157–166. https://doi.org/10.1007/s13670-021-00366-6

Acquati, C., Chen, T. A., Martinez Leal, I., Connors, S. K., Haq, A. A., Rogova, A., Ramirez, L. R., & McNeill, L. H. (2021). The impact of the COVID-19 pandemic on cancer care and health-related quality of life of non-Hispanic Black/African American, Hispanic/Latina and non-Hispanic White women diagnosed with breast cancer in the U.S.: A mixed-methods study protocol. *International Journal of Environmental Research and Public Health*, *18*(24), 13084. https://doi.org/10.3390/ijerph182413084

American Cancer Society (2022). Cancer facts and figures. Retrieved from https://www.cancer.org/content/dam/cancer-org/research/cancer-facts-and-statistics/annual-cancer-facts-and-figures/2022/2022-cancer-facts-and-figures.pdf

American Cancer Society Cancer Action Network (ACSCAN). (n.d.). COVID-19 pandemic impact on cancer patients and survivors: Survey findings summary. *American Cancer Society Cancer Action Network.* Retrieved January 3, 2022, from https://www.fightcancer.org/sites/default/files/National%20Documents/Survivor%20Views.COVID19%20Polling%20Memo.Final.pdf

Boucher, N. A., & Johnson, K. S. (2021). Cultivating cultural competence: How are hospice staff being educated to engage racially and ethnically diverse patients? *American Journal of Hospice and Palliative Care, 38*(2), 169–174. https://pubmed.ncbi.nlm.nih.gov/32734763/

Brooks, M. P., & Houck, D. W. (Eds.). (2013). *The speeches of Fannie Lou Hamer: To tell it like it is.* University Press of Mississippi.

Bullock, K., & Allison, H. (2015). Access to medical treatment for African American populations: The current evidence base. In G. Christ, C. Messner, & L. Behar (Eds.), *Handbook of oncology social work* (pp. 293–298). Oxford University Press.

Bullock, K., Gray, T. F., Tucker, R., & Quest, T. E. (2022, February 10). Race roundtable series: Structural racism in palliative care. *Journal of Pain and Symptom Management, 63*(5), E455–E459. https://doi.org/10.1016/j.jpainsymman.2022.01.015

Bullock-Johnson, R., & Bullock, K. (2020). *Exploring mental health treatment and prevention among homeless older adults.* IntechOpen Access. https://doi.org/10.5772/intechopen.89731

Cadet, T., Burke, S. L., Naseh, M., Grudzien, A., Kozak, R. S., Romeo, J., Bullock, K., & Davis, C. (2021). Examining the family support role of older Hispanics, African Americans, and non-Hispanic Whites and their breast cancer screening behaviors. *Social Work in Public Health, 36*(1), 38–53. https://doi.org/10.1080/19371918.2020.185299

Centers for Disease Control and Prevention. (n.d.). *An update on cancer deaths in the United States.* Retrieved November 17, 2020, from https://www.cdc.gov/cancer/dcpc/research/update-on-cancer-deaths/index.htm

Crawley, L., Payne, R., Bolden, J., Payne, T., Washington, P., Williams, S., & Initiative to Improve Palliative and End-of-Life Care in the African American Community. (2000). Palliative and end-of-life care in the African American community. *Journal of the American Medical Association, 284*(19), 2518–2521. https://doi.org/10.1001/jama.284.19.2518

Curseen, K., & Bullock, K. (2022). Response to Fitzgerald Jones et al., Top ten tips palliative care clinicians should know about delivering antiracist care to Black Americans. *Journal of Palliative Medicine.* https://doi.org/10.1089/jpm.2021.0622

Ejem, D. B., Barrett, N., Rhodes, R. L., Olsen, M., Bakitas, M., Durant, R., Elk, R., Steinhauser, K., Quest, T., Dolor, R. J., & Johnson, K. (2019). Reducing disparities in the quality of palliative care for older African Americans through improved advance care planning: Study design and protocol. *Journal of Palliative Medicine, 22*(S1), 90–100. https://doi.org/10.1089/jpm.2019.0146

Elbaum, A. (2020). Black lives in a pandemic: Implications of systemic injustice for end-of-life care. *Hastings Center Report.* https://doi.org/10.1002/hast.1135

Hooper, M. W., Nápoles, A. M., & Pérez-Stable, E. J. (2020). COVID-19 and racial/ethnic disparities. *Journal of the American Medical Association, 323*(24), 2466–2467.

Kamal, A. H., Bull, J., Wolf, S. P., Portman, D., Strand, J., Johnson, K. S. (2017). Unmet needs of African Americans and Whites at the time of palliative care consultation. *American Journal of Hospice and Palliative Care, 34*(5), 461–465. https://pubmed.ncbi.nlm.nih.gov/26888883/

Mattison, D. (2015). Vicarious resilience: Sustaining a career over the long haul. In G. Christ, C. Messner, & L. Behar (Eds.), *Handbook of oncology social work* (pp. 737–744). Oxford University Press.

National Association of Social Workers. (2017). *Code of Ethics of the National Association of Social Workers*. Retrieved October 18, 2022, from the National Association of Social Workers website: https://www.socialworkers.org/About/Ethics/Code-of-Ethics/Code-of-Ethics-English

Patt, D., Gordan, L., Diaz, M., Okon, T., Grady, L., Harmison, M., Markward, N., Sullivan, M., Peng, J., & Zhou, A. (2020). Impact of COVID-19 on cancer care: How the pandemic is delaying cancer diagnosis and treatment for American seniors. *Journal of Clinical Oncology: Clinical Cancer Informatics*, *4*, 1059–1071. https://doi.org/10.1200/CCI.20.00134

Sanders, J. J., Robinson, M. T., & Block, S. D. (2016). Factors impacting advance care planning among African Americans: Results of a systematic integrated review. *Journal of Palliative Medicine*, *19*(2), 202–227. http://doi.org/10.1089/jpm.2015.0325

Siker, M. L., Deville, C., Suneja, G., & Winkfield, K. (2020). Lessons from COVID-19: Addressing health equity in cancer care. *International Journal of Radiation: Oncology Biology Physics*, *108*, 475–478.

Venkatesulu, B. P., Chandrasekar, V. T., Girdhar, P., Advani, P., Sharma, A., Elumalai, T., Hsieh, C., Elghazawy, H. I., Verma, V., & Krishnan, S. (2021). A systematic review and meta-analysis of cancer patients affected by a novel coronavirus. *Journal of the National Cancer Institutes Cancer Spectrum*, *5*(2), 1–11. http://doi.org/10.1093/jncics/pkaa102

Wang, H., & Li, Z. (2020). Risk of COVID-19 for patients with cancer. *Lancet Oncology*, *21*(4). https://doi.org/10.1016/S1470-2045(20)30150-9

Wang, M. L., Behrman, P., Dulin, A., Baskin, M. L., Buscemi, J., Alcaraz, K. I., Goldstein, C. M., Carson, T. L., Shen, M., & Fitzgibbon, M. (2020). Addressing inequities in COVID-19 morbidity and mortality: Research and policy recommendations. *Translational Behavioral Medicine*, *10*, 516–519.

Washington, H. A. (2006). *Medical apartheid: The dark history of medical experimentation on Black Americans from colonial times to the present*. Random House.

6

Beyond Survival

Survivorship, Integrative Programs, Lifestyle, and Rehabilitation

Randi Lyn Hornyak, Yvette Colón, and Mary Lou Galantino

Key Concepts

- Domains of cancer rehabilitation include treatment, follow-up care, and survivorship.
- The role of the interprofessional care team is vital.
- Social determinants of health throughout the cancer care continuum must be considered.
- Addressing disparities via community-based exercise and knowledge transfer can improve quality of life.

Keywords: cancer survivorship, disparities, integrative programs, mindfulness, pain management, psychosocial distress, rehabilitation, social determinants of health

Cancer survivorship has changed significantly in the decades since Mullan (1985) wrote about the "seasons of survival" and launched a movement, defining it as a process that begins at diagnosis and continues throughout the rest of life. Diagnostic and treatment advances have led to a significant increase in the number of cancer survivors in the United States; in January 2019, there were an estimated 16.9 million (National Cancer Institute, 2020). Although its use has become widespread, the term *cancer survivor* is by no means uniformly accepted. Berry et al. (2019) express, "Using a single term for people who share in common a cancer diagnosis is convenient. But in the interest of *simplifying* communication, can any term do justice to a population as large and heterogeneous as those who have lived with cancer?" (p. 414). We use the term *cancer survivor* in this chapter with that caveat fully in mind.

Randi Lyn Hornyak, Yvette Colón, and Mary Lou Galantino, *Beyond Survival* In: *Oncology and Palliative Social Work*.
Edited by: Susan Hedlund, Bryan Miller, Grace Christ, and Carolyn Messner, Oxford University Press.
 DOI: 10.1093/oso/9780197607299.003.0006

Among cancer survivors, psychosocial distress (e.g., depression, anxiety, sadness, fear, overwhelm) is common (Carlson et al., 2019). Between 2010 and 2013, cancer survivors in the United States took medications to treat depression and anxiety at twice the rate of the general population (Hawkins et al., 2017). Experiences that a survivor perceives as physically or emotionally harmful or life-threatening can have long-lasting adverse effects on their physical, psychological, social, and spiritual well-being and functioning. Survivors may perceive their cancer experience as traumatic, or they may have experienced trauma from adverse events prior to their cancer diagnosis and treatment. Rowland (2021) stressed the need for researchers and clinicians to acquire skills to help cancer survivors prevent and manage the physical, emotional, and social challenges they often face, to promote rehabilitation as a necessary part of ongoing care, and to improve quality of life at every opportunity.

What We Have Learned So Far

Treatment for cancer has significantly improved survival across all cancer types; however, these interventions may compromise function and quality of life. Despite recommended guidelines for physical activity, a considerable number of cancer survivors experience various comorbidities that hamper daily activities and compromise work capacity and social engagement. Specific models for rehabilitation in oncology care emphasize the importance of prospective surveillance to screen appropriately and treat accordingly. Here, we present a physical, psychological, and spiritual approach to optimizing lifestyle behaviors from a nonpharmacologic perspective; additionally, we explore integrative oncology strategies and evidence-based approaches for various cancer populations.

Addressing Symptoms Following Cancer Care—The Role of the Interprofessional Care Team

With different disease and recovery courses, multiple treatment approaches, and varying side-effects, cancer survivorship is inherently an individual and multifaceted experience. Therefore, a cancer care team should comprise a multitude of health care professionals at points of intervention to improve function and quality of life. During and upon completion of acute management of cancer, the interprofessional health care team plays a vital role in connecting the patient/client to rehabilitative and community-based providers for continued care throughout cancer survivorship.

Many physical impairments and pain symptoms may emerge during treatment and linger after, negatively affecting an individual's health-related quality of life. Impairments not only stem from the disease process itself but also may arise from various treatments. For example, radiation therapy may result in skin irritation, pain, and fatigue (Borrelli et al., 2019); survivors with a history of chemotherapy may have adverse effects including damage to nerves and muscles and nutritional deficits that may contribute to frailty and fall risk (Galantino et al., 2019). Various surgical interventions may also lead to significant pain and impaired function. Unfortunately, these impairments may go undetected and untreated, resulting in disability and distress. Early detection of physical decline followed by prompt intervention can help reduce the possible sequalae of impairments following cancer treatment, including pain, physical limitations, disability, impaired function, and decreased participation in work and social roles. Rehabilitation professionals involved in this detection and treatment include physiatrists, nurses, nutritionists, social workers, and psychologists, as well as speech, occupational, and physical therapists. Interprofessional practice among these rehabilitation professionals, along with oncologists, primary care providers, and other experts in behavior change can help patients live longer, healthier lives throughout the cancer care continuum. With support from an interdisciplinary rehabilitation care team, rehabilitation can act as an effective transition between active cancer treatment and post-treatment lifestyle to promote continued health and wellness maintenance (McNeely et al., 2016).

At the center of every care team, the patient is the focal point throughout the cancer care and survivorship continuum. Team members should always explain plans of care and discuss intervention options, and patients should play a primary role in decision-making regarding their care. Communication among patient, health care providers, and integrative practitioners is vital to optimal health and well-being outcomes for patients with a cancer diagnosis (Lopez et al., 2017).

Pain Management and Psychologically Informed Physical Therapy

Cancer survivors may experience pain from postoperative loss of function, chemotherapy-induced peripheral neuropathy (CIPN), and radiation fibrosis. Proper physical therapy assessment and treatment can improve range of motion, reduce pain, and manage lymphedema.

Patients with cancer use many strategies to manage pain. Whereas those who catastrophize often report increased pain, those who prioritize self-efficacy report lower levels of pain. Therefore, it is important for social workers and others on the care team to assess domains of capability to execute a plan of care including health literacy and self-efficacy. Cognitive-behavioral therapies and mind-body interventions can positively impact anxiety, stress, depression, or mood disturbances, and massage, acupuncture, healing touch, hypnotherapy, and music therapy can reduce cancer pain. Other mind-body therapies have shown trends in reducing the severity of cancer pain and improving treatment-related distress, and they include education through coping skills training, yoga, tai chi, qigong, guided imagery, virtual reality, and cognitive-behavioral therapy alone or combined (Maindet et al., 2019). Evidence demonstrates that psychoemotional distress, anxiety, uncertainty, depression, and hopelessness interact with pain and can increase a survivor's perception of pain. Knowing these interrelationships between pain and a patient's psychoemotional state indicates just how essential an interprofessional approach to pain management is.

Although exercise can mitigate pain, it is important to address impairment prior to engaging in an exercise program. Yoga, tai chi, hypnotherapy, and exercise show promise for controlling pain. Although some of these treatments effectively reduce pain for patients with advanced disease, few have been evaluated in patients at the end of life. Psychological factors affect cancer pain, behavioral treatments are effective in reducing varying types of pain for patients with active disease, and multidisciplinary teams are important in oncology settings to foster holistic pain management strategies and expertise in psychological and behavioral interventions (Maindet et al., 2019).

Lifestyle Medicine: Exercise and Nutrition

Increasing evidence supports the use of lifestyle medicine—combined exercise and nutrition—for individuals throughout the cancer care continuum and across the lifespan. Achieving and maintaining a healthy weight throughout life, adopting a physically active lifestyle, and consuming a healthy diet with an emphasis on plant sources is important. Presence and severity of treatment-related side effects, the individual's cognitive functioning, psychological status, and coping capacity, and external factors including social determinants of health (SDOH) and other environmental and behavioral considerations must be considered when designing lifestyle intervention plans (Stout et al., 2021). Rehabilitation interventions that include social workers and nutrition professionals can assist in appropriate guidance to individuals to ensure safety and efficacy of these behavior modifications.

Physical activity prescription helps improve common cancer treatment-related impairments including fatigue, lymphedema, physical function, anxiety, depression, and health-related diminishment of a patient's quality of life. A rehabilitation specialist can assist individuals in designing and monitoring progression of an exercise plan while also considering the individual's personal and environmental factors to ensure the greatest benefit with minimal to no adverse effects.

Growing evidence supports the importance of exercise, physical activity, and weight management in the prevention of cancer. Spending at least 150 minutes per week in moderate activity has the potential to reduce the risk of colon, breast, kidney, liver, lung, myeloid leukemia, myeloma, head and neck, rectal, endometrial, bladder esophageal, and stomach cancers (Moore et al., 2016). This benefit of physical activity is a critical component of cancer recurrence prevention and healthy lifestyle practice.

Nutrition and weight management is an important part of the plan of care for cancer survivors. Individuals with advanced cancer, especially older adults, often experience a reduction in weight, bone density, and muscle mass, resulting in frailty. Specific nutrition guidelines regarding caloric intake and specific nutrient and/or supplement recommendations can address these changes.

Professional consultation before making diet changes is highly encouraged. Nutrition specialists, including registered dieticians, can modify recommendations for cancer survivors to ensure safety and effectiveness. Additional considerations after certain procedures and treatments involving the neck, throat, and mouth may affect chewing and swallowing and the patient should discuss this with a health care professional, such as a speech-language therapist.

Integrative Oncology Strategies: Mindfulness, Yoga, and Tai Chi

Along with lifestyle medicine approaches, integrative oncology and mindfulness practices may ease physical and psychological symptoms following cancer and cancer treatment. Integrative oncology is an evidence-based, patient-centered, comprehensive intervention method that involves lifestyle modifications, mind-body practices, and use of natural products from various traditions in combination with conventional cancer treatments

(Latte-Naor & Mao, 2019). Mindfulness, yoga, and tai chi interventions provide symptom management and allow for a holistic approach to wellness. Connecting individuals with community-based practitioners who offer these integrative interventions has the potential to help cancer survivors reach optimal outcomes throughout cancer survivorship.

The goal of mindfulness meditation is to notice and acknowledge physical sensations, breath, emotions, and thoughts without judgment. Mindfulness is an essential underpinning for yoga and tai chi and adds a unique dynamic to movement therapies. Various clinical trials have shown evidence in support of mindfulness-based stress reduction (MBSR) improving psychological health, including reducing both emotional symptoms like anxiety, stress, and fear of recurrence and physical symptoms, including chronic pain and fatigue (Lengacher et al., 2016; Paice et al., 2016). Body awareness and presence without judgment can foster moment-to-moment experiences for cancer survivors, especially during moments of uncertainty.

The many styles of yoga center around meditation, physical postures (asanas), and breathing techniques based in Ayurvedic medicine. Research highlights moderate evidence for yoga interventions as a supportive strategy for various cancer diagnoses to improve health-related quality of life and reduce fatigue and sleep disturbances. Furthermore, yoga can help reduce anxiety and depression in cancer survivors and serve to manage chronic cancer pain (Cramer et al., 2017). Somatic yoga focuses on meditation and aims to increase body and mind sensitivity; it has the potential to reduce persistent CIPN and improve fall risk, flexibility, balance, and quality of life in cancer survivors (Galantino et al., 2019). If a cancer survivor experiences fatigue due to treatments or is unable to access a gym or community group to exercise, yoga (which is easily done at home) may be an effective alternative to other forms of physical activity.

Tai chi is a practice that originates in Chinese martial arts and focuses on coordinating slow, flowing movement sequences with focused grounding, attention, and breathing techniques. Elements of traditional Chinese medicine, including acupuncture, tu ina, tai chi, or qigong, may serve as effective adjunctive therapies to improve quality of life and address adverse symptoms, including fatigue, among cancer survivors (Wayne et al., 2018). Tai chi may serve especially well for deconditioned or older cancer survivors, providing them a gentle way in which to both increase their physical activity and reduce fall risk due to frailty and CIPN (Klein et al., 2019).

For lifestyle medicine and integrative oncology approaches to be effective and sustainable, an individual must remain committed to these changes. Ongoing monitoring, surveillance, and feedback can maximize long-term adherence to the exercise, nutrition, and integrative interventions discussed in this chapter.

Behavior-change interventions and the resulting formation of long-term habits can help individuals effectively adopt and glean the benefits of these approaches.

Brenda, a 64-year-old woman, presented to outpatient physical therapy (PT) with lower back and pelvic pain. She worked as a high school principal and had been highly active until her pain symptoms began to limit her mobility. Twenty years earlier, she received a diagnosis of invasive carcinoma of the breast; her medical history included treatment with surgical modified radical mastectomy and chemotherapy including Adriamycin, Cytoxan, and Taxol. She received PT at that time to improve shoulder movement due to restrictive postoperative axillary scarring and expander implant discomfort but was discharged in four weeks. Physical therapy also addressed her peripheral neuropathy from Taxol through desensitization, exercise, and balance activities, which increased her overall safety. Prior to presenting with her current back pain, this had been Brenda's only encounter with PT.

According to the clinical assessment, Brenda presented with "Significant limitations in spine movement in all directions due to pain in this second episode of care. Visual analog pain scale (VAS) score: 7/10; Oswestry Disability Score: 34% indicating moderate disability. Posture: forward head and shoulders. Muscle Strength: 4/5 throughout upper and lower extremities. Neurological exam: unremarkable." Brenda stated she experienced more pain and difficulty with activities of daily living and was able only to work part-time now due to pain. The physical therapist provided various manual therapy techniques to reduce her muscle spasms but was concerned this was a breast cancer recurrence and consulted the interprofessional team. The physical therapist requested a diagnostic workup and imaging studies that revealed multiple lytic and blastic lesions in the lumbar and thoracic vertebrae, ribs, and sternum. Brenda returned to her oncologist, who confirmed metastatic disease, prescribed additional pain medication, and ordered radiation to reduce the lytic lesions and lessen her pain. Brenda was overwhelmed and depressed about her diagnosis, and social work support was initiated after the physical therapist measured these domains on the patient-reported distress scale (National Comprehensive Cancer Network, 2022).

Brenda's team initiated palbociclib (Ibrance) along with an aromatase inhibitor (letrozole) as first-line treatment for estrogen receptor-positive, HER2-negative metastatic breast cancer. Because the risks of this regimen include lowered white blood cells, the interprofessional team had to address optimal hand hygiene and environmental cleaning when interacting with Brenda.

The social worker met concurrently with Brenda to cultivate coping strategies while the physical therapist continued to provide pain modulation techniques and strategies for activities of daily living and work-related postural adaptations over the course of radiation and medication treatment. A licensed dietician was consulted to address weight reduction and improved eating habits. Overall, the team addressed Brenda's new diagnosis and prognosis with several different coping strategies over the course of various sessions. After three months of radiation, PT, social work, and nutrition Interventions, Brenda joined a community support group and was able to begin a gentle yoga class after discharge from PT. Although her disease required targeted interventions as necessary, Brenda continued to work, resumed many of her usual activities, and lived with metastatic disease for another five years after her second diagnosis.

Social Determinants of Health Throughout the Cancer Care Continuum

Social determinants of health (SDOH), as defined by Healthy People 2030, include "the conditions in the environments where people are born, live, learn, work, play, worship, and age that affect a wide range of health, functioning, and quality-of-life outcomes and risks" (Office of Disease Prevention & Health Promotion [ODPHP], 2022). The ODPHP categorizes SDOH into five components: neighborhood and built environment, education access and quality, health care access and quality, social and community context, and economic stability. Each category can produce either facilitators or barriers to healthy behaviors that are related to health outcomes, including physical activity level, quality of life, and mortality rates (Pronk et al., 2021).

Social inequities function as upstream factors that can lead to downstream effects, including personal risk factors, biomarkers, tumor characteristics, comorbidities, and access or lack of access to quality health care. The Social Determinants Framework for Cancer Equity identifies and addresses these upstream health inequities and disparities, including social and community context, institutional environments, and living environments (Alcaraz et al., 2020). For the most optimal design of lifestyle and integrative interventions, an interprofessional team must consider and address SDOH .

Social constructs—elitism, racism, sexism, homophobia, and other forms of discrimination—are immensely negative SDOH. Provider or implicit bias hinders communication between the patient and their care team, diminishes a patient's ability to share in decision-making, and reduces a patient's confidence in treatment recommendations and symptom management. Black breast cancer survivors have reported an increased need to advocate for access to quality information about their own care (Ozdemir & Finkelstein, 2018).

Cancer survivors identifying as sexual and gender minorities, including lesbian, gay, bisexual, or transgender individuals, report difficulty with care coordination and team members' lack of attention to gender identity, gender expression, or specific life needs (Kamen, 2018).

Addressing Disparities via Community-Based Exercise and Knowledge Transfer

Community-Based Exercise Programs

One way to address health disparities affecting individuals within various communities is by implementing community-based interventions, which can serve as an excellent resource to improve quality of life in adult cancer survivors and facilitate sustainable behavior change. Working in conjunction with community organizations—for example, churches, community centers, and support groups—located within marginalized communities can be an effective strategy in promoting lifestyle interventions. Relationships forged through participation in community programs such as health coaching and peer support groups significantly improve long-term adherence to healthy behaviors (Adlard et al., 2019). Community organizations can serve as trusted messengers to minimize distrust and skepticism and promote active engagement in these programs. Furthermore, these organizations may be essential to recruit for various clinical trials to serve minority populations.

Health and Wellness Coaching

Health and wellness coaching is an effective strategy of knowledge transfer to address barriers in health literacy via patient education, wellness plan development, and goal setting. Once an individual understands the impact of adopting a healthy lifestyle and sustainable behavior changes on quality of life, the goal for the health care and community teams is to promote consistency and positively reinforce the positive lifestyle changes. With careful consideration of barriers at the patient, provider, and health system levels, health and wellness coaches can help individuals create a personalized nutrition and physical activity plan throughout the cancer care continuum; the earlier that wellness is promoted, the better the possible outcomes. Fostering goal setting in concert with patient education can effectively reduce cancer pain and depression and anxiety in cancer survivors (Hawkins et al., 2017).

This chapter has presented various approaches to optimize cancer survivorship with a focus on community-based sustainable checkpoints. It is important to consistently explore the evidence for rehabilitation and apply accordingly for several types of cancer, treatment interventions, and psychosocial challenges in the context of survivors' SDOH. Furthermore, the importance of interdisciplinary health care professionals using best practices for the well-being of both the oncology team and all patients is highlighted.

Guiding Best Practices for the Future

Without proper and effective communication, patient-centered care is impossible, resulting in poor health outcomes. The interprofessional care team must consider SDOH when determining appropriate and effective lifestyle or integrative medicine approaches to meet the nuanced needs of each individual cancer survivor. Allyship (the use of one's privilege or power to advocate for all underrepresented and vulnerable individuals and groups) is necessary to address health inequities; challenging systemic structures that create and maintain these inequities is a moral imperative (Nixon, 2019). Advocacy, community trust, specific outreach, and health literacy are key in clinical practice to produce the most optimal health and wellness outcomes for cancer survivors.

Pearls

- Cancer survivorship has increased significantly in the last four decades.
- Interprofessional collaboration is vital to successfully achieving goals of survivorship care.
- Psychologically informed pain management, physical therapy, and integrative oncology strategies are needed to address patient needs in a holistic way.

Pitfalls

- Patients can experience psychosocial distress through all phases of treatment and survivorship.
- Treatment for cancer has significantly improved survival across all cancer types, but these interventions may compromise physical function and quality of life.

- Health inequities will have a negative effect on treatment and survivorship outcomes.

Additional Resources

Academy of Oncologic Physical Therapy: www.oncologypt.org
Cancer.gov: www.cancer.gov/resources-for/patients
Cancer*Care*: www.cancercare.org/publications/60-finding_resources_in_your_community
Cancer Support Community: www.cancersupportcommunity.org/
Centers for Disease Control & Prevention: www.cdc.gov/cancer/health-care-providers/index.htm

References

Adlard, K. N., Jenkins, D. G., Salisbury, C. E., Bolam, K. A., Gomersall, S. R., Aitken, J. F., Chambers, S. K., Dunn, J. C., Courneya, K. S., & Skinner, T. L. (2019). Peer support for the maintenance of physical activity and health in cancer survivors: The PEER trial—a study protocol of a randomised controlled trial. *BMC Cancer*, *19*(1), 656. https://doi.org/10.1186/s12885-019-5853-4

Alcaraz, K. I., Wiedt, T. L., Daniels, E. C., Yabroff, K. R., Guerra, C. E., & Wender, R. C. (2020). Understanding and addressing social determinants to advance cancer health equity in the United States: A blueprint for practice, research, and policy. *CA: A Cancer Journal for Clinicians*, *70*(1), 31–46. https://doi.org/10.3322/caac.21586

Berry, L. L., Davis, S. W., Godfrey Flynn, A., Landercasper, J., & Deming, K. A. (2019). Is it time to reconsider the term "cancer survivor"? *Journal of Psychosocial Oncology*, *37*(4), 413–426.

Borrelli, M. R., Shen, A. H., Lee, G. K., Momeni, A., Longaker, M. T., & Wan, D. C. (2019). Radiation-induced skin fibrosis: Pathogenesis, current treatment options, and emerging therapeutics. *Annals of Plastic Surgery*, *83*(4S Suppl 1), S59–S64. https://doi.org/10.1097/SAP.0000000000002098

Carlson, L. E., Zelinski, E. L., Toivonen, K. I., Sundstrom, L., Jobin, C. T., Damaskos, P., & Zebrack, B. (2019). Prevalence of psychosocial distress in cancer patients across 55 North American cancer centers. *Journal of Psychosocial Oncology*, *37*(1), 5–21.

Cramer, H., Lauche, R., Klose, P., Lange, S., Langhorst, J., & Dobos, G. J. (2017). Yoga for improving health-related quality of life, mental health, and cancer-related symptoms in women diagnosed with breast cancer. *Cochrane Database of Systematic Reviews*. https://doi.org/10.1002/14651858.CD010802.pub2

Galantino, M. L., Tiger, R., Brooks, J., Jang, S., & Wilson, K. (2019). Impact of somatic yoga and meditation on fall risk, function, and quality of life for chemotherapy-induced peripheral neuropathy syndrome in cancer survivors. *Integrative Cancer Therapies*, *18*. https://doi.org/10.1177/1534735419850627

Hawkins, N. A., Soman, A., Lunsford, N. B., Leadbetter, S., & Rodriguez, J. L. (2017). Use of medications for treating anxiety and depression in cancer survivors in the United States. *Journal of Clinical Oncology*, *35*(1), 78–87.

Kamen, C. (2018). Lesbian, gay, bisexual, and transgender (LGBT) survivorship. *Seminars in Oncology Nursing*, *34*(1), 52–59. https://doi.org/10.1016/j.soncn.2017.12.002

Klein, P. J., Baumgarden, J., & Schneider, R. (2019). Qigong and tai chi as therapeutic exercise: Survey of systematic reviews and meta-analyses addressing physical health conditions. *Alternative Therapies in Health and Medicine*, *25*(5), 48–53.

Latte-Naor, S., & Mao, J. J. (2019). Putting integrative oncology into practice: Concepts and approaches. *Journal of Oncology Practice*, *15*(1), 7–14.

Lengacher, C. A., Reich, R. R., Paterson, C. L., Ramesar, S., Park, J. Y., Alinat, C., Johnson-Mallard, V., Moscoso, M., Budhrani-Shani, P., Miladinovic, B., Jacobsen, P. B., Cox, C. E., Goodman, M., & Kip, K. E. (2016). Examination of broad symptom improvement resulting from mindfulness-based stress reduction in breast cancer survivors: A randomized controlled trial. *Journal of Clinical Oncology*, *34*(24), 2827–2834. https://doi.org/10.1200/JCO.2015.65.7874

Lopez, G., Mao, J. J., & Cohen, L. (2017). Integrative oncology. *Medical Clinics of North America*, *101*(5), 977–985. https://doi.org/10.1016/j.mcna.2017.04.011

Maindet, C., Burnod, A., Minello, C., George, B., Allano, G., & Lemaire, A. (2019). Strategies of complementary and integrative therapies in cancer-related pain-attaining exhaustive cancer pain management. *Supportive Care in Cancer*, *27*(8), 3119–3132. https://doi.org/10.1007/s00520-019-04829-7

McNeely, M. L., Dolgoy, N., Al Onazi, M., & Suderman, K. (2016). The interdisciplinary rehabilitation care team and the role of physical therapy in survivor exercise. *Clinical Journal of Oncology Nursing*, *20*(6 Suppl), S8–S16. https://doi.org/10.1188/16.CJON.S2.8-16

Moore, S. C., Lee, I. M., Weiderpass, E., Campbell, P. T., Sampson, J. N., Kitahara, C. M., Keadle, S. K., Arem, H., DeGonzalez, A. B., Hartge, P., & Adami, H. O. (2016). Association of leisure-time physical activity with risk of 26 types of cancer in 1.44 million adults. *JAMA Internal Medicine*, *176*(6), 816–825. https://doi.org/10.1001/jamainternmed.2016.1548

Mullan, F. (1985). Seasons of survival: Reflections of a physician with cancer. *New England Journal of Medicine*, *313*(4), 270–273.

National Cancer Institute. (2020, September 25). *Cancer statistics*. Retrieved from https://www.cancer.gov/about-cancer/understanding/statistics

National Comprehensive Cancer Network. (2022). *Guidelines for patients: Distress during cancer care*. Retrieved from www.nccn.org/docs/default-source/patient-resources/nccn_distress_thermometer.pdf?sfvrsn=ef1df1a2_4

Nixon, S.A. (2019). The coin model of privilege and critical allyship: Implications for health. *BMC Public Health*, *19*(1), 1–13.

Office of Disease Prevention & Health Promotion. (2022). *Social determinants of health*. Retrieved from https://health.gov/healthypeople/objectives-and-data/social-determinants-health

Ozdemir, S., & Finkelstein, E. A. (2018). Cognitive bias: The downside of shared decision making. *JCO Clinical Cancer Informatics*, *2*, 1–10. https://doi.org/10.1200/cci.18.00011

Paice, J. A., Portenoy, R., Lacchetti, C., Campbell, T., Citron, M., Constine, L. S., Cooper, A., Glare, P., Keefe, F., & Koyyalagunta, L. (2016). Management of chronic pain in survivors of adult cancers: American Society of Clinical Oncology clinical practice guideline. *Journal of Clinical Oncology*, *34*(27), 3325–3345. https://doi.org/10.1200/JCO.2016.68.5206

Pronk, N., Kleinman, D. V., Goekler, S. F., Ochiai, E., Blakey, C., & Brewer, K. H. (2021). Promoting health and well-being in healthy people 2030. *Journal of Public Health Management & Practice*, *27*(6), S242–S248. https://doi.org/10.1097/PHH.0000000000001254

Rowland, J. (2021). Survivorship in the next era of cancer control: Three key foci for pursuit. *Journal of Cancer Rehabilitation*, *4*(1), 259–262. https://doi.org/10.48252/JCR42

Stout, N. L., Santa Mina, D., Lyons, K. D., Robb, K., & Silver, J. K. (2021). A systematic review of rehabilitation and exercise recommendations in oncology guidelines. *CA: A Cancer Journal for Clinicians*, *71*(2), 149–175. https://doi.org/10.3322/caac.21639

Wayne, P. M., Lee, M. S., Novakowski, J., Osypiuk, K., Ligibel, J., Carlson, L. E., & Song, R. (2018). Tai chi and qigong for cancer-related symptoms and quality of life: A systematic review and meta-analysis. *Journal of Cancer Survivorship*, *12*(2), 256–267. https://doi.org/10.1007/s11764-017-0665-5

7
Innovative Models in Palliative Care in Oncology

Jennifer J. Halpern and Eunju Lee

Key Concepts

- Innovations in biopsychosocial fields are measured by the extent to which they address the needs of historically marginalized populations and require input from the communities they hope to serve.
- Innovations in palliative care tend to be general to the field without reference to a particular medical specialty.
- Use of digital telehealth models is a strategy for managing health care's financial challenges.
- Population-based or grassroots models, such as those emerging in tribal lands and in faith-based communities, respond to the unique cultural needs of the community.
- Awareness of biomedicine's cultural biases and assumptions will help mitigate its authoritative power over culturally divergent groups.
- Trauma-informed and pluralistic approaches to care can widen palliative care's reach to populations that previously experienced discrimination.

Keywords: digital platforms, grassroots models, innovation, palliative care, race-based traumatic stress, telehealth, trauma-informed care

The global pandemic of COVID-19 and racial conflict have revealed the fundamental role of racism in American institutions and systems. In response, leaders in the allied fields of medicine, psychology, and social work have publicly acknowledged their complicity in propagating and maintaining systems of racial injustice through their culture, training, policies, and clinical practices. This wider movement for health equity dictates that whatever innovations develop in the field of palliative care social work (PCSW), they be measured by the extent to which they improve access, decrease structural

Jennifer J. Halpern and Eunju Lee, *Innovative Models in Palliative Care in Oncology* In: *Oncology and Palliative Social Work*. Edited by: Susan Hedlund, Bryan Miller, Grace Christ, and Carolyn Messner, Oxford University Press.
 DOI: 10.1093/oso/9780197607299.003.0007

inequalities, and reduce inequities in palliative health care (Nelson et al., 2021). This chapter examines structural and clinical innovations in PCSW that specifically address issues of racial inequity. When examined from a health equity perspective, some innovations, such as telehealth, may in fact be technocratic advancements. Other innovations, such as community-based collaborations, despite having been pioneered a decade ago, remain important to the work of equity and warrant renewed attention. Palliative care innovations also include aspirational directions for clinical practice that integrate race-based trauma-informed care and challenge conventional Eurocentric biomedical models.

Innovations in Delivery

Palliative care faces several challenges, including a lack of patient and clinician awareness and appreciation of the specialty, a shortage of qualified and certified team members, and most importantly, a plethora of financial constraints and regulations, including a lack of billing codes specific to palliative care. As one chief medical officer reminded one of the authors as she developed a proposal for a palliative care unit for their hospital, "We follow the money" (P. Llobet, personal communication, April 14, 2016). From the hospital's perspective, palliative care saves money but is not a profit center. The following section demonstrates how financial concerns and advances continue to dominate and define the sustainability of innovations in palliative care.

Digital Platforms and Their Financial Implications

Responding to the needs of patients for palliative care and hospitals' need to receive appropriate reimbursement for services, health care analytics companies have created digital platforms that shoulder the administration and much of the risk involved in determining which procedures are most appropriate for palliative care. Coders develop algorithms that, among other functions, match patients to palliative care service delivery methods. Palliative care physicians may then be encouraged to work with specific patient populations at outpatient clinics or in private homes, helping prevent costly hospital visits.

Digital platforms also collect payment from insurers, reducing patients' confusion about which palliative services are covered by Medicare and Medicaid. Votive Health, one such platform provider, proclaims that it eases the process with "better payer-provider integration through value-based agreements" (Votive Health, 2021).

The algorithms underlying these platforms predetermine the point beyond which palliative care physicians must discontinue their professional relationship with a patient and transfer them to specialists considered more cost-effective. Cost concerns thus seem to extinguish the relationship-based team approach so fundamental to palliative care. Impersonal algorithms are unlikely to give appropriate weight to the important psychosocial and cultural concerns that affect patient healing.

Another kind of digital platform advancing palliative care focuses on patient-reported outcomes (PROs), an emerging paradigm that attempts to capture the patient's self-assessed health status in order to provide a more personal perspective on a treatment's efficacy. PRO platforms keep the patient an active member of the palliative care decision-making team, which is especially important for cancer and other chronic conditions (Finucane et al., 2021). MyPal, a European PRO platform, was developed with input from and validated by the broad community of patients it serves, is provided in five languages, and conforms to European privacy regulations (Koumakis et al., 2021).

At-Home Palliative Care Services

Palliative care at home, like hospice, can involve regular home visits by various team members. Telehealth and home-based palliative care services emerged from hospitals' struggles to manage patients during the COVID-19 pandemic. In addition to simplifying the financial and logistical aspects of this work, the approach incorporates remote monitoring and provision of complex care in the patient's home, supplemented by in-person medical staff home visits. Many families find relief in knowing that the digital solution can coordinate service, accept payment, and navigate insurance, which allows family members to focus on the emotional care of their loved ones (Gajarawala et al., 2021). Hospitals are experimenting with integrating home-based palliative programs into their service lines; notable among these are the Contessa/Mt. Sinai collaboration in New York City as well as similar programs in North Dakota, Georgia, Missouri, and Michigan.

Hospitals' and insurers' financial motivations drive this seemingly patient-home-centered approach. Hospices, currently providing about 50% of home-based palliative care services, find themselves in competition with the new hospital lines of service for palliative care at home (Vossel, 2021). The strong financial motivation is discernible in that Amedisys, an established in-home care provider, recently acquired Contessa for over $250 million (Khan, 2022).

Advances enabling the delivery of in-home services may appear at first glance to represent the epitome of palliative care. While in-home care feels personalized and caring to many, others, including those lacking trust in the medical system, may instead find it depersonalized and uncaring. Contessa reports that they use evidence-based procedures to create their treatment decision algorithms (Khan, 2022). Important questions include on what evidence these procedures are based and how representative this evidence is of traditionally underserved communities receiving treatment. Individuals who feel historically marginalized by the medical system may question whether they are in fact receiving the best possible care if they are out of sight of the providers. Additionally, some patients who might otherwise benefit from palliative telecare may experience technical and social challenges to access, including no or limited access to high-speed Internet or cell service; lack of skill or comfort with using technology; and barriers to developing remote relationships, particularly when the patient is also experiencing visual or hearing impairment. As Zimlichman et al. (2021) comment in their future-oriented *NEJM Catalyst* essay, patient and family needs are rarely the focus of care by many modern health systems. Business and social models support the increased use of these innovations—their distinctions are worthy of further examination.

Government-Driven and Grassroots-Based Palliative Care Models

Innovations are extending the reach of community-based palliative care through both clinics and home visits (Cohn et al., 2017). Some models are driven by and receive funding from U.S. governmental organizations; others are motivated by grassroots approaches of the people affected and tend to be grant funded.

Government-Driven Models

New government-driven strategies seek to identify and support patients to decrease the likelihood of their bouncing back to the hospital. The category includes the provision of palliative care in medical offices and clinics, in long-term care facilities, and in patients' homes as discussed above.

One promising innovation that may increase access to and provide more equal distribution of palliative care by geographically isolated populations is the forthcoming introduction of rural emergency hospitals (REHs), which Medicare is scheduled to begin covering in January 2023. This model intends to stabilize and expand access to health care services in rural America, transforming hospitals with fewer than 50 beds to emergency and outpatient care facilities. The approach supports local communities in embarking on a community needs assessment that involves the input of an array of stakeholders. Consequently, palliative care in REHs may become an option for those in need (Olsen, 2021).

From the perspective of systemic health equity, stakeholders are attempting to address the social determinants of health and holding REHs accountable for equitable health access and outcomes. For example, the Rural Policy Research Institute health panel reported to the Center for Medicare and Medicaid Services (CMS) that the needs of a diverse population require support on both micro and macro levels through education about barriers to access, recruitment of a diverse staff, and creation of an inclusive health care environment (Olsen, 2021). Time will tell if CMS responds with funding to support appropriate workforce development.

Grassroots-Based Models

Grassroots forms of palliative care have developed in a number of different contexts. For example, in some prisons, volunteer inmates receive training to provide psychosocial support to dying inmates (Coyle, 2018). A grassroots model from Canada worthy of imitation in the United States is the Paramedics Providing Palliative Care at Home program. Canada, which adopted the provision of palliative care to patients who need it as a health care goal many years before the United States, has made paramedic palliative care (Carter et al., 2019) a growth area, shifting its emphasis away from acute trauma and emergency management. The initial implementation of the program began in Nova Scotia and Prince Edward Island in 2017 (Carter et al., 2019). This study revealed that the program reduced emergency department visits, ensured reliable care, and reduced patient and family stress, and further found that the paramedics support the concept of supplying palliation and believe palliative care should fall within their scope of practice. A subsequent program was introduced in Edmonton, Canada. There is increasing global attention to integrating palliative care into the provision of paramedic practice in other countries, including Germany, Great Britain, Australia, and the United States (Juhrmann et al., 2021).

This Canadian model may solve a rural health care challenge in the United States, where distance and the CMS payment model for ambulances make transportation to rural hospitals a barrier to care. Currently, Medicare sets fee-for-service payments to ambulance agencies based on dense urban environments, where hospitals are easier to access because of their comparative proximity to the populations they serve. High unreimbursed costs for readiness to respond and a lack of call volume over which to spread these costs have caused many agencies to close. The Canadian example holds possibilities for increasing patient well-being in their homes, while supporting the essential rural ambulance corps.

Perhaps the most distinctively grassroots model is the growth of palliative care and hospice on Native American lands. The health care access challenges faced by individuals living in many rural areas are exacerbated on tribal lands by a lack of infrastructure and underfunding for preventive care, let alone for specialty palliative care. Wherever palliative care has been introduced following the introduction of broadband and telemedicine or using trained community health workers, life with serious illness and dying has become more bearable.

The Lakota people have welcomed palliative care and hospice programs supporting several tribes in South Dakota, as have the Zuni in New Mexico. Grant-funded programs focus on overcoming infrastructure issues and the equally important goal of developing trust among palliative providers and people in tribal communities. Palliative care services for Native Americans living on tribal lands must be culturally congruent with tribal life in order to develop much-needed trust. Needs and messaging may vary among tribal communities. For example, some elders express discomfort with chaplains from a different faith or social workers, whose association with governmental agencies perceived as disruptive can make them appear threatening (Isaacson & Lynch, 2018).

Alaska Native Tribal Health Consortium communities welcome the use of technology to support rural providers with palliative care through telehealth and telemonitoring programs and resources throughout the state. A visiting registered nurse, for example, may only be able to reach patients by small plane, so having alternative methods of accessing patients is crucial to effective palliative care. A unique innovation for communities served by one of the programs involves end-of-life (EOL) training to the family and village (Decourtney et al., 2010).

As if these obstacles for tribal land palliative care programs were not enough, they are further compounded by hurdles created by federal regulations that revolve around the requirement for nurse visits within a specified period and requirements for frequent physical, occupational, and recreational therapy.

Another challenge is staff turnover and the availability of local staff trained in palliative or EOL care.

In 2013, the Alameda County Care Alliance in California partnered with five churches in a faith-based program providing critical support for predominantly African American adults with advanced illness and their caregivers. Through this innovative program, faith leaders learn to help congregants prepare for end of life through not only spiritual guidance and support but also practical assistance in navigating resources related to advanced illness. The program has since expanded to over 20 African American churches in neighboring counties. Subsequent programs have likewise found that community health workers can markedly support advance care planning and EOL options for African American patients; assistance of this type leads to better outcomes, including a statistically significant drop in symptom severity across numerous palliative care domains (Sedhom et al., 2021).

Innovations in Clinical Practice

Trauma-Informed Care and Race-Based Traumatic Stress

Since the early 2000s, there has been an increasing awareness of the relevance of trauma-informed care (TIC) in medicine, mental health, and social services (Becker-Blease, 2017) and with it, a growing interest in the link between racial discrimination and post-traumatic stress disorder (PTSD) (Williams et al., 2018). In the setting of the COVID-19 pandemic and related trauma, "TIC in health care has become increasingly essential" (Brown et al., 2020, p. e27), prompting both the National Hospice and Palliative Care Organization and CAPC to call for greater integration of TIC at EOL (Parker, 2020). Because TIC aligns closely with core palliative care values, "trauma-informed health care should be seen as a tool to realize the vision of palliative care" (Meier & Machtinger, 2020) for patients with trauma, including race-based traumatic stress (RBTS).

Palliative care's holistic vision of care tends to the lived experience of patients whose RBTS symptoms can manifest in hypervigilance, diminished concentration, or defensive behaviors. Due to underlying implicit bias, these trauma response behaviors in the health care setting can stigmatize patients of color as uncooperative, noncompliant, combative, or worse, lead to misdiagnosis of depression or substance abuse (Williams et al., 2018). Despite growing awareness of trauma, RBTS lags in both awareness and acceptance partially because it does not fit neatly into the *Diagnostic and Statistical Manual of Mental Disorders* (DSM) criteria of PTSD. Although symptoms of RBTS may overlap with PTSD, the DSM frame fails to capture the psychological impact and type of stress unique to RBTS and better conceptual models are needed (Carter & Pieterse, 2020). This work is slowly emerging, but as a nascent concept, empirically validated treatments for RBTS have yet to be identified (Williams et al., 2018). As RBTS models develop, they are likely to exist at the intersection of what health care practitioners know about the protective factors against the detrimental effects of racism and the six principles of TIC (Substance Abuse and Mental Health Services Administration, 2014).

It is important to note that trauma, especially RBTS, is "inextricably linked to systems of power and oppression" (Becker-Blease, 2017, pp. 131–132). Without engagement at the macro systems level, there is a risk of diminishing TIC into just another mental health tool aimed at fixing so-called individual pathology. Acknowledging the inextricable connection between the individual experience of RBTS and racism in wider social systems begins with acceptance that palliative care and the larger biomedical system are inherently embedded in the racial and cultural biases of the broader society. Too often, the role of the clinicians' culture is obscured as if health care providers were blank slates of cultural neutrality. In doing so, clinicians may be masking their own culpability, thus negating the historical and social location in which the clinician and patient interaction is situated.

Challenges to Conventional Biomedicine: Medical and Epistemological Pluralism

Despite its seeming universal applicability as irrefutable value-free science, biomedicine is not objective knowledge but rather shaped and driven by philosophies and ideologies "woven into Western culture and its power dynamics . . . [and its] social systems and economies" (Valles, 2020, p. 1). Coming into its own in industrialized Western countries following World War II, biomedicine as a sociotechnical system is based in culturally specific epistemology and practices situated in a uniquely Western historical and social context (Lock & Nguyen, 2018; Valles, 2020). Among the epistemological foundations of biomedicine is that of reductionism, presumed value-neutrality of science, mind–body dualism, and a decontextualized individualistic orientation—in other words, a "narrowly individualistic and highly biological approach" to care (Davis & González, 2016, p. 2). Biomedicine reduces disease to specific somatic malfunctions whose treatment comprises specific individual-level technological interventions in contrast to a holistic approach to disease as complex, interdependent, and multicausal (Davis & González, 2016). This reductionist versus holistic approach parallels a distinction made by cross-cultural psychiatrist Arthur Kleinman (1988) between disease and illness, where *disease* refers to the "practitioner's perspective . . . in narrow biological terms . . . as an alteration in biological structure or functioning" (pp. 5–6) and *illness* to "the innately human experience of symptoms and suffering" (p. 3). Healing the lived, embodied experience of suffering rather than focusing narrowly on curing disease exemplifies the philosophy of palliative care. Despite this, the practice of palliative care can be difficult to distinguish from traditional biomedicine, not only because the culture of biomedicine is powerful but also because people fail to recognize that biomedicine itself is a culture. This failure blinds people to how they might be inadvertently contributing to cultural imperialism in health care.

Socially and legally separated for centuries, racial groups in the United States are more segregated in 2019 than they were in 1990 (Beckett, 2021). Racial residential segregation determines not only the institutions of daily life but also distinct cultural patterns and preferences developed according to racial identities outside the dominant White culture (Carter & Pieterse, 2020). Dominant American culture is based in White ethnic values and beliefs, including individualism, independence, control, future orientation, directness and honesty, and objectivity and informality (Carter & Pieterse, 2020). Within this cultural context have developed biomedical practices focused on individual autonomy, informed consent, advance directives, and "truth" telling. That biomedicine's values are culturally bound explains why patients of color may not share the belief that biomedicine's values are the moral absolutes that health care systems tend to portray them to be. It reveals the moral relevance of culture and argues for cultural humility as essential in providing person-centered care concordant with the culture, values, and worldview of the patient and family.

Cultural humility also creates an openness to medical practices that do not conform to conventional Western biomedicine, such as the use of complementary or integrative medicine or medical pluralism. Those who research integrative medicine have noted that patients are more likely to seek complementary approaches when they distrust doctors and the health care system, face economic constraints, are positively inclined toward local health practices and beliefs, and have greater risk tolerance (Penkala-Gawęcka & Rajtar, 2016). Whatever the impetus, patients are increasingly seeking complementary approaches, as illustrated by a 2018 survey that reported nearly

40% of Americans believe cancer can be cured by alternative therapies alone (American Society of Hematology [ASH], 2019). While caution is warranted against the unvalidated claims of some alternative therapies, palliative care practitioners must remain open-minded about nonconventional healing practices not only because many patients are likely to continue to seek them but also because palliative care practitioners recognize there are diverse epistemologies of illness and human knowledge is far from absolute. Indeed, integrative medicine and clinical trials of numerous complementary therapies are being increasingly advanced (National Cancer Institute, n.d.). Large treatment centers, including Memorial Sloan Kettering's Bendheim Integrative Medicine Center, are working to mainstream integrative medicine (ASH, 2019). The United States is unlikely to develop a plural medical environment such as that found in Germany, where a wide range of therapeutic options are supported and biomedicine is not the ultimate and only approach (Penkala-Gawęcka & Rajtar, 2016). However, greater integration of complementary therapies will further the practice of holistic healing and expand the reach of palliative care to a more multicultural population.

Recent palliative care innovations seeking to address the important problems of disparities in health care access and outcome, especially racial disparity, are encouraging. Innovations in palliative care delivery seek to increase care to historically marginalized communities through public and private initiatives. Similar efforts are being pursued in clinical practice by advancing TIC and increasing responsiveness to epistemologies, values, and practices outside the conventional biomedical model in order to meet the needs of the lived experiences of our multicultural pluralistic population. Palliative care's ability to pursue creative solutions, however, continues to be thwarted by financial and regulatory obstacles. This has increased reliance on grassroots communities to care for their own, which comes at the risk of further burdening resource-strapped populations while absolving government of its responsibilities. More than ever, palliative care must anchor itself in its values to navigate the complex landscape of health care in the United States.

Guiding Best Practices for the Future

Future innovations should address not only where and how palliative care is delivered but also the aspirations and identity of the field itself. The field's foundational values of whole person–centered care of total pain—somatic, emotional, psychological, spiritual, social, and cultural—must remain as its weather vane, affirming the social work view of person-in-environment. In its embrace of holistic care, palliative care acknowledges a history embedded in a legacy of White supremacy and patriarchy, and its resultant inequities in the prevalence, treatment, and outcomes for disease and pain. Palliative care practitioners must seek to redress the biopsychosocial suffering of this legacy.

Pearls

- Some innovations in palliative care have targeted the increasingly important problem of disparities in health care access and outcome for historically marginalized communities.
- Grassroots and government innovations in palliative care delivery focus on increasing access to marginalized communities via the introduction of a CMS category of rural emergency hospitals, care on tribal lands, faith-based alliances, and in Canada, the use of paramedics as palliative care providers.
- RBTS is an emerging perspective that provides an innovative lens to TIC in palliative care to address the legacy and current practice of medical racism.
- Mainstreaming integrative medicine will increase the reach of palliative care to patients with diverse cultural views on healing.

Pitfalls

- Expanding the use of digital platforms and other remote technologies may not reflect the needs and concerns of the communities they purport to serve.
- Government regulatory barriers challenge rural and urban communities differently.
- Relying on grassroots communities to care for their own absolves government of its responsibilities in health care, which is a public good, and continues a legacy of negligence of historically discriminated communities.

Additional Resources

Center for the Advancement of Palliative Care. (2021). *The case for community-based palliative care: A new paradigm for improving the care of serious illness.* https://www.capc.org/documents/download/867/

Centers for Medicare and Medicaid Services. (2021). *Hospice and palliative care.* https://www.cms.gov/Outreach-and-Education/American-Indian-Alaska-Native/AIAN/LTSS-TA-Center/ltss-focus-areas/hospice-and-palliative-care

National Advisory Committee on Rural Health and Human Services. (2021). *Rural emergency hospital policy brief and recommendations to the secretary.* https://www.hrsa.gov/sites/default/files/hrsa/advisory-committees/rural/2021-rural-emergency-hospital-policy-brief.pdf

Substance Abuse and Mental Health Services Administration. (2014). *SAMHSA's concept of trauma and guidance for a trauma-informed approach* (HHS Publication No. [SMA] 14-4884). https://store.samhsa.gov/product/SAMHSA-s-Concept-of-Trauma-and-Guidance-for-a-Trauma-Informed-Approach/SMA14-4884

References

American Association of Hematology. (2019, December). Mainstreaming alternative and complementary medicine. *ASH Clinical News.* https://ashpublications.org/ashclinicalnews/news/4801/Mainstreaming-Alternative-and-Complementary

Becker-Blease, K. A. (2017). As the world becomes trauma-informed, work to do. *Journal of Trauma & Dissociation, 18*(2), 131–138. https://doi.org/10.1080/15299732.2017.1253401

Beckett, L. (2021, June 28). "Where you live determines everything": Why segregation is growing in the U.S. *Guardian: U.S. Edition.* https://www.theguardian.com/us-news/2021/jun/28/us-racial-segregation-study-university-of-california-berkeley

Brown, C., Peck, S., Humphreys, J., Schoenherr, L., Saks, N. T., Sumser, B., & Elia, G. (2020). COVID-19 lessons: The alignment of palliative medicine and trauma-informed care. *Journal of Pain and Symptom Management, 60*(2), e26–e30. https://doi.org/10.1016/j.jpainsymman.2020.05.014

Carter, A. J. E., Arab, M., Harrison, M., Goldstein, J., Stewart, B., Lecours, M., Sullivan, J., Villard, C., Crowell, W., Houde, K., Jensen, J. L., Downer, K., & Pereira, J. (2019). Paramedics providing palliative care at home: A mixed-methods exploration of patient and family satisfaction and paramedic comfort and confidence. *Canadian Journal of Emergency Medicine, 21*(4), 513–522. https://doi.org/10.1017/cem.2018.497

Carter, R. T., & Pieterse, A. L. (2020). *Measuring the effects of racism: Guidelines for the assessment and treatment of race-based traumatic stress injury.* Columbia University Press.

Cohn, J., Corrigan, J., Lynn, J., Meier, D., Miller, J., Shega, J., & Wang, S. (2017). *Community-based models of care delivery for people with serious illness: NAM Perspectives* [Discussion paper]. National Academy of Medicine. https://doi.org/10.31478/201704b

Coyle, S. (2018). End-of-life care in prison. *Social Work Today, 18*(6), 16.

Davis, J. E., & González, A. M. (2016). *To fix or to heal: Patient care, public health, and the limits of biomedicine.* New York University Press.

Decourtney, C. A., Branch, P. K., & Morgan, K. M. (2010). Gathering information to develop palliative care programs for Alaska's Aboriginal peoples. *Journal of Palliative Care, 26*(1), 22–31. https://pubmed.ncbi.nlm.nih.gov/20402181/

Finucane, A. M., O'Donnell, H., Lugton, J., Gibson-Watt, T., Swenson, C., & Pagliari, C. (2021). Digital health interventions in palliative care: A systematic meta-review. *Nature Partner Journals: Digital Medicine, 4*(1), 64. https://doi.org/10.1038/s41746-021-00430-7

Gajarawala, S. N., & Pelkowski, J. N. (2021). Telehealth benefits and barriers. *Journal for Nurse Practitioners, 17*(2), 218–221. https://doi.org/10.1016/j.nurpra.2020.09.013

Isaacson, M. J., & Lynch, A. R. (2018). Culturally relevant palliative and end-of-life care for U.S. Indigenous populations: An integrative review. *Journal of Transcultural Nursing, 29*(2), 180–191. https://doi.org/10.1177/1043659617720980

Juhrmann, M., Vandersman, P., Butow, P. N., & Claayton, J. M. (2021). Paramedics delivering palliative and end-of-life care in community-based settings: A systematic integrative review with thematic synthesis. *Palliative Medicine*, 1–17. https://doi.org/10.1177/02692163211059342

Khan, G. (2022). *Care convergence: Contessa's one-of-a-kind healthcare technology platform*. Retrieved from https://contessahealth.com/care-convergence-contessas-healthcare-technology-platform/

Kleinman, A. (1988). *The illness narratives: Suffering, healing, and the human condition*. Basic.

Koumakis, L., Schera, F., Parker, H., Bonotis, P., Chatzimina, M., Argyropaidas, P., Zacharioudakis, G., Schäfer, M., Kakalou, C., Karamanidou, C., Didi, J., Kazantzaki, E., Scarfo, L., Marias, K., & Natsiavas, P. (2021, December 17). Fostering palliative care through digital intervention: A platform for adult patients with hematologic malignancies. *Frontiers in Digital Health* (3), 186–188. https://doi.org/10.3389/fdgth.2021.730722

Lock, M. M., & Nguyen, V. K. (2018). *An anthropology of biomedicine*. Wiley.

Meier, D. E., & Machtinger, E. (2020, February 14). *Re: An interview with Dr. Edward Machtinger: Lessons of trauma-informed care*. Center to Advance Palliative Care. https://www.capc.org/blog/palliative-pulse-the-palliative-pulse-october-2018-an-interview-with-dr-edward-machtinger-lessons-of-trauma-informed-care/

National Cancer Institute. (n.d.) *Complementary and alternative medicine*. Retrieved from https://www.cancer.gov/about-cancer/treatment/cam

Nelson, K. E., Wright, R., Fisher, M., Koirala, B., Roberts, B., Sloan, D. H., Wu, D. S., & Davidson, P. M. (2021). A call to action to address disparities in palliative care access: A conceptual framework for individualizing care needs. *Journal of Palliative Medicine*, *24*(2), 177–180.

Olsen, A. T. (2021). *NRHA outlines new rural emergency hospital* model. Rural Health Voices. https://www.ruralhealth.us/blogs/ruralhealthvoices/april-2021/nrha-outlines-new-rural-emergency-hospital-model

Parker, J. (2020, November 17). Growing numbers of hospices pursue trauma-informed-care. *Hospice News*. https://hospicenews.com/2020/11/17/growing-number-of-hospices-pursuing-trauma-informed-care/

Penkala-Gawęcka, D., & Rajtar, M. (2016). Introduction to the special issue "Medical pluralism and beyond." *Anthropology & Medicine*, *23*(2), 129–134. https://doi.org/10.1080/13648470.2016.1180584

Sedhom, R., Nudotor, R., Freund, K. M., Smith, T. J., Cooper, L. A., Owczarzak, J. T., & Johnston, F. M. (2021). Can community health workers increase palliative care use for African American patients? A pilot study. *JCO Oncology Practice*, *17*(2), e158–e167. https://doi.org/10.1200/OP.20.00574

Valles, S. (2020, April 9). Philosophy of biomedicine. In Edward N. Zalta (Ed.), *Stanford encyclopedia of philosophy* (Summer 2020 ed.). Retrieved from https://plato.stanford.edu/archives/sum2020/entries/biomedicine/

Vossel, H. (2021, June 11). Value-based models could promote palliative care integration. *Hospice News*. https://hospicenews.com/2021/06/11/value-based-models-could-promote-palliative-care-integration/

Votive Health raised $2,500,000 / seed from Andrew Lasher and 14 other investors. (2021, April 28.) *Healthcare Weekly Pulse Check* Issue #17 Apr 26–May 1, LXL Capital. Retrieved from https://lxl-capital.com/newsletter-subscribe-1/f/healthcare-weekly-pulse-check-issue-17-apr-26--may-1

Williams, M. T., Metzger, I. W., Leins, C., & DeLapp, C. (2018). Assessing racial trauma within a DSM–5 framework: The UConn Racial/Ethnic Stress & Trauma Survey. *Practice Innovations*, *3*(4), 242–260. https://doi.org/10.1037/pri0000076

Zimlichman, E., Nicklin, W., Aggarwal, R., & Bates, D. W. (2021, March 3). Health Care 2030: The coming transformation. *NEJM Catalyst*. https://doi.org/10.1056/CAT.20.0569

SECTION II

CLINICAL ISSUES AND INTERVENTIONS

Cecilia L. W. Chan

As a patient embarks on their journey with cancer, the oncology and palliative social worker's (OPSW) job is first to build a relationship with the patient and then to conduct comprehensive assessments of their emotional, psychosocial, practical, and materials needs. Despite the fact that most humans will develop cancer at some point in their lives, most patients are shocked when they receive the diagnosis. The traumatic combination of physical, psychosocial, and spiritual distress among patients often results in debilitating pain and suffering, which the authors of Chapters 8 and 9 explore.

Besides providing a solid discussion on critical clinical issues, the chapters in this section discuss state-of-the-art interventions in oncology social work and provide a comprehensive overview on the most recent evidence-based interventions available from diagnosis to treatment to palliation to bereavement. The chapters address how OPSWs can empower individuals, families, and communities. The authors of Chapters 10 and 12 introduce holistic interventions, such as trauma-informed and collaborative care, and examine best practices for supporting patients on the path of cancer treatment, especially as they grapple with complex choices and decisions about various treatments, such as chemotherapy, immunotherapy, targeted therapies, and radiation. The topic of Chapter 11 is how cancer patients with special needs, such as persons with severe mental illness, can suffer even further hardships in access to care and clinical trial resources and how OPSWs can foster better quality of care for this group of people. Chapter 13 presents a balanced perspective from the informal caregivers and interventions to serve them during their journey.

One-third of deaths in developed countries are cancer related. Advancements in cancer treatment that have led to the development and increase in the use of targeted drugs and immunotherapy have led to an increasing number of patients living with advanced cancers or an end-stage diagnosis. Chapters 14 and 15 illuminate interventions for alleviating pain, symptoms, and side effects of prolonged treatment, as well as the demand on clinical interventions during palliative and bereavement phases. They also address ways to assess levels and intensity of distress among informal caregivers and offer interventions for family members and caregivers.

8

Beyond Distress Screening

The Future of Psychosocial Oncology and Palliative Care

Brad Zebrack, Meredith Doherty, and Katrina R. Ellis

Key Concepts

- Adherence to distress management protocols improves patients' quality of life; reduces distress, anxiety, and depression; achieves medical cost offsets; and reduces emergency department visits and hospitalizations.
- Addressing patients' material needs, as well as their psychological and emotional concerns, is critical for reducing distress and delivering high-quality cancer care, particularly for patients from socially marginalized and historically oppressed populations.
- Structural competency—understanding and acknowledging how social and environmental factors influence vulnerability—can enhance efforts to adequately mitigate distress among cancer patients and achieve health equity.

Keywords: social determinants of health, social risk, structural vulnerability, trauma-informed care

Managing distress in cancer patients is an evidence-informed component of whole-person care that can optimize a range of health and quality-of-life outcomes. Distress management (DM) is a comprehensive system of screening, assessment, triage, intervention, and outcome monitoring related to patient distress. Distress management involves proactive use of standardized patient-reported outcome (PRO) measures to identify and triage distressed patients with specific care needs. A systematic approach to distress management aims to address identified symptoms and needs by implementing evidence-informed interventions with demonstrated efficacy (Jacobsen, 2009). Adherence to distress management protocols in cancer care reduces distress, decreases anxiety and depression, achieves medical cost

Brad Zebrack, Meredith Doherty, and Katrina R. Ellis, *Beyond Distress Screening* In: *Oncology and Palliative Social Work*. Edited by: Susan Hedlund, Bryan Miller, Grace Christ, and Carolyn Messner, Oxford University Press.
 DOI: 10.1093/oso/9780197607299.003.0008

offsets, minimizes emergency department visits and hospitalizations, and improves patients' quality of life (Deshields et al., 2021).

In recent years, multidisciplinary cancer care teams have developed and implemented standardized distress screening procedures in response to the American College of Surgeons' Commission on Cancer standards for patient-centered care. In addition, clinical researchers have developed and tested novel and effective interventions to promote adherence to therapy, enhance shared decision-making, and improve patients' symptom management, quality of life, and long-term survival (Faller et al., 2013). Despite these advances, many patients do not receive needed psychosocial support services, which may reflect ineffective screening or lack of access; patients with the greatest needs are often not identified, and those who may benefit the most from services often do not use them. These shortcomings are likely attributable to societal and structural conditions and not personal or individual choices or character flaws. Furthermore, needs detected through distress management protocols are most often a function of stressors occurring within families, communities, and broader societal contexts. Thus, potential solutions must be systemic and multilevel in nature and focused on the social conditions that structure people's lives, choices, and behaviors, and contribute to their vulnerability.

Structural Vulnerability Screening

In 2019, the National Academies of Sciences, Engineering, and Medicine emphasized the importance of addressing social needs within the context of health care delivery in the United States (National Academies of Sciences, 2019). This was driven in part by a recognition that achieving high-quality, high-value health care for all requires attention to nonmedical factors such as housing, food, and transportation—the social determinants of health. Physicians have recently raised awareness of the importance and relevance of social determinants as well as their own limitations in addressing them (Maani & Galea, 2020). Social workers in health care settings, however, have been keenly aware of and acting on social needs and their influences on health behaviors and outcomes for patients, families, and communities for over 100 years (Gehlert et al., 2021). Ida Cannon established the first hospital social work department at Massachusetts General Hospital in 1905. Recognized as the founder of the field of medical social work, Cannon described the important interrelationship between medical practice and patients' social conditions. She argued that a hospital social worker must be assigned to represent the patient's point of view and work with physicians to determine the best medical treatment considering each patient's specific social conditions.

The ability to address patients' material needs as well as their psychological and emotional concerns is critical to reducing distress and delivering high-quality cancer care, particularly to patients from socially marginalized and historically oppressed populations. Unlike mental health interventions, evidence-based social-needs interventions delivered in a cancer care setting are limited in availability. When faced with seemingly intractable problems related to poverty and vulnerability and in the absence of sound guidance on how to address them, health care providers can experience moral distress and burnout (Bernhardt et al., 2021). Efforts on the part of clinical care providers to adequately mitigate distress among cancer patients and thus achieve better outcomes and health equity can be enhanced via structural competency, defined as understanding and acknowledging the social conditions that produce vulnerability within a population (Bourgois et al., 2017).

Social-Risk Screening and Referral

Oncology and palliative care programs are beginning to implement social-risk screening and referral protocols. A variety of screening tools are available, and evidence of their validity and utility in the clinical care context is growing (Billioux et al., 2017; Henrikson et al., 2019). A recent pilot study examining the use of a novel social-risk screening tool found that patients with cancer reported an average of 2.5 social risk factors. The most reported risk factor was financial hardship, followed by problems accessing the Internet, social isolation, and housing instability. Although most patients were comfortable disclosing social risks to their provider, most did not want the information stored in the electronic health record or shared with other clinicians (Davis et al., 2021).

It is important to note that social-risk screening could have unintended negative consequences. Patients could experience trauma through exposing their sensitive information. These potential downsides are particularly intolerable if the hospital or clinic does not have adequate resources to effectively address the patient's needs once they are surfaced. Health care providers are ethically bound to assist identified patient needs. Social workers are the most adequately trained clinicians prepared to sensitively assess and address social risks.

Social workers are the providers most likely to have knowledge of support resources available in the institution and wider community. These resources can come from government assistance programs, local and national nonprofit organizations, pharmaceutical companies, and an institution's own charitable programs. Assistance programs have a range of eligibility requirements, application processes, and deadlines. Social workers may use websites or digital platforms that aggregate program information to identify and match patients to programs.

Caregiver and Family Involvement and Support

Patients may identify family members, friends, and significant others as critical to supporting their health and well-being after a cancer diagnosis. These caregivers provide a range of assistance, including symptom management, care coordination, and emotional support. Yet, caregivers often feel unprepared for these tasks, indicating that they lack information and the skills necessary to meet desired or expected obligations. They often experience their own emotional distress. Too often, institutional leaders make assumptions regarding the availability and capability of caregivers and families to conduct supportive tasks outside medical settings (Gallagher-Thompson et al., 2020). These assumptions further exacerbate patient distress and burden for patients and families.

Clinical assessments can help determine the resources and constraints of caregivers and families so that clinicians and other health service providers can offer appropriate support. While assessment tools exist, barriers to their use include lack of staff to administer measures, inadequate resources to meet identified needs, and insufficient reimbursement for clinical time with caregivers (Ratcliff et al., 2019). All these challenges call for system-level solutions. Practitioners, researchers, and policymakers have proposed opportunities for increasing funding to support work with caregivers, such as value-based payment systems that incorporate care-management fees for caregiver services, and employer-backed programs driven by an urgency to maintain a productive and healthy workforce (Berry et al., 2017). Given the known associations between patient and family well-being, supporting their collective needs is of immense importance.

The Future of Oncology and Palliative Care Social Work

The future of oncology and palliative care social work lies in the profession's capacity to respond to structural vulnerability—the social and environmental conditions that place people and families at risk and that contribute to disparities in outcomes and care. Realizing the need for more guidance on integrating social care into the delivery of health care, the National Academies of Science, Engineering, and Medicine (2019) introduced the 5As model, which describes five categories of health and social care integration activities: awareness, adjustment, assistance, alignment, and advocacy. *Awareness* requires identifying the social needs and assets of individual patients, their families, and their communities. This includes screening individual patients for social risks and conducting regular needs assessments of the catchment area communities served by the hospital or provider. *Adjustment* refers to adapting clinical care to accommodate identified barriers to care; for example, a patient with high transportation costs may be able to receive the same treatment with fewer monthly clinic visits or may be transferred to a clinic closer to their house. Social workers provide *assistance* with patients' social needs by connecting patients to available resources, such as copayment assistance programs that can reduce the burden of high-cost medications, for example. *Alignment* refers to strategies that health care organizations use to understand and interact with the communities they serve via collaboration with "anchor" institutions—community-based agencies engaged in long-term strategies to support local economic ecosystems through employment and community investment. And *advocacy* refers to the ways in which health care organizations (usually in coalition with social care and political organizations) promote federal, state, and local policies that address the fundamental social determinants of health inequity. Many industry associations, such as the American Hospital Association, develop advocacy agendas to advance policies that directly address health-related social needs.

Some oncology and palliative care social workers in direct practice may have the latitude to engage in activities across each of the 5As categories; however, clinical social work practice to date typically has involved activities related to awareness, assistance, and to some extent, adjustment. The future is ripe for considering innovative approaches to oncology and palliative social work in terms of alignment and advocacy activities that can lead to the restorative allocation of resources directly to the communities where patients and their families live, work, and receive health care.

Trauma- and Liberation-Informed Care

Trauma-informed care focuses on understanding trauma that individuals experience, directly or indirectly, with appropriate attention to culture and context, meaning-making, and the potential impact of trauma across time and place (Center for Substance Abuse Treatment, 2014). Key principles of trauma-informed care include safety, trustworthiness, and transparency, collaboration and peer support, empowerment, choice, and the intersectionality of identity characteristics (Bowen & Murshid, 2016). An intersectional approach to trauma-informed care aims to help patients and families heal from experiences directly or indirectly connected to cancer care and to enhance their overall physical and psychological well-being.

Poverty, stigma, and discrimination are forms of trauma known to contribute to cumulative and substantial disadvantages across the life course. When individuals engage in the cancer care system, it is important to recognize the trauma they may already be experiencing. They may feel vulnerable when relying on healing and comfort from systems and/or individuals with whom they may associate trauma and harm. Individual and collective trauma related to health care, such as harm associated with experiences accessing or receiving care, may pose challenges to patient and family engagement. In addition, various social identities influence patient and family experiences with cancer care in ways that privilege and benefit some and oppress or harm others.

Trauma-informed care can also be considered from a policy and systems perspective (Bowen & Murshid, 2016). Collaboration in cancer care through a trauma-informed lens would view patients and families as partners in care and experts in their own health and health needs. From this perspective, clinical providers would strive to collaborate with patients and families, aiming to best integrate knowledge and expertise as they work to implement and carry out treatment plans. Empowerment, from a trauma-informed lens, would lead to cancer prevention and control efforts that deeply involve patients and families, recognizing that those closely affected by policies and practices that influence cancer outcomes can make valuable contributions to the success of this work.

Liberation psychology aligns with structural competency in that it aims to increase awareness of the causes of marginalization, including how inequitable social structures and long-standing ideologies (e.g., meritocracy, individualism, racism) perpetuate oppression. Liberation-informed care moves beyond individual level causes, interpretations, and solutions to address the challenges marginalized groups face. Instead, it raises consciousness among patients and families as to how broader social and structural factors outside their control affect their health and well-being. The results can be empowering for members of marginalized groups, enhance positive self-perceptions, and strengthen internal coping mechanisms. Liberation-informed care offers a lens through which social workers can advocate for the dismantling of White supremacy and other forms of institutionalized discrimination (Shin, 2015).

Confronting Implicit Bias in Clinical Practice

Implicit biases are thoughts, attitudes, beliefs, and behaviors that unconsciously and unfairly advantage or disadvantage others. They are often based on stereotypes associated with social categories and statuses and can affect cancer care service delivery throughout a continuum of care. Implicit bias is more likely to be activated in situations where there is stress on one's cognitive capacity, such as feeling physically or mentally depleted, having to make a quick decision, or within an emotionally charged situation. Implicit biases can influence clinicians' decision-making and judgments. For example, stereotypes about illicit drug use, drug dependency, or pain tolerance can lead to inappropriate pain management.

Efforts to confront implicit bias in clinical care must involve interventions at the individual, group, and systems levels. At the individual level, evidence-based strategies to reduce biases include perspective taking, finding individualizing information, and increasing exposure/contact with individuals outside one's own social grouping (Devine et al., 2012). At the group level, clinic staff can work together to create a culture in which discussing and collaborating to address biases is purposeful and productive, not punitive. In addition, implicit bias training and assessments can help health professionals understand and reflect on their own biases, though these activities likely work best when included in broader conversations and institutionally sponsored initiatives tied to actionable steps aimed at organizational culture change. At the systems level, clinics and institutions can promote efforts to diversify their workforce (including management and leadership positions), collect and analyze data to identify disparities in care, and ensure that there is accountability for mitigating bias at all levels.

Patient- and Family-Centered Care Policy

Alcaraz and colleagues (2020) developed a conceptual framework for understanding and addressing the social determinants of health to advance cancer health equity. The framework identified upstream cancer inequities due to social structural factors (e.g., marginalization, laws, living environments) and disparities in cancer risk factors, biomarkers, morbidity, and mortality that are consequences of those upstream factors. Addressing broader social structural factors through policy and practice can reduce exposure to risk factors associated with an increased likelihood of cancer and increase exposure to protective factors associated with cancer prevention, early detection, and better outcomes for patients and families during treatment and survivorship.

Policies that enhance the ability of patients and caregivers to participate fully in care and decision-making can also have a positive impact on their psychosocial well-being. A family's ability to mobilize resources to meet their cancer-related needs will likely mirror broader social inequities (Ellis et al., 2020). For example, patients and caregivers may maintain employment during cancer treatment to avoid changes to their income or insurance that could negatively affect their well-being. Increasing the availability of paid family leave from work for treatment and caregiving can enable more families, particularly those in vulnerable economic positions, to focus on cancer care without compromising their financial stability.

Community Organizing and Cancer

Community organizing, a foundational principle of social work history and practice, has long been used as a vehicle to address social and structural inequities. Limited attention, however, has been given to the role of community organizing to improve cancer outcomes. Some community-driven efforts to address cancer outcomes and disparities have focused on investigating and resolving environmental toxins and injustice linked to increased cancer incidence in specific geographic areas (e.g., along southern portions of the Mississippi River often referred to as "Cancer Alley"). Community action to address inequities in the physical environment such as housing instability and lack of access to healthy foods, parks, and recreational spaces can drive changes that ultimately help decrease cancer risk, morbidity, and mortality (Alcaraz et al., 2020).

Other community-driven efforts have focused on specific cancer sites. For example, the Accountability for Cancer Care through Undoing Racism and Equity (ACCURE) project was developed through a partnership between the Greensboro Health Disparities Collaborative, researchers at the University of North Carolina, cancer center clinicians and administrators, and other key community and academic stakeholders (Black et al., 2019). The impetus for this project was community-identified racial disparities in cancer outcomes. Together, using an antiracism approach, the multifaceted, system-based ACCURE intervention successfully documented and addressed treatment-related disparities among Black and White lung and breast cancer patients. The intervention included training for nurse navigators to use a racial equity lens in patient interactions, a real-time warning system to alert nurse navigators to deviations in care, race-specific feedback to clinical teams, and health equity education and training for cancer center providers and staff. Common threads among these examples and others are significant investments in time and resources to nurture and build the relationships and capacity necessary to address the identified issues. Several leading health organizations (e.g., National Cancer Institute, U.S. Centers for Disease Control) have invested in community partnerships. Moving forward, efforts that prioritize community empowerment and ownership and foster connections among community coalitions for resource sharing and mobilization can help build momentum and support for broader structural change.

We cannot consider a future for psychosocial oncology without accounting for the direct effects of COVID-19 as well as the social, environmental, and structural factors that have and will continue to create inequities in health outcomes, service access, and utilization for persons of marginalized communities and identities. Achieving enhanced patient experience, improved population health, and cost containment—the Institute for Healthcare Improvement's "Triple Aim" (Whittington et al., 2015)—will require a transformation of medical care, in general, and cancer care, specifically, including role delineation and standardization of competencies for oncology and palliative care social workers. Furthermore, the COVID-19 pandemic has underscored the need to consider and enhance patient-, family-, and caregiver-focused approaches to care. Challenges with accessing care have led to a rapid expansion of telemedicine services. There is a potential to build on the resources more widely available and reimbursed through telemedicine to expand the support provided to caregivers and improve their ability to access services and support in a timely and effective manner.

Within and across various domains of health, mental health, and behavioral health, the global COVID-19 pandemic has even further highlighted long-standing inequities in medical care and health outcomes in the United States. It has pushed the U.S. health care infrastructure beyond its capacity to provide safe, efficient, effective, timely, patient-centered, and equitable care. Specifically related to cancer care, COVID-19 has created delays in the use of and access to cancer prevention and detection services and challenges to the delivery of treatment for active disease. For example, disruptions in cancer screening and treatment that are attributable to COVID-19 are projected to result in approximately 10,000 excess deaths per year from breast and colorectal cancer alone by 2030 (Sharpless, 2021).

We can expect the consequences of COVID-19 on cancer care and cancer outcomes to be disproportionately borne by the most vulnerable and socially marginalized populations in the United States, which include persons of color, children, women, veterans, and people with both physical disabilities and mental disorders. The pandemic has highlighted how race, gender, class, age, ability, geographical location, and other axes of inequality intersect. It is altering the conditions under and environments in which people are born, live, learn, work, play, worship, and age in ways that will continue to affect health, functioning, and quality-of-life outcomes and risks for years to come.

Guiding Best Practices for the Future

Oncology and palliative social workers can help set clear communication about expectations for visits and assessments for distress and racial trauma (Dhawan & LeBlanc, 2021). To enhance trust and transparency, care teams can improve the quality of interactions with patients and families by being fully present during visits, minimizing distractions, and working to build relationships with them. Acknowledging the uncertainty inherent to cancer experiences and underscoring a commitment to the patient and their care (i.e., nonabandonment) reflect a trauma-informed lens. Service providers can also support system-level policies and practices that guard against inequitable treatment and mitigate bias.

Pearls

- Social workers are and have been the primary providers of psychosocial care in cancer for decades; they have been attending to the social determinants of health for over a century.
- There is a potential to build on the resources more widely available and reimbursed through telemedicine to expand the support provided to caregivers and improve their ability to access services and support in a timely, and effective manner.
- A liberation-informed approach to social work has the potential to extend the impact of social work service delivery by advancing patients' understanding of and ability to respond to the social environmental conditions contributing to their health, well-being, and ability to cope with cancer.

Pitfalls

- Many patients do not receive needed supportive care services; those most likely to benefit from support services often are the least likely to use them.
- Some patients may not want information about their social risks stored in their electronic health records; plans for storing and sharing this information need to consider patient concerns about confidentiality.
- Collecting information from patients about their social risks and conditions may be traumatizing. Care and sensitivity are required when assessing these risks and conditions.

Additional Resources

Protocol for Responding to and Assessing Patient Assets, Risks, and Experiences (PRAPARE): https://prapare.org

Structural Vulnerability Assessment Tool: https://www.ncbi.nlm.nih.gov/pmc/articles/PMC5233668/

Centers for Medicare and Medicaid Services' Accountable Health Communities Health-Related Social Needs Screening Tool: https://innovation.cms.gov/files/worksheets/ahcm-screeningtool.pdf

References

Alcaraz, K. I., Wiedt, T. L., Daniels, E. C., Yabroff, K. R., Guerra, C. E., & Wender, R. C. (2020). Understanding and addressing social determinants to advance cancer health equity in the United States: A blueprint for practice, research, and policy. *CA: A Cancer Journal for Clinicians*, *70*(1), 31–46. https://doi.org/10.3322/caac.21586

Bernhardt, C., Forgetta, S., & Sualp, K. (2021). Violations of health as a human right and moral distress: Considerations for social work practice and education. *Journal of Human Rights and Social Work*, *6*(1), 91–96. https://doi.org/10.1007/s41134-020-00150-0

Berry, L. L., Dalwadi, S. M., & Jacobson, J. O. (2017). Supporting the supporters: What family caregivers need to care for a loved one with cancer. *Journal of Oncology Practice*, *13*(1), 35–41.

Billioux, A., Verlander, K., Anthony, S., & Alley, D. (2017, May 30). *Standardized screening for health-related social needs in clinical settings: The Accountable Health Communities screening tool* [Discussion paper]. National Academy of Medicine perspectives. https://nam.edu/standardized-screening-for-health-related-social-needs-in-clinical-settings-the-accountable-health-communities-screening-tool/

Black, K. Z., Baker, S. L., Robertson, L. B., Lightfoot, A. F., Alexander-Bratcher, K. M., Befus, D., Cothern, C., Dixon, C. E., Ellis, K. R., Guerrab, F., Schaal, J. C., Simon, B., Smith, B., Thatcher, K., Wilson, S. M., Yongue, C. M., Eng, E., Ford, C. L., Griffith, D. M., . . . Gilbert, K. L. (2019). Health care: Antiracism organizing for culture and institutional change in cancer care. In *Racism: Science and tools for the public health professional*. American Public Health Association. https://doi.org/10.2105/9780875533049ch14

Bourgois, P., Holmes, S. M., Sue, K., & Quesada, J. (2017). Structural vulnerability: Operationalizing the concept to address health disparities in clinical care. *Academic Medicine, 92*(3), 299–307.

Bowen, E. A., & Murshid, N. S. (2016, July 20). Trauma-informed social policy: A conceptual framework for policy analysis and advocacy. *American Journal of Public Health, 106*(2), 223–229.

Center for Substance Abuse Treatment. (2014). *Trauma-informed care in behavioral health services*. U.S. Department of Health and Human Services, Substance Abuse and Mental Health Administration.

Davis, J., Zinck, L., Kelly, S., Sangha, H., Shulman, L. N., Aakhus, E., . . . Chaiyachati, K. (2021). Screened social risk factors and screening acceptability among oncology patients in Philadelphia. *Journal of Clinical Oncology, 39*(no. 15 suppl.), 12125. https://doi.org/10.1200/JCO.2021.39.15_suppl

Deshields, T., Wells-Di Gregorio, S., Flowers, S., Irwin, K., Nipp, R., Padgett, L., & Zebrack, B. (2021). Addressing distress screening challenges: Recommendations from the Consensus Panel of the American Psychosocial Oncology Society. *CA: A Cancer Journal for Clinicians, 71*, 407–436. https://doi.org/10.3322/caac.21672

Devine, P. G., Forscher, P. S., Austin, A. J., & Cox, W. T. L. (2012). Long-term reduction in implicit race bias: A prejudice habit-breaking intervention. *Journal of Experimental Social Psychology, 48*(6), 1267–1278. https://doi.org/10.1016/j.jesp.2012.06.003

Dhawan, N., & LeBlanc, T. W. (2021). Lean into the uncomfortable: Using trauma-informed care to engage in shared decision-making with racial minorities with hematologic malignancies. *American Journal of Hospice and Palliative Medicine, 39*(1), 4–8. https://doi.org/10.1177/10499091211008431

Ellis, K. R., Black, K. Z., Baker, S., Cothern, C., Davis, K., Doost, K., Goestch, C., Griesemer, I., Guerrab, F., & Lightfoot, A. F. (2020). Racial differences in the influence of health care system factors on informal support for cancer care among black and white breast and lung cancer survivors. *Family and Community Health, 43*(3), 200–212.

Faller, H., Schuler, M., Richard, M., Heckl, U., Weis, J., & Kuffner, R. (2013). Effects of psycho-oncologic interventions on emotional distress and quality of life in adult patients with cancer: Systematic review and meta-analysis. *Journal of Clinical Oncology, 31*(6), 782–793.

Gallagher-Thompson, D., Choryan-Bilbrey, A., Apesoa-Varano, E. C., Ghatak, R., Kim, K. K., & Cothran, F. (2020). Conceptual framework to guide intervention research across the trajectory of dementia caregiving. *Gerontologist, 60*, S29–S40. https://doi.org/10.1093/geront/gnz157

Gehlert, S., Hudson, D., & Sacks, T. (2021, May 21). A critical theoretical approach to cancer disparities: Breast cancer and the social determinants of health. *Frontiers in Public Health, 9*, 1–8. https://doi.org/10.3389/fpubh.2021.674736

Henrikson, N. B., Blasi, P. R., Dorsey, C. N., Mettert, K. D., Nguyen, M. B., Walsh-Bailey, C., & Lewis, C. C. (2019). Psychometric and pragmatic properties of social risk screening tools: A systematic review. *American Journal of Preventive Medicine, 57*(6), S13–S24.

Jacobsen, P. B. (2009). Promoting evidence-based psychosocial care for cancer patients. *Psycho-Oncology, 18*, 6–13.

Maani, N., & Galea, S. (2020). The role of physicians in addressing social determinants of health. *Journal of the American Medical Association, 323*(16), 1551–1552.

National Academies of Sciences, Engineering, and Medicine. (2019). *Integrating social care into the delivery of health care: Moving upstream to improve the nation's health*. National Academies Press. https://doi.org/10.17226/25467

Ratcliff, C. G., Vinson, C. A., Milbury, K., & Badr, H. (2019). Moving family interventions into the real world: What matters to oncology stakeholders? *Journal of Psychosocial Oncology, 37*(2), 264–284. https://doi.org/10.1080/07347332.2018.1498426

Sharpless, N. E. (2021). COVID-19 and cancer. *Science, 368*(6497), 1290–1291. https://doi.org/10.1126/science.abd3377

Shin, R. Q. (2015). The application of critical consciousness and intersectionality as tools for decolonizing racial/ethnic identity development models in the fields of counseling and psychology. In R. D. Goodman & P. C. Gorski (Eds.), *Decolonizing "multicultural" counseling through social justice* (pp. 11–22). Springer.

Whittington, J., Nolan, K., Lewis, N., & Torres, T. (2015). Pursuing the triple aim: The first 7 years. *Milbank Quarterly, 93*(2), 263–300. https://doi.org/10.1111/1468-0009.12122

9

Psychosocial Aspects of Cancer

Angelique Caba, Maria Chi, and Stewart B. Fleishman

Key Concepts

- Research shows that individuals with cancer experience an array of psychosocial, supportive, and psychopharmacology needs.
- Social support can improve quality of life, protect against post-traumatic stress, and decrease depression and anxiety.
- The psychosocial concerns that arise from a cancer diagnosis occur in a sociocultural context.

Keywords: assessment, cancer, distress, intervention, oncology, psychological, psychosocial

Psychosocial and Existential Distress, and Clinical Depression

Until the COVID-19 pandemic of 2020, cancer mortality rates in the United States were on the decline, driven by advances in treatment (Henley et al., 2020). As fewer people attended cancer screening appointments for fear of COVID exposure, the cancer mortality rate will likely increase due to later detection and delayed treatment (Fedewa et al., 2022). One study estimates that screening delays will cause an additional 2,500 deaths from breast cancer over the next 10 years, although the total impact is yet unknown (Alagoz et al., 2021).

Psychosocial distress, or the painful psychological, social, and/or spiritual feelings that may impede cancer coping is highly prevalent: In one study of over 4,000 cancer patients, almost half reported significant distress (Carlson et al., 2019). Against the background of a worldwide pandemic, the natural fear of death in response to a cancer diagnosis may have been heightened. Potentially life-threatening, cancer amid COVID may have created an amplified existential crisis, evoking terror, dread, isolation, and demoralization.

Angelique Caba, Maria Chi, and Stewart B. Fleishman, *Psychosocial Aspects of Cancer* In: *Oncology and Palliative Social Work*. Edited by: Susan Hedlund, Bryan Miller, Grace Christ, and Carolyn Messner, Oxford University Press.
 DOI: 10.1093/oso/9780197607299.003.0009

Existential distress is qualitatively distinct from general anxiety, depression, and other types of distress (Philipp et al., 2021).

Under "normal" circumstances (i.e., prepandemic), distress was considered a "normal" response to a diagnosis of cancer. Feelings of grief, fear, sadness, and confusion are common for people newly diagnosed with cancer. As time goes on, most patients establish a new equilibrium and begin to adapt to new routines that include treatment. The distress may extend into the survivorship period and may involve fear of recurrence, feelings of lack of control, and at times, anxiety or depression. Over time, most cancer survivors report an ability to adapt, to find resilience, and in some cases, to create new priorities and meaning either because of or in spite of a cancer diagnosis (Hedlund, 2018).

If a recurrence occurs, patients may revisit their distress and attempt to adapt and reevaluate priorities. Some patients also report that they have learned new skills and develop the ability to cope, despite the uncertainty that accompanies cancer.

Social workers and other mental health professionals need to recognize symptoms of anxiety and depression. Anxiety exists for approximately 30% of cancer patients and depression for approximately 25% of cancer patients (Naser et al., 2021). Additionally, it is important to evaluate for preexisting experiences of major depression, anxiety, and post-traumatic stress disorder (PTSD). Treatments such as cognitive behavioral therapy (CBT), acceptance and commitment therapy (ACT), and other supportive interventions can be very helpful in alleviating distress. Treatment of mental health issues can assist patients in complying with medical treatment and promote quality of life (Berchuck et al., 2020).

Existential distress is more prevalent among those with a terminal cancer (Bovero et al., 2018). Moreover, the inherent uncertainty of a cancer diagnosis may initiate a review of one's core identity and values and a search for meaning and purpose in one's life (Philipp et al., 2021). Treatment approaches such as life review, dignity therapy, and meaning-centered therapy can be helpful for patients dealing with the existential issues that may accompany end of life.

M. T. is a 50-year-old man living with non-Hodgkin lymphoma. His optimism at the start of treatment gradually faded with the onset of COVID-19, heightening his sense of isolation. His compromised immune system made him feel more vulnerable. Our work, which began with obtaining home health care services, centered around his desire to spend more time with his family. He dreamed of feeling well enough to work on an old car with his favorite nephew and that brought him great joy. He learned to focus on the present and not dwell on cancer's uncertainties. Each day he asked himself: How do I feel? What can I do today? How can I make the best use of my time?

Clinical Depression

Depression is common in the general population, and studies have shown that between 17%–25% of cancer patients will experience symptoms suggestive of depression (e.g., Krebber et al., 2014; Roth & Nelson, 2021). While feelings of loss and sadness are common at diagnosis, depression may have a burdensome effect on an individual's quality of life and a negative impact on treatment outcomes.

Screening of emotional distress among cancer patients along the disease trajectory is important in helping identify patients who may need further assessment, clinical intervention, and support. For patients with cancer and depressive symptoms, determining the need for professional psychosocial support may be challenging due to the overlap between depressive symptoms and the physical sequelae (e.g., fatigue or appetite changes) associated with the disease and treatment side effects (Bickel et al., 2021). While a patient's initial emotional distress may be normal and expected, major depression may be considered as a differential diagnosis when specific clinical criteria are met as indicated in the American Psychiatric Association's (2013) *Diagnostic and Statistical Manual of Mental Disorders* (5th ed.). Assessment and management of depressive symptoms require an understanding of the diagnostic criteria, cancer itself, cancer treatments, and evidence-based psychosocial treatment options. Major depression is correctly diagnosed when the symptoms are not due to medications (including cancer treatments), metabolic abnormalities, pain or tumors in the brain, or brain metastases (Valentine, 2014). Sorting through those variables may require the guidance of a (specialist-level provider) neurologist, psychiatrist, or palliative care physician with expertise in oncology.

Need for Social and Emotional Support

Research shows that individuals with cancer experience an array of psychosocial, supportive, and psychopharmacology care needs (Adler et al., 2008). These needs vary by type of cancer, treatment, the life stages of individuals and their families, and underlying sociodemographic, environmental, and living circumstances. Social and emotional support systems can significantly mitigate feelings of distress and enhance quality of life and emotional well-being (Zamanian et al., 2021).

Accessing Cancer-Related Information

With the advent of the Internet and the ubiquitous availability of portable devices such as cell phones on which to access it, people now have access to seemingly endless amounts of cancer information. Material from reliable and vetted sources such as the National Cancer Institute (NCI), American Cancer Society (ACS), and Cancer*Care*, and several professional advocacy organizations supplement and clarify the education a patient and family get from their providers and treatment team. Cancer information is available in text, audio, and video formats that are responsive and adapted to address variabilities in patients' health literacy. Interactive, real-time electronic platforms may quickly provide answers to individual questions. Ratings, rankings, and reviews of hospitals and providers are also readily available.

Such convenient and wide-ranging access to cancer-related information does not ensure that the information is correct, unbiased, or applicable to a person's specific health situation. Without regulation or the imprimatur of a trusted source, seemingly helpful information may be created to sell certain products or services with the motive of profit over medical safety, efficacy, and security. Others may tout unproven remedies or echo disappointments of unsuccessful treatment or unmet expectations. For example, online posts often promote the idea that "positive thinking" is necessary for chemotherapy or radiation therapy to be effective—a belief that can be more burdensome than helpful for patients (Holland & Lewis, 2001). Social workers should take care to direct patients and caregivers to trusted websites (e.g., National Health Center for Complementary and Integrative Health) and professionally moderated online communities.

The rise of remote access between providers and patients during the COVID-19 pandemic has had some unintended helpful consequences for cancer care. Many services suddenly became available from home, such as genetic, nutritional, and psychosocial counseling, and even support groups and physical therapy. Telehealth/telemedicine and remote consultations or visits may endure even as the public health crisis wanes (Weiner, 2021). However, if the shift to more telehealth persists after the pandemic, providers will be forced to address a main concern providers have with the system. Unfortunately, although telehealth offers access to patients who either are too sick to come to the clinic in person (e.g., palliative care patients) or live a long distance from cancer centers, insurance companies do not reimburse these visits at the same rates of reimbursement as in-person visits. This fact has led to concern that telehealth for certain service lines—which has proven to be a positive outcome of the pandemic—may be phased out as the crisis wanes.

Initial Client Meeting and Biopsychosocial Assessment

Starting Where the Client Is

The health care professional's initial encounter with a patient or caregiver is an opportunity to identify which psychological factors are most salient for the individual at a current point in time. One of the most fundamental tenets of social work practice is "starting where the client is," allowing them to set the pace, define the problem, and establish their own goals (Vakharia & Little, 2017). For example, someone newly diagnosed with metastatic lung cancer may not be ready to engage in advance care planning but might welcome a problem-solving approach for certain needs: How will she get to treatment? How will she pay for it? An open and collaborative stance encourages patients to prioritize their psychosocial needs.

Establishing a strong therapeutic alliance with people facing cancer is especially important because the stakes are so high. Failing to fully assess patients' needs and honor their priorities may result in missed opportunities for intervention. For example, if a patient cannot afford cancer-related costs, they are more likely to miss treatment, which can lead to greater mortality (Gilligan, 2018).

Assessment as Intervention: Psychological and Social Factors

After oncology providers conduct their initial medical evaluation, social workers can screen patients and caregivers for distress. They should also evaluate patients' and caregivers' psychosocial health needs to help determine whether someone needs further assessment to identify relevant interventions and/or referrals to desired psychosocial and supportive care services. The National Comprehensive Cancer Network's *NCCN Guidelines* version 2.2022, on distress management, provides information on patients at increased risk for distress and periods of increased vulnerability. Specifically, concerns related to health, finances, access to care, and other psychosocial factors can create additional distress for patients (NCCN, 2022). Screening and assessment may include using standardized and validated screening instruments for distress, depression, anxiety, trauma, suicide risk, and other issues. Clinical assessment interviews can enhance the client's understanding of their situation as it relates to the evolution of the disease, the treatment plan, potential side effects, and cancer's potential impact on their overall coping and needs. Building on clients' strengths can improve functioning. The oncology social worker bears witness, validates, and normalizes client experiences, promoting an active process of change. When uncertainty intensifies psychosocial distress, one can convey realistic hope and identify areas of functioning needing specialized assistance. This approach combined with reflective listening can have positive and clinically meaningful effects (Grassi et al., 2015).

Relationship building, which begins with screening and assessment, is important in establishing a trusting alliance among the social worker, the patient, and the family, loved ones, or friends who surround the patient. In oncology settings, relationship building encompasses members of the interdisciplinary team who work to identify and address the adjustment challenges a patient faces, to understand a patient's treatment stressors, emotional needs, relationships, and caregiving issues, and to help the patient cope with pain and other symptoms.

Social workers should be aware that a person receiving an initial cancer diagnosis is not in the same emotional circumstance as someone who has just been informed of a recurrence or relapse (Leano et al., 2019). A patient's psychosocial needs and concerns can differ at each juncture of the illness trajectory. Being compassionate and genuine is important in forging a therapeutic alliance.

Psychosocial Interventions

Psychosocial interventions include case management, resource referrals, and advocacy around concrete needs such as treatment-related financial assistance. When social workers address such practical needs early in the cancer trajectory, they are more likely to develop a stronger rapport and sense of trust with patients and families. In turn, clients and providers may work together to problem-solve practical barriers to accessing quality care. Patients may need assistance with navigating health insurance options, transportation, housing, or finances. Aiding these efforts may increase patients' hope and sense of self-efficacy and make it possible to tackle other issues (Vakharia & Little, 2017).

Helping patients resolve concrete obstacles can be a segue to a deeper focus on their psychological experience with cancer. The emotional distress that comes along with cancer can be a hindrance to quality of life but may be ameliorated with psychotherapy or counseling. Clinicians may help identify the psychological meaning of their diagnosis and their need for support. Integrated care among primary oncology care teams, social workers, and palliative care providers is especially effective when they provide services from the time of diagnosis through survivorship or end of life (Fleishman, 2011).

Clinical Interventions

Individual Counseling

Individual supportive counseling is usually time-limited and provides one-to-one focused collaboration. Counseling encourages patients to express emotions, validates individuals' experiences, and offers emotional support through empathetic listening. Counselors emphasize the individual's strengths and encourage their use of adaptive coping techniques. In psycho-oncology, specifically, counseling may be used to integrate the physical, practical, emotional, and spiritual changes that result from diagnosis and treatment to improve overall mood, coping, and functional adjustment.

One common struggle patients face is adjusting to the "new normal"—the changes a person faces because of a cancer diagnosis and treatments (NCI, 2019). Physical or emotional changes, differing routines, changed relationships, and functional limitations are some challenges the new normal might encompass. Helping patients adapt through individual counseling is a central task for oncology social workers.

The post-treatment period can be equally unsettling for patients who often have mixed emotions. Feelings of relief can be coupled with worry about the unknown path ahead. Fostering resilience and positive adaptation may help many patients improve their overall quality of life once their cancer treatments have concluded (Seiler & Jenewein, 2019).

Evidence-Based Therapies

Evidence-based therapies that have been shown to be helpful for managing anxiety and distress from cancer include CBT, ACT, dialectical behavior therapy (DBT), and motivational interviewing (MI). CBT is a therapeutic approach that emphasizes the significance of how our thinking affects both the way we feel and our behavior (Daniels, 2015). It may help cancer patients challenge cognitive errors in how they conceptualize or cope with their illness, such as believing that they solely caused their cancer or that they must suffer with it on their own. ACT offers a model of healthy adaptation to difficult circumstances. ACT uses mindfulness strategies along with commitment and behavioral strategies to increase flexibility in processing dynamic emotions of cancer adjustment (Fashler et al., 2017). DBT offers four core behavioral interventions: mindfulness, distress tolerance, interpersonal effectiveness, and emotion regulation. This therapy aims to teach people how to live in the moment, develop healthy ways to cope with stress, regulate their emotions, and improve their relationships with others (Stuntz & Linehan, 2021). The use of MI helps clients resolve ambivalence about behavior change, such as quitting smoking, increasing exercise, or joining a support group. MI techniques such as reflective statements and summarizing can reduce a patient's resistance to accepting help and support, expressing their feelings, or adhering to treatment. MI can also foster a greater sense of autonomy in the face of cancer, which may seem like a situation outside one's control (Spencer & Wheeler, 2016).

Finding Professional Psychosocial Oncology Assistance for Patients

Practitioners deliver cancer treatment in a variety of settings: a solo physician's office, a multiprovider ambulatory center, accredited interdisciplinary cancer centers, NCI-designated cancer centers, or all-cancer specialty hospitals. Specialist-level psychosocial interventions may be available within a solo practice, a cancer facility, or in the community. Working with a mental health therapist with familiarity with cancer and cancer treatment can help patients and families cope. Patients can find practitioners in subspecialty disciplines within cancer centers, and external organizations can also be helpful. Organizations such as the American Psychosocial Oncology Society, Association of Oncology Social Work, Oncology Nursing Society, ACS, Cancer*Care*, and Cancer Support Community all provide resources to help patients locate practitioners with psycho-oncology expertise.

Trauma-Informed Care and the Risk of Suicide

PTSD is a type of anxiety disorder. Some people develop PTSD after experiencing a frightening or life-threatening situation. PTSD symptoms may include anxiety, flashbacks, nightmares, fear, anger, or difficulty concentrating. Cancer and cancer treatment can also cause PTSD for both patients and caregivers. One study showed that nearly 1 in 4 women who had been told they had breast cancer had PTSD (Swartzman et al., 2017). Past trauma may also resurface during diagnostic procedures or cancer treatments. Routine scans, radiation therapy, or physical exams may trigger flashbacks. Awareness of a trauma history may help providers avoid unpleasant reactions in cancer patients. Offering treatment approaches such as psychotherapy, medication, support groups, and mindfulness-based stress reduction can help mitigate the distress of PTSD.

Recent data suggests that while suicide rates in people with cancer remain higher than in the general public, the rates are declining (NCI, 2021). Researchers believe this is due to greater access to supportive care and mental health treatment. Thoughts of suicide without intent or plan are often a surrogate for hopelessness and physical and emotional suffering (Kolva et al., 2020).

Building a Support Network

Support Groups

Support groups provide an environment in which people with the common experience of cancer (whether as patients, loved ones, or caregivers) can share and receive emotional understanding with others. Groups both lessen one's sense of isolation and provide valuable information. Additional benefits include a sense of kinship, an expanded perspective, the opportunity to share resources, exposure to new ideas and normalization, sharing medical knowledge, the opportunity to learn new coping techniques, increased insight, and a safe place to express fear and anger (Cipolletta et al., 2019). Potential cons of participating in a support group may include the triggering of feelings of hopelessness and discouragement if group members' similar experiences are overwhelming.

Family and Friends

In the context of a serious illness like cancer, one's sources of practical and emotional support are critical. Family, friends, the health care team, and other people in other communities, such as faith communities or other cancer survivors can be sources of support. Overall, social support improves quality of life, protects against PTSD, and decreases depression and anxiety among people with cancer (Zamanian et al., 2021).

Cancer is a biopsychosocial illness. Treatment can be complex and technical, which makes forging a collaborative and understanding relationship among providers, patients, families, and partners is essential. A burgeoning understanding of the emotional components of cancer draws from modern concepts of mental health as well as cancer subspecialties. When social workers focus on the intrapsychic and interpersonal aspects of cancer, they enrich the quality of patient care throughout the trajectory of illness.

Pearls

- An interdisciplinary approach is essential for providing optimal care to cancer patients and their loved ones.
- Knowledge of the psychosocial impact of cancer is imperative to supporting patients through treatment.
- The use of screening, assessment, and therapeutic interventions can identify and assist patients in need of greater care and support.

Pitfalls

- Minimizing the psychosocial distress of patients can lead to "missing" critical issues such as anxiety and depression.
- Not all cancer programs have professionals trained in the psychosocial aspects of cancer care.
- As new treatments are developed, more research is needed on approaches that optimize coping.

Additional Resources

American Psychosocial Oncology Society: www.apos-society.org
Association of Oncology Social Work: www.aosw.org
American Society of Clinical Oncology: www.cancer.net
Cancer*Care*: www.cancercare.org
National Center for Complementary and Integrative Health: www.nccih.nih.gov

References

Adler, N. E., Page, A. E. K., & Institute of Medicine Committee on Psychosocial Services to Cancer Patients/Families in a Community Setting (Eds.). (2008). *Cancer care for the whole patient: Meeting psychosocial health needs*. National Academies Press.

Alagoz, O., Lowry, K. P., Kurian, A. W., Mandelblatt, J. S., Ergun, M. A., Huang, H., Lee, S. J., Schechter, C. B., Tosteson, A., Miglioretti, D. L., Trentham-Dietz, A., Nyante, S. J., Kerlikowske, K., Sprague, B. L., Stout, N. K., & the CISNET Breast Working Group. (2021). Impact of the COVID-19 pandemic on breast cancer mortality in the U.S.: Estimates from collaborative simulation modeling. *Journal of the National Cancer Institute, 113*(11), 1484–1494. https://doi.org/10.1093/jnci/djab097

American Psychiatric Association. (2013). *Diagnostic and statistical manual of mental disorders* (5th ed.). APA. https://doi.org/10.1176/appi.books.9780890425596

Berchuck, J. E., Meyer, C. S., Zhang, N., Berchuck, C. M., Trivedi, N. N., Cohen, B., & Wang, S. (2020, June 4). Association of mental health treatment with outcomes for U.S. veterans diagnosed with non-small cell lung cancer. *JAMA Oncology*, *6*(7), 1055–1062. https://doi.org/10.1001/jamaoncol.2020.1466

Bickel, E. A., Auener, A. M., Ranchor, A. V., Fleer, J., & Schroevers, M. J. (2021). Understanding care needs of cancer patients with depressive symptoms: The importance of patients' recognition of depressive symptoms. *Psycho-Oncology*, *31*(1), 62–69. https://doi.org/10.1002/pon.5779

Bovero, A., Sedghi, N. A., Opezzo, M., Botto, R., Pinto, M., Ieraci, V., & Torta, R. (2018). Dignity-related existential distress in end-of-life cancer patients: Prevalence, underlying factors, and associated coping strategies. *Psycho-Oncology*, *27*(11), 2631–2637. https://doi.org/10.1002/pon.4884

Carlson, L. E., Zelinski, E. L., Toivonen, K. I., Sundstrom, L., Jobin, C. T., Damaskos, P., & Zebrack, B. (2019). Prevalence of psychosocial distress in cancer patients across 55 North American cancer centers. *Journal of Psychosocial Oncology*, *37*(1), 5–21. https://doi.org/10.1080/07347332.2018.1521490

Cipolletta, S., Simonato, C., & Faccio, E. (2019, February 18). The effectiveness of psychoeducational support groups for women with breast cancer and their caregivers: A mixed methods study. *Frontiers in Psychology*, *10*. https://doi.org/10.3389/fpsyg.2019.00288

Daniels, S. (2015). Cognitive behavior therapy for patients with cancer. *Journal of the Advanced Practitioner in Oncology*, *6*(1), 54–56. https://doi.org/10.6004/jadpro.2015.6.1.5

Fashler, S. R., Weinrib, A. Z., Azam, M. A., & Katz, J. (2017). The use of acceptance and commitment therapy in oncology settings: A narrative review. *Psychological Reports*, *121*(2), 229–252. https://doi.org/10.1177/0033294117726061

Fedewa, S. A., Star, J., Bandi, P., Minihan, A., Han, X., Yabroff, K. R., & Jemal, A. (2022, June 3). Changes in cancer screening in the U.S. during the COVID-19 pandemic. *JAMA Network Open*, *5*(6). https://doi.org/10.1001/jamanetworkopen.2022.15490

Fleishman, S. B. (2011). *Manual of cancer treatment recovery*. Demos Medical.

Gilligan, A. M., Alberts, D. S., Roe, D. J. & Skrepnek, G. H. (2018). *Death or debt? National estimates of financial toxicity in persons with newly-diagnosed cancer*. American.

Grassi, L., Caruso, R., Sabato, S., Massarenti, S., & Nanni, M. G. (2015, January 7). Psychosocial screening and assessment in oncology and palliative care settings. *Frontiers in Psychology*, *5*. https://doi.org/10.3389/fpsyg.2014.01485

Hedlund, S. (2018). Building a team to improve cancer survivorship: Integrative care's increasing role. In P. Hopewood & M. Milroy (Eds.), *Quality cancer care* (pp. 149–160). Springer. https://doi.org/10.1007/978-3-319-78649-0_10

Henley, S. J., Ward, E. M., Scott, S., Ma, J., Anderson, R. N., Firth, A. U., Thomas, C. C., Islami, F., Weir, H. K., Lewis, D. R., Sherman, R. L., Wu, M., Benard, V. B., Richardson, L. C., Jemal, A., Cronin, K., & Kohler, B. A. (2020). Annual report to the nation on the status of cancer, Part I: National cancer statistics. *Cancer*, *126*, 2225–2249.

Holland, J. C., & Lewis, S. (2001). *The human side of cancer: Living with hope, coping with uncertainty*. HarperCollins.

Kolva, E., Hoffecker, L., & Cox-Martin, E. (2020). Suicidal ideation in patients with cancer: A systemic review of prevalence, risk factors, intervention, and assessment. *Palliative and Supportive Care*, *18*(2), 206–219. https://doi.org/10.1017/S14789515190000610

Krebber, A., Buffart, L. M., Kleijn, G., Riepma, I. C., de Bree, R., Leemans, C. R., Becker, A., Brug, J., van Straten, A., Cuijpers, P., & Verdonck-de Leeuw, I. M. (2014). Prevalence of depression in cancer patients: A meta-analysis of diagnostic interviews and self-report instruments. *Psycho-Oncology*, *23*(2), 121–130. https://doi.org/10.1002/pon.3409

Leano, A., Korman, M. B., Goldberg, L., & Ellis, J. (2019). Are we missing PTSD in our patients with cancer? Part I. *Canadian Oncology Nursing Journal*, *29*(2), 141–146.

Naser, A. Y., Hameed, A. N., Mustafa, N., Alwah, H., Dahmash, E. Z., Alyami, H. S., & Khalil, H. (2021). Depression and anxiety in patients with cancer: A cross-sectional study. *Frontiers in Psychology*, *12*, 585534. https://doi.org/10.3389/fpsyg.2021.585534

National Cancer Institute. (n.d.). *Cancer stat facts: Cancer disparities*. Surveillance, Epidemiology, and End Results Program. Retrieved November 14, 2022, from https://seer.cancer.gov/statfacts/html/disparities.html

National Cancer Institute. (2019, June 17). *A* new *normal*. Retrieved from https://www.cancer.gov/about-cancer/coping/survivorship/new-normal

National Cancer Institute. (2021, February 17). Rate of suicide related to cancer is declining. *Cancer Currents*. Retrieved from https://www.cancer.gov/news-events/cancer-currents-blog/2021/cancer-related-suicide-rate-declining

National Comprehensive Cancer Network. (2022, January 27). *NCCN Guidelines version 2.2022, Distress management*. Retrieved from https://www.nccn.org/professionals/physician_gls/pdf/distress.pdf

Philipp, R., Kalender, A., Härter, M., Bokemeyer, C., Oechsle, K., Koch, U., & Vehling, S. (2021). Existential distress in patients with advanced cancer and their caregivers: Study protocol of a longitudinal cohort study. *BMJ Open*, *11*(4), e046351. https://doi.org/10.1136/bmjopen-2020-046351

Roth, A. J., & Nelson, C. J. (2021). *Psychopharmacology in cancer care: A guide for non-prescribers and prescribers*. Oxford University Press.

Seiler, A., & Jenewein, J. (2019). Resilience in cancer patients. *Frontiers in Psychiatry*, *10*, 1–35. https://doi.org/10.3389/fpsyt.2019.00208

Spencer, J. C., & Wheeler, S. B. (2016). A systematic review of motivational interviewing interventions in cancer patients and survivors. *Patient Education and Counseling*, *99*(7), 1099–1105. https://doi.org/10.1016/j.pec.2016.02.003

Stuntz, E., & Linehan, M. M. (2021). *Coping with cancer: DBT skills to manage your emotions and balance hope with uncertainty*. Guilford.

Swartzman, S., Booht, A., Munro, A., & Sani, F. (2017). Posttraumatic stress disorder with cancer diagnosis in adults: A meta-analysis. *Depression and Anxiety*, *34*(4), 327–329. https://doi.org/10.1002/da.22542

Vakharia, S. P., & Little, J. (2017). Starting where the client is: Harm reduction guidelines for clinical social work practice. *Clinical Social Work Journal*, *45*, 65–76. https://doi.org/10.1007/s10615-016-0584-3

Valentine, A. D. (2014). Mood disorders. In J. C. Holland, M. Golant, D. B. Greenberg, M. K. Hughes, J. A. Levenson, M. J. Loscalzo, & W. F. Pirl (Eds.), *Psycho-oncology: A quick reference on the psychosocial dimensions of cancer symptom management* (2nd ed., pp. 53–62). Oxford University Press. https://doi.org/10.1093/med/9780199988730.003.0006

Weiner, S. (2021, October 21). What happens to telemedicine after COVID-19? *AAMC News*. https://www.aamc.org/news-insights/what-happens-telemedicine-after-covid-19

Zamanian, H., Amini-Tehrani, M., Jalali, Z., Daryaafzoon, M., Ala, S., Tabrizian, S., & Foroozanfar, S. (2021, February). Perceived social support, coping strategies, anxiety, and depression among women with breast cancer: Evaluation of a mediation model. *European Journal of Oncology Nursing*, *50*, 101892. https://doi.org/10.1016/j.ejon.2020.101892

10

Finding Comfort

Pain, Symptom, and Treatment-Related Toxicity Management

Sara Taub, Kamel Abou Hussein, Victoria Puzo, and Jason A. Webb

Key Concepts

- Pain, associated with a cancer diagnosis, is an individual experience, affected by a person's social experiences, psychological state and history, spiritual supports, and existential concerns.
- Psychological symptoms are highly comorbid with physical symptoms for patients with cancer, and often, addressing a patient's physical symptoms improves psychological outcomes.
- The evolution of cancer therapies from chemotherapy and radiation to newer agents such as immunotherapy and targeted therapies has drastically changed the lived experience and symptom experience of patients undergoing advanced cancer therapies.

Keywords: anxiety, depression, pain, post-traumatic stress, symptom management

Pain and symptom management is a fundamental goal of palliative care services for patients with cancer (National Comprehensive Cancer Network, 2022). Cancer itself, cancer treatments, and the toxicities associated with certain treatments often lead to significant decrements in function and quality of life. In this chapter, we describe the role of the interdisciplinary palliative care team in tending to the whole person through the lens of a biopsychosocial-spiritual model to assess and manage pain and non-pain-related symptoms. We explore ways oncology and palliative care social workers can integrate their expertise and skills for pain and symptom management in collaboration with other members of the interprofessional care team. We also offer an

Sara Taub, Kamel Abou Hussein, Victoria Puzo, and Jason A. Webb, *Finding Comfort* In: *Oncology and Palliative Social Work.*
Edited by: Susan Hedlund, Bryan Miller, Grace Christ, and Carolyn Messner, Oxford University Press.
 DOI: 10.1093/oso/9780197607299.003.0010

overview of medical concepts underlying interdisciplinary symptom management and treatment-related toxicities.

Mrs. Carson is a 56-year-old woman Spiritual Inter metastatic breast cancer whose disease has spread to her thoracic spine and lungs. She is on her fourth line of treatment with an investigational endocrine therapy. She has been suffering from back pain due to her thoracic metastases, which has also limited her mobility. Her pain, nausea, and vomiting caused her to stop working as a high school teacher. She is married with two children in college. Her husband has been avoiding coming to appointments due to his distress with her physical decline and her symptoms. Recently, her oncologist referred her for a palliative care consultation to help manage her pain and treatment-induced nausea and vomiting.

Oncology and palliative social workers have a vital role in the multidimensional screening and assessment, interventions, management, and care coordination for patients with pain and nonpain symptoms. For patients such as Mrs. Carson, social workers can help identify inadequately managed physical symptoms like pain, nausea and vomiting, and loss of physical function and communicate this to appropriate members of the interprofessional team. In addition, the social worker can screen and assess for clinically significant behavioral or psychological symptoms, social, relational, spiritual, and practical issues that may occur in a patient whose life has changed significantly over the course of her disease trajectory.

The Nature of Pain and Pain Definitions

In 2020, the International Association for the Study of Pain updated its definition of *pain* to "an unpleasant sensory and emotional experience associated with . . . actual or potential tissue damage" (Raja et al., 2020). The new definition (the first since 1979) underscores that pain is a personal experience (although we need not rely on a person's ability to describe the experience). Globally, health care professionals and pain researchers have accepted the new definition; additionally, professional, governmental, and nongovernmental organizations across the world have adopted it.

Many people perceive having cancer as synonymous with being in pain. Cancer pain is prevalent but not universal. Cancer itself can cause pain when a tumor presses on nerves or when the cancer is in the bone. Treatments themselves can cause pain as well, with chemotherapies causing some nerve-ending pain, radiation therapy irritating tissues or making them less elastic, and surgical sutures causing pain (Cherny, 2021). Most of these types of pain can be prevented or reduced with medications as well as a variety of modalities such as massage, acupuncture, exercise or movement, and nutritional and psychosocial interventions. The evaluation and management of pain before, during, and after a cancer diagnosis and treatment is part of the comprehensive "whole person" approach to care. Comprehensive care relies on an interdisciplinary team, whether at accredited treatment centers or in local oncology practices.

Total Pain

Though pain often is thought of as a physical symptom, we must remember that it can take many different forms. Beyond biological manifestations of visceral, somatic, or neuropathic pain, individuals often experience exacerbations of pain due to distress around the instability cancer causes in their social lives, psychological anguish when mental health symptoms arise, a spiritual crisis if deeply held beliefs come into question, or existential torment for those no longer able to make meaning of their life story. Taken together, the various layers of pain that often coexist in combination and exacerbate one another, are referred to as *total pain*, a concept that Dame Cicely Saunders first described (Clark, 1999). Total pain emphasizes that we are more than the sum of our parts. Discrete co-occurring experiences that disrupt various facets of ourselves affect us holistically.

Cancer Pain Types and Physical Symptoms

Nociceptive pain results from ongoing tissue injury, which activates the somatosensory systems that alert us to noxious events and ultimately leads to the perception of pain. Nociceptive pain can be divided into two categories: *somatic* and *visceral*. Somatic pain involves injury to somatic structures, such as bone, joints, or muscles. Patients often describe this type of pain as "aching," "stabbing," "throbbing," or "pressure-like" in quality. Visceral pain involves injury to viscera and is usually characterized as "gnawing" or "crampy" when arising from the obstruction of a hollow viscus (e.g., the bowel lumen) and "aching" or "stabbing" when arising from other visceral structures, such as organ capsules, myocardium, or pleura.

Pain is defined as *neuropathic* if the results of a pain evaluation suggest that it is sustained by abnormal somatosensory processing caused by a lesion or disease affecting the peripheral or central somatosensory system (Finnerup et al., 2016). Neuropathic mechanisms are involved in approximately 40% of cancer pain syndromes and can be caused by either the disease or its treatment (Caraceni et al., 1999). Physical examination of a patient with neuropathic pain may identify findings of allodynia (pain induced by nonpainful stimuli), hyperalgesia (increased perception of painful stimuli), or other sensory findings. Patients may have other concomitant neurologic findings like weakness, numbness, or changes in reflexes along with autonomic dysfunction within the anatomic distribution of the pain.

Acute or Chronic Cancer Pain Syndromes

In many cases, the constellation of symptoms and signs that a patient reports can suggest a specific cancer pain syndrome (Caraceni et al., 1999). Identifying the appropriate syndrome may help elucidate the etiology of the pain, direct the diagnostic evaluation, clarify the prognosis for the pain, and guide therapeutic intervention. Cancer pain syndromes can be divided into acute and chronic. Whereas acute pain syndromes usually accompany diagnostic or therapeutic interventions, chronic pain syndromes usually are directly related to the neoplasm itself or treatment (Cherny, 2010).

Breakthrough pain is typically defined as a transient flare of moderate to severe pain occurring in the background of controlled pain. Usually, the flare is short-lived and directly associated with a feature of the cancer or cancer treatment. A substantial proportion of chronic pain syndromes are directly due to the neoplasm (Portenoy, 2011). However, patients might develop chronic pain secondary to cancer treatment as well (Paice et al., 2016).

Physical Pain as a Treatment-Related Toxicity

Cancer treatment modalities such as surgery, radiation therapy, cytotoxic chemotherapy, and endocrine therapy can lead to pain-like symptoms even after completion of a treatment plan. In chemotherapy-induced peripheral neuropathy, chemotherapeutic agents cause direct damage to peripheral sensory fibers causing tingling and numbness. The sensation might be in the tips of the toes and fingers or might extend in a “stocking/glove” distribution. For many patients, peripheral neuropathy can be prevented or self-limiting with dose reduction of certain cytotoxic chemotherapeutic agents. However, many others may go on to develop chronic and debilitating neuropathic pain syndrome.

Two common postsurgical pain syndromes are post-thoracotomy pain syndrome and postradical neck dissection syndrome. Postsurgical pain is typically secondary to nerve injury at the time of surgery with evidence of neuropathic pain or phantom sensation following limb amputation (Richardson & Kulkarni, 2017). Lymphedema following lymph node dissection is a common cause of localized pain to an extremity after cancer surgery. In addition to physical pain, lymphedema can cause psychological pain associated with disfigurement and cosmetic changes in the aftermath of treatment.

Postradiation pain syndromes occur when patients develop chronic pain following radiation therapy. This is seen, for instance, when the thorax or brachial plexus are in radiation field, as is the case for women undergoing breast radiation.

Measuring Pain and Pain Assessment

Addressing pain in a biopsychosocial-spiritual framework that uses the concept of total pain allows for a deeper focus on patient needs in the cancer diagnosis setting. This approach honors the patient as a whole person and increases the sense of partnership in decisions and planning. Social workers can support a patient's pain experience by exploring and clarifying their subjective and emotional experience and framework of understanding—as shaped by the patient's lived experience, which multiple variables can influence. Talking with the patient should help identify how pain is causing them distress and disruption. Screening for comorbid disorders such as depression is important since the underlying condition may affect the pain experience and affect overall quality of life. An example of a multipurpose self-administered tool is the Patient Health Questionnaire-9 (PHQ-9). The PHQ-9 is a nine-item depression scale that serves as a screening tool, aids in differential diagnosis, and serves as a symptom-tracking tool (Anderson et al., 2014). Taking a thorough spiritual history may also inform how to take a person-centered approach in identifying management and coping strategies. The FICA (faith/belief, importance, community, and address in care) or HOPE (hope, organized religion, personal spirituality/practices, and effects) spiritual history assessment tools can assist social workers and the medical team in understanding how spirituality and/or religion play a part in the patient's perception of illness and decision-making throughout treatment (Borneman et al., 2010).

A comprehensive biopsychosocial-spiritual assessment includes learning about the patient's social support system. Social workers can help identify concrete roles for willing and available family or friends; for example, some may be able to provide transportation to appointments or assist with childcare while others are more adept at providing emotional support. Social workers can also educate patients about pertinent community groups and professional resources available to them such as local volunteers or foundations that help people with cancer. Supporting primary caregivers is another domain around which the social worker can provide valuable information, for example, steering them to support groups, home care, respite options, and other related resources. Both patients and caregivers may benefit from referrals to counseling and support groups to address social and emotional needs.

Pediatric and Adult Pain Assessment Tools

Because pain is subjective, researchers have developed various scales to rate symptoms as an individual experiences them. At least two dozen such tools have been clinically tested and validated; among these, most rely on self-reporting. One of the most frequently used scales in the United States is the VAS (visual analog scale), which invites a person to choose a point on a 100-millimeter line (score 1–10) that best describes their pain. Other scales rely on observation by health care professionals or family members, like the FLACC (face, legs, activity, cry, consolability) scale used in children ages 2 months to 7 years or individuals who are unable to communicate their pain. While most pain scales are geared toward adults, others are specific to children, such as the Wong-Baker FACES scale that asks children to identify which of six faces best represents their pain experience (Crellin et al., 2015; Price et al., 1983).

Whereas most scales focus on intensity of pain, some try to assess a person's ability to function with pain. Finally, some scales have been created for pain localized to certain areas (e.g., Dallas Pain Questionnaire [DPQ] for adults with chronic spinal pain), pain that is particular to certain diseases (Palliative Care Outcome Scale [PCOS] for adult palliative cancer patients), or pain that is experienced chronically (McGill Pain Questionnaire [MPQ]) for adults with various pain syndromes (Hearn & Higginson, 1999; Lawlis et al., 1989; Melzack, 1975).

Beyond the scales themselves, traditional measures for describing physical pain include such characteristics as provoking/relieving factors, quality of the pain, region of the pain and its propensity to radiate, severity of the pain, and timing of the pain (summarized by the mnemonic acronym PQRST). Other measures include how pain is affecting a patient's daily life and ability to perform quotidian activities independently (Webb & LeBlanc, 2018).

Social Work Role With Patients and Caregivers

Social workers' comprehensive biopsychosocial-spiritual assessments of patients help provide insights into patients' experiences as a whole, taking into account their family structure, living environment, finances, social supports, cultural influences, core values, and presenting concerns. Social workers should include caregivers during these assessments to learn about the patients' support systems and available resources. In-depth interviews can help a patient, caregiver, and social worker build trust. The patient may find comfort in knowing that their social worker and treatment team are taking the time to get to know them, to understand their preferences, beliefs, and values, and to elucidate their needs.

Another particularly useful tool for social workers is the Pain Disability Index, which measures how pain interferes with a patient's day-to-day living (work, home, self-care, sexual activity, social activity, recreation, etc.) (Tait et al., 1990). How a patient responds to each of these questions will give additional guidance on the how to address pain and other symptoms.

Symptoms Associated With Cancer and Treatments

Pulmonary

Pulmonary symptoms in the setting of cancer diagnosis can occur with a primary lung malignancy or metastatic disease or secondary to a malignant pleural effusion. They could also be a side effect of treatment, like pneumonitis from chemotherapy, immunotherapy, or radiation therapy. Symptom complexes can involve shortness of breath, whether with activity or at rest. Dyspnea can be improved with cancer-directed therapies, supplemental oxygen, or with medications such as low-dose opioids. Opioids are frequently used for patients with advanced cancer who have refractory dyspnea to manage this life-limiting symptom (Mahler et al., 2010). Social workers can counsel patients about relaxation techniques and biofeedback regarding dyspnea.

Gastrointestinal (Nausea, Constipation, Dysphagia, and Cachexia)

Gastrointestinal (GI) symptoms can manifest due to primary disease or treatment-related toxicities. Assessing underlying structural or metabolic abnormalities, which may contribute to symptoms, is important. Nausea and emesis are the most common GI symptoms for patients undergoing cancer therapies. In fact, nausea and vomiting are typically managed as part of the standard of care for patients receiving chemotherapy regimens to avoid treatment intolerance. Radiation therapy—in particular, therapies that include the central nervous system, hollow viscera, or solid tissue—also frequently leads to nausea. Nausea and vomiting can occur secondary to malignant bowel obstruction, which can be a surgical emergency or a terminal complication for patients with solid tumors, and secondary to gastroparesis (or delayed transit) in association with peritoneal metastasis.

Constipation is a common symptom seen in up to 90% of patients (Clark et al., 2011, 2012; Erichsén et al., 2015; Hoekstra et al., 2006). It can be a medication side effect (e.g., opioid- or chemotherapy-induced) or a disease complication (e.g., in spinal-cord compression or metabolic abnormalities). Addressing the underlying etiology is essential to clarifying whether there are any reversible nonpharmacologic factors. Stool softeners, laxatives, enemas, and opioid antagonists can be helpful to patients with refractory opioid-induced constipation. There is no evidence to support that certain laxatives were more effective than others or caused fewer adverse events (Candy et al., 2015).

Dysphagia and xerostomia (dry mouth) are especially prevalent after radiation therapy in patients with head and neck cancers. Xerostomia can also be an anticholinergic medication side effect. Altered taste sensation is a frequent symptom that can make it challenging for patients to eat and swallow appropriately (Sweeney & Bagg, 2000). Dietary changes, good oral hygiene, rinsing with salt water, and using ice chips and artificial saliva can be helpful interventions. Some patients may require placement of enteral feeding tubes, which can lead to psychological distress. Social workers can help guide patients who are adjusting to the physical and psychological changes that can occur with GI symptoms and disordered eating due to their cancer or its treatments.

Commonly seen in patients with advanced chronic diseases, including cancer, cachexia is a hypercatabolic state that results in a significant loss of skeletal muscle and often predisposes patients to infections, causing general decline. Patients and their caregivers may struggle as weight loss and debility progress, requiring reassurance that loss of interest in food is a natural expectation of disease progression. A consultation with a nutritionist can be helpful in navigating dietary adjustments and finding ways to help patients continue to enjoy the taste of food in addition to its nutritional benefits (Hutton et al., 2006). Nutritional supplementation, including enteral feeding tubes or parenteral administration, may be a goal-concordant desire for patients, though there is no evidence that artificial nutrition prolongs life or improves the patient's overall functional status (Good et al., 2008). Discussions among the patient, family, social worker, oncology, and palliative care team should include thoughtful consideration of the trade-offs of such interventions (Brard et al., 2006; Bruera et al., 2013; Good et al., 2008; Hoda et al., 2005).

Cutaneous

Lymphedema, which occurs when there is disruption of the lymphatic flow, may be seen either after surgery and radiation therapy or as a complication of the cancer itself. The patient will display swelling, most commonly in the extremities, with the potential for deleterious effects on mobility, function, and body image (Frid et al., 2006; Pyszel et al., 2006). Exercise and physical therapy, along with manual lymphatic drainage and skin care, may help. These may be offered under the auspices of specialized lymphedema programs where available.

Psychological/Psychiatric

The experience of patients with both solid tumors or hematologic malignancies often involves loss and trauma, along with associated grief. These may occur against a backdrop of preexisting mental health conditions, given the high prevalence of depression and anxiety in the general U.S. population. In this section, we explore some of the common mental health–related comorbidities of patients with cancer, with a focus on manageable symptoms.

Depression

Depression symptoms vary across cancer types, diagnostic experiences, and treatment phases (Li et al., 2016). At times, they can be difficult to distinguish from manifestations of the cancer itself or ramifications of treatments. Depressed mood and anhedonia are more specific for major depression than neurovegetative symptoms (fatigue, sleep disturbance, low appetite, psychomotor slowing) and neurocognitive manifestations (guilt, poor concentration/memory deficits), which can sometimes be attributed to the cancer itself or treatment side effects.

Depression symptom management may involve a combination of psychotherapeutic intervention, and medication management and can be guided by

American Society for Clinical Oncology guidelines for depression that rely on use of the PHQ-9. While no specific psychotherapy modalities have been validated specific to depression in cancer, cognitive behavioral therapy (CBT), acceptance and commitment therapy (ACT), and dignity therapy have been studied and show efficacy (Li et al., 2016).

Regarding pharmacologic interventions, selective serotonin reuptake inhibitors (SSRIs, including escitalopram, sertraline) or selective serotonin and norepinephrine reuptake inhibitors (SNRIs, including duloxetine, venlafaxine) are first-line therapies for depression. These come with their own side effects and complications that warrant monitoring: GI side effects (nausea, vomiting, and diarrhea) and sexual side effects (anorgasmia, low libido) can negatively affect quality of life and adherence. In patients over the age of 65, depression itself and these medications can increase the risks of falls and medication-related osteoporosis.

Anxiety

Irrespective of premorbid mental health disorders, worry and fear accompany much of the cancer care trajectory for patients, as a normative psychological response to a life-threatening illness. Screening with the 7-item Generalized Anxiety Disorder Questionnaire (GAD-7) at the time of diagnosis and at any point during the care trajectory with a treatment change or disease progression is warranted (Anderson et al., 2014).

Psychotherapeutic interventions, such as supportive psychotherapy and CBT, should be the first-line treatment for anxiety. Patients with high symptom burdens interfering with quality of life, sleep, and treatment adherence should be treated with first-line pharmacotherapy including SSRIs, SNRIs, and low-dose antihistaminergic medications FDA approved for anxiety. Benzodiazepines (BZDs) can play a role in the short-term treatment of anxiety, especially ahead of procedures and scans or in the case of sleep disturbances due to corticosteroid therapy. We recommend either lorazepam or clonazepam at the lowest effective dosage. BZDs can increase the risks for delirium, tolerance, dependence, and in particular, risks for respiratory depression in patients on concomitant opioids for pain. The same formulations of BZDs are also used routinely as antiemetics.

Post-Traumatic Stress

The shock of a cancer diagnosis, the burdens of many available therapies, prolonged hospitalizations, and associated disruptions on life trajectory make cancer an intensely traumatic experience for many patients. This shock comes in addition to any premorbid illness or trauma experiences that can be reactivated by the threat responses inherent to cancer care. Recent research demonstrates that early palliative care integration can decrease post-traumatic stress disorder (PTSD) symptoms through symptom management and improvements in adaptive coping (El-Jawahri et al., 2021).

Social work team members can help with both the diagnosis and psychotherapeutic management of PTSD or trauma. Supportive psychotherapy, CBT, ACT, and trauma-focused therapies should be first-line treatments where available. Pharmacotherapy can also be considered when treating PTSD symptoms.

Delirium

Delirium, an acute change in awareness, attention, concentration, perception, and orientation, can occur because of the cancer itself, cancer treatments, and toxicities associated with treatments. All three subtypes of delirium (hypoactive, hyperactive, and mixed) can cause intense distress in patients and caregivers.

Social workers play a key role in listening to patients and families. They also offer anticipatory guidance around the distress associated with delirium and how to cope with it. Social workers should coordinate closely with the interdisciplinary health care team in their interventions with families and patients. Medications such as haloperidol, olanzapine, quetiapine, and risperidone may be used to help with symptom control particularly if delirium is accompanied by psychosis or agitation. Some patients and families may opt for increased sedation (palliative sedation) toward the end of life if delirium symptoms are severe and intractable.

Pediatric

A full overview of pediatric symptoms and considerations is beyond the scope of this chapter. However, it may be valuable for social workers to keep some unique considerations in mind when working with pediatric patients. Some symptoms ensue from biological and physiological characteristics associated with certain phases of growth. For instance, young children whose brains are actively developing may be more sensitive to brain radiation. The potential impact of therapies on reproductive health should also be explored in pediatric patients.

Other symptoms are more unique to children's developmental status and conceptions of the world. These might include heightened distress associated with changing body image (weight gain with steroids, cachexia, hair loss) during a phase of life when appearance in the eyes of peer may feel closely intertwined with acceptance and notions of identity/self-worth.

Compromised independence for children who derive tremendous pride from having achieved new milestones or for adolescents committed to being their own person may be experienced as significant setbacks. Existential distress surrounding having to come to terms with one's own mortality, even as one is seen as not yet having lived their life, may be overwhelming.

Additional complications may ensue from the fact that young children or children who are neurocognitively atypical may not understand that they have cancer, what cancer even is, and why they must be in the hospital apart from family and friends and/or subjected to painful treatments. They also may not be able to verbalize the pain and discomfort they are experiencing in association with disease and associated therapies. Finally, they may be especially sensitive to witnessing distress in their parents, guardians, or other meaningful figures in their lives.

Toxicities of Cancer-Directed Therapies

We think of cancer treatments as either local (including surgery and radiation therapy) or systemic (including cytotoxic chemotherapy, endocrine therapy, targeted therapies, and immunotherapy, among others). Each type of treatment has its own side effects.

Chemotherapy/Radiation Therapy

Cytotoxic chemotherapy plays an integral part in the management of multiple types of cancers. Side effects from chemotherapy are dependent on factors that include the type of chemotherapy, dose, and mode of administration. In addition to side effects already discussed above (fatigue, GI issues, neuropathy), hair loss, low blood counts, fever, and cardiac, renal, or hepatic toxicity are also common. Radiation therapy often causes fatigue, nausea, loss of appetite, diarrhea, and skin changes such as radiation dermatitis.

Endocrine Therapy

Endocrine therapies are essential treatments for hormonally driven cancers (such as breast and prostate cancer). The most common side effects are hot flashes, joint or muscle pain and stiffness, decreased libido, weight gain, excessive fatigue, headaches, loss of bone mineral density, and changes in lipid profile. Endocrine therapy can also cause significant mood and sleep disturbances.

Immunotherapy/Targeted Therapies

Immunotherapy and targeted therapies focus on improving the immune system's ability to target cancer cells. In the process, the immune system can also target healthy cells, causing adverse events. Treatment toxicities include varying degrees of skin rash, colitis, myositis (muscle inflammation), pneumonitis, hepatitis, and endocrine-related problems, including thyroiditis and diabetes, among others.

Targeted therapies are cancer treatments that target specific genes or proteins involved in the growth and survival of cancer cells. They include monoclonal antibodies and small molecule drugs. Diarrhea and liver toxicities are common with this class of drugs; however, patients can also experience worsening hypertension, fatigue, mouth sores, and skin and nail changes.

The "Opioid Crisis"

The current "opioid crisis" has adversely affected many communities, who have seen the largest substance abuse epidemic ever. This complex biopsychosocial-spiritual crisis has adversely affected those experiencing cancer. Patients are often loath to take the proper amount of pain relievers on a schedule that reflects the duration of time the medication affords the most relief, cutting back to avoid becoming drug dependent. Exact schedules to start, maintain, and then reduce opioid medications can be complex but teachable. Many different forms of opioid and nonopioid medications can and should be mixed to provide the most relief with the least risk of dependence. The fear that once opioids are started they will become permanent is unfounded. The small subset of cancer patients that develop an opioid dependence have likely had substance dependence in their precancer background or a close blood relative with substance abuse (Bruera & Paice, 2015), depression, or trauma.

An obstacle to receiving specialist-level pain relief with cancer comes when the team most experienced to do so is mistakenly misperceived to be "end of life" specialists. The palliative care team (Brown et al., 2019) or anesthesia pain team are available at most treatment centers but underutilized from the time of diagnosis through long-term cancer survivorship because of the stigma associated with end-of-life care. Overcoming this obstacle is occurring, however slowly.

Access to the variety of pain-reducing care is yet another obstacle. Many local pharmacies do not keep supplies of opioids inventoried due to storage and regulatory demands. Physical therapists, acupuncturists, massage therapists, and oncology nutritionists are often not available in underserved communities. Some pain management services may be provided remotely, such as exercise programs or visits with members of the interdisciplinary treatment team. However, telehealth pain services can be limited in underserved communities or groups caused by inaccessible broadband internet service or a lack of electronic devices that connect to the internet.

Guiding Best Practices for the Future

Advanced cancer causes intense and debilitating symptoms related to the primary disease process as well as the toxicities associated with cancer-directed therapies. Impeccable attention to the biopsychosocial-spiritual model of care is the standard of care approach to palliative care and symptom management. Patients who have been marginalized and exposed to systemic racism in health care are at higher risk for poor symptom control as well as social and psychological distress. Palliative care social work interventions to address symptoms and identify barriers to safe and equitable care are first-line interventions to ensure comprehensive supportive and palliative care for all patients with advanced cancer.

Pearls

- Oncology and palliative care social workers are integral members of the interprofessional cancer care team.
- Collaborative, interprofessional care team symptom screening, assessment, and intervention can result in early identification and improved management of symptoms affecting overall quality of life.
- Psychological interventions, such as supportive therapy, can substantially improve pain, sleep, anxiety, and depressive symptoms among people living with cancer.

Pitfalls

- Screening tools for psychological symptoms can overestimate depression symptoms for patients with cancer, which makes an expert diagnostic assessment key (Grapp et al., 2019; Thekkumpurath et al., 2011).
- Physical symptoms such as pain should be managed as the primary symptom before initiating pharmacotherapy for mood and anxiety disorders as these symptoms may improve with direct pain control.
- Access to primary palliative care for patients and families facing life-threatening illnesses remains extremely limited.

Additional Resources

NCCN Clinical Practice Guidelines in Oncology—Supportive Care: www.nccn.org/guidelines/category_3

Center to Advance Palliative Care—Social Work Serious Illness Designation Foundational Skills: www.capc.org/training/learning-pathways/social-work-serious-illness-designation/

OncoLink Resources for More Information, Cancer Pain Management: www.oncolink.org/support/side-effects/pain-management/resources-for-more-information-cancer-pain-management

References

Andersen, B. L., DeRubeis, R. J., Berman, B. S., Gruman, J., Champion, V. L., Massie, M. J., Holland, J. C., Partridge, A. H., Bak, K., Somerfield, M. R., & Rowland, J. H. (2014). Screening, assessment, and care of anxiety and depressive symptoms in adults with cancer: An American Society of Clinical Oncology guideline adaptation. *Journal of Clinical Oncology*, *32*(15), 1605–1619. https://doi.org/10.1200/JCO.2013.52.4611

Borneman, T., Ferrell, B., & Puchalski, C. M. (2010). Evaluation of the FICA tool for spiritual assessment. *Journal of Pain and Symptom Management*, *40*(2), 163–173. https://doi.org/10.1016/j.jpainsymman.2009.12.019

Brard, L., Weitzen, S., Strubel-Lagan, S. L., Swamy, N., Gordinier, M. E., Moore, R. G., & Granai, C. O. (2006). The effect of total parenteral nutrition on the survival of terminally ill ovarian cancer patients. *Gynecologic Oncology*, *103*(1), 176–180. https://doi.org/10.1016/j.ygyno.2006.02.013

Brown, T. J., Smith, T. J., & Gupta, A. (2019). Palliative care. *JAMA Oncology*, *5*(1), 126. https://doi.org/10.1001/jamaoncol.2018.4962

Bruera, E., & Paice, J. A. (2015). Cancer pain management: Safe and effective use of opioids. In *American Society of Clinical Oncology Educational Book. American Society of Clinical Oncology. Annual Meeting* (pp. e593–e599). https://doi.org/10.14694/EdBook_AM.2015.35.e593

Bruera, E., Hui, D., Dalal, S., Torres-Vigil, I., Trumble, J., Roosth, J., Krauter, S., Strickland, C., Unger, K., Palmer, J. L., Allo, J., Frisbee-Hume, S., & Tarleton, K. (2013). Parenteral hydration in patients with advanced cancer: A multicenter, double-blind, placebo-controlled randomized trial. *Journal of Clinical Oncology*, *31*(1), 111–118. https://doi.org/10.1200/JCO.2012.44.6518

Candy, B., Jones, L., Larkin, P. J., Vickerstaff, V., Tookman, A., & Stone, P. (2015). Laxatives for the management of constipation in people receiving palliative care. *Cochrane Database of Systematic Reviews*. https://doi.org/10.1002/14651858.CD003448.pub4

Caraceni, A., Portenoy, R. K., & Working Group of the IASP Task Force on Cancer Pain. (1999). An international survey of cancer pain characteristics and syndromes: IASP Task Force on Cancer Pain: International Association for the Study of Pain. *Pain*, *82*(3), 263–274. https://doi.org/10.1016/S0304-3959(99)00073-1

Cherny, N. I. (2010). Pain assessment and cancer pain syndromes. In G. Hanks, N. I. Cherny, N. Christakis, M. Fallon, S. Kaasa, & R. K. Portenoy (Eds.), *Oxford Textbook of Palliative Medicine* (4th ed., pp. 599–626). Oxford University Press.

Cherny, N. I. (2021, August 1). Chronic cancer pain syndromes. In *Oxford Textbook of Palliative Medicine* (pp. 345–363) (online edition). Retrieved from https://doi.org/10.1093/med/9780198821328.003.0037

Clark, D. (1999). "Total pain," disciplinary power and the body in the work of Cicely Saunders, 1958–1967. *Social Science & Medicine*, *49*(6), 727–736. https://doi.org/10.1016/s0277-9536(99)00098-2

Clark, K., Lam, L., & Currow, D. C. (2011). Exploring the relationship between the frequency of documented bowel movements and prescribed laxatives in hospitalized palliative care patients. *American Journal of Hospice and Palliative Care*, *28*(4), 258–263. https://doi.org/10.1177/1049909110385548

Clark, K., Smith, J. M., & Currow, D. C. (2012). The prevalence of bowel problems reported in a palliative care population. *Journal of Pain and Symptom Management*, *43*(6), 993–1000. https://doi.org/10.1016/j.jpainsymman.2011.07.015

Crellin, D. J., Harrison, D., Santamaria, N., & Babl, F. E. (2015). Systematic review of the Face, Legs, Activity, Cry, and Consolability scale for assessing pain in infants and children: Is it reliable, valid, and feasible for use? *Pain*, *156*(11), 2132–2151. https://doi.org/10.1097/j.pain.0000000000000305

El-Jawahri, A., LeBlanc, T. W., Kavanaugh, A., Webb, J. A., Jackson, V. A., Campbell, T. C., O'Connor, N., Luger, S. M., Gafford, E., Gustin, J., Bhatnagar, B., Walker, A. R., Fathi, A. T., Brunner, A. M., Hobbs, G. S., Nicholson, S., Davis, D., Addis, H., Vaughn, D., . . . Temel, J. S. (2021). Effectiveness of integrated palliative and oncology care for patients with acute myeloid leukemia: A randomized clinical trial. *JAMA Oncology*, *7*(2), 238–245. https://doi.org/10.1001/jamaoncol.2020.6343

Erichsén, E., Milberg, A., Jaarsma, T., & Friedrichsen, M. J. (2015). Constipation in specialized palliative care: Prevalence, definition, and patient-perceived symptom distress. *Journal of Palliative Medicine*, *18*(7), 585–592. https://doi.org/10.1089/jpm.2014.0414

Finnerup, N. B., Haroutounian, S., Kamerman, P., Baron, R., Bennett, D., Bouhassira, D., Cruccu, G., Freeman, R., Hansson, P., Nurmikko, T., Raja, S. N., Rice, A., Serra, J., Smith, B. H., Treede, R. D., & Jensen, T. S. (2016). Neuropathic pain: An updated grading system for research and clinical practice. *Pain*, *157*(8), 1599–1606. https://doi.org/10.1097/j.pain.0000000000000492

Frid, M., Strang, P., Friedrichsen, M. J., & Johansson, K. (2006). Lower limb lymphedema: Experiences and perceptions of cancer patients in the late palliative stage. *Journal of Palliative Care*, *22*(1), 5–11.

Good, P., Cavenagh, J., Mather, M., & Ravenscroft, P. (2008). Medically assisted nutrition for palliative care in adult patients. *Cochrane Database of Systematic Reviews*. https://doi.org/10.1002/14651858.CD006274.pub2

Grapp, M., Terhoeven, V., Nikendei, C., Friederich, H. C., & Maatouk, I. (2019). Screening for depression in cancer patients using the PHQ-9: The accuracy of somatic compared to non-somatic items. *Journal of Affective Disorders*, *254*, 74–81. https://doi.org/10.1016/j.jad.2019.05.026

Hearn, J., & Higginson, I. J. (1999). Development and validation of a core outcome measure for palliative care: The palliative care outcome scale. Palliative Care Core Audit Project Advisory Group. *BMJ Quality & Safety*, *8*(4), 219–227. https://doi.org/10.1136/qshc.8.4.219

Hoda, D., Jatoi, A., Burnes, J., Loprinzi, C., & Kelly, D. (2005). Should patients with advanced, incurable cancers ever be sent home with total parenteral nutrition? A single institution's 20-year experience. *Cancer*, *103*(4), 863–868. https://doi.org/10.1002/cncr.20824

Hoekstra, J., de Vos, R., van Duijn, N. P., Schadé, E., & Bindels, P. J. (2006). Using the symptom monitor in a randomized controlled trial: The effect on symptom prevalence and severity. *Journal of Pain and Symptom Management*, *31*(1), 22–30. https://doi.org/10.1016/j.jpainsymman.2005.06.014

Hutton, J. L., Martin, L., Field, C. J., Wismer, W. V., Bruera, E. D., Watanabe, S. M., & Baracos, V. E. (2006). Dietary patterns in patients with advanced cancer: Implications for anorexia-cachexia therapy. *American Journal of Clinical Nutrition*, *84*(5), 1163–1170. https://doi.org/10.1093/ajcn/84.5.1163

Lawlis, G. F., Cuencas, R., Selby, D., & McCoy, C. E. (1989). The development of Dallas pain questionnaire. *Spine*, *14*, 515–516.

Li, M., Kennedy, E. B., Byrne, N., Gérin-Lajoie, C., Katz, M. R., Keshavarz, H., Sellick, S., & Green, E. (2016). Management of depression in patients with cancer: A clinical practice guideline. *Journal of Oncology Practice*, *12*(8), 747–756. https://doi.org/10.1200/JOP.2016.011072

Mahler, D. A., Selecky, P. A., Harrod, C. G., Benditt, J. O., Carrieri-Kohlman, V., Curtis, J. R., Manning, H. L., Mularski, R. A., Varkey, B., Campbell, M., Carter, E. R., Chiong, J. R., Ely, E. W., Hansen-Flaschen, J., O'Donnell, D. E., & Waller, A. (2010). American College of Chest Physicians consensus statement on the management of dyspnea in patients with advanced lung or heart disease. *Chest*, *137*(3), 674–691. https://doi.org/10.1378/chest.09-1543

Melzack, R. (1975). The McGill Pain Questionnaire: Major properties and scoring methods. *Pain*, *1*(3), 277–299. https://doi.org/10.1016/0304-3959(75)90044-5

National Comprehensive Cancer Network. (2022). *Adult cancer pain*. Retrieved from https://www.nccn.org/login?ReturnURL=https://www.nccn.org/professionals/physician_gls/pdf/pain.pdf

Paice, J. A., Portenoy, R., Lacchetti, C., Campbell, T., Cheville, A., Citron, M., Constine, L. S., Cooper, A., Glare, P., Keefe, F., Koyyalagunta, L., Levy, M., Miaskowski, C., Otis-Green, S., Sloan, P., & Bruera, E. (2016). Management of chronic pain in survivors of adult cancers: American Society of Clinical Oncology clinical practice guideline. *Journal of Clinical Oncology*, *34*(27), 3325–3345. https://doi.org/10.1200/JCO.2016.68.5206

Portenoy, R. K. (2011). Treatment of cancer pain. *Lancet*, *377*(9784), 2236–2247. https://doi.org/10.1016/S0140-6736(11)60236-5

Price, D. D., McGrath, P. A., Rafii, A., & Buckingham, B. (1983). The validation of visual analogue scales as ratio scale measures for chronic and experimental pain. *Pain*, *17*(1), 45–56. https://doi.org/10.1016/0304-3959(83)90126-4

Pyszel, A., Malyszczak, K., Pyszel, K., Andrzejak, R., & Szuba, A. (2006). Disability, psychological distress, and quality of life in breast cancer survivors with arm lymphedema. *Lymphology*, *39*(4), 185–192.

Raja, S. N., Carr, D. B., Cohen, M., Finnerup, N. B., Flor, H., Gibson, S., Keefe, F. J., Mogil, J. S., Ringkamp, M., Sluka, K. A., Song, X. J., Stevens, B., Sullivan, M. D., Tutelman, P. R., Ushida, T., & Vader, K. (2020). The revised International Association for the Study of Pain definition of pain: Concepts, challenges, and compromises. *Pain*, *161*(9), 1976–1982. https://doi.org/10.1097/j.pain.0000000000001939

Richardson, C., & Kulkarni, J. (2017). A review of the management of phantom limb pain: Challenges and solutions. *Journal of Pain Research*, *10*, 1861–1870. https://doi.org/10.2147/JPR.S124664

Sweeney, M. P., & Bagg, J. (2000). The mouth and palliative care. *American Journal of Hospice and Palliative Care*, *17*(2), 118–124. https://doi.org/10.1177/104990910001700212

Tait, R. C., Chibnall, J. T., & Krause, S. (1990). The Pain Disability Index: Psychometric properties. *Pain*, *40*(2), 171–182. https://doi.org/10.1016/0304-3959(90)90068-O

Thekkumpurath, P., Walker, J., Butcher, I., Hodges, L., Kleiboer, A., O'Connor, M., Wall, L., Murray, G., Kroenke, K., & Sharpe, M. (2011). Screening for major depression in cancer outpatients. *Cancer*, *117*, 218–227. https://doi.org/10.1002/cncr.25514

Webb, J. A., & LeBlanc, T. W. (2018). Evidence-based management of cancer pain. *Seminars in Oncology Nursing*, *34*(3), 215–226. https://doi.org/10.1016/j.soncn.2018.06.003

11

A Novel Collaborative Care Model for People With Cancer and Serious Mental Illness

Amy Corveleyn, Vilmarie Rodriguez, and Kelly Irwin

Key Concepts

- Though not more likely to be diagnosed with cancer, people with serious mental illness (SMI) are more likely to die from cancer due to inequities in cancer care.
- Early mental health involvement may protect against disruptions in cancer care for people with SMI.
- A collaborative care model approach to treating people with SMI who have cancer is acceptable and feasible to patients, caregivers, and clinicians.
- Caregivers of patients with SMI may be spouses, siblings, or adult children; community mental health workers may also be caregivers.
- Individuals with SMI experience barriers to accessing palliative care and are more likely to die in skilled nursing facilities.

Keywords: collaborative care, health inequities, psycho-oncology, serious mental illness (SMI), social work, stigma

More than 14 million adults are affected by serious mental illness (SMI) in the United States. SMI can be defined as a mental health disorder that significantly affects functioning and commonly includes schizophrenia/schizoaffective disorder, bipolar disorder, and severe major depression (NIMH, 2008). Individuals with SMI experience premature mortality from medical illness (Olfson et al., 2015). Adults with SMI are significantly more likely to die from common cancers in part because of delays to cancer diagnosis and inequities in care across the cancer continuum. Approximately one in four

Amy Corveleyn, Vilmarie Rodriguez, and Kelly Irwin, *A Novel Collaborative Care Model for People With Cancer and Serious Mental Illness* In: *Oncology and Palliative Social Work*. Edited by: Susan Hedlund, Bryan Miller, Grace Christ, and Carolyn Messner, Oxford University Press. © Oxford University Press 2024. DOI: 10.1093/oso/9780197607299.003.0011 women with breast cancer have a preexisting mental health disorder (Haskins et al., 2018). More than 40% of clinical trials exclude people with SMI because of their mental illness (Humphreys et al., 2015). This may cause fewer people with SMI to be approached for clinical trials and limit their access to care.

Cancer caregivers often experience higher levels of distress than the patient (Applebaum & Breitbart, 2013). Caregivers of people with schizophrenia also experience increased depression and anxiety (Awad & Voruganti, 2008). Caregivers of people with SMI have unique needs and have reported that a lack of resources for caregivers is challenging (Murphy et al., 2022).

Early mental health involvement is associated with fewer disruptions in cancer care among adults with SMI, and team-based models demonstrate promise in this underserved population (Irwin et al., 2019). However, integrated psychosocial services for patients with cancer remain inadequate and fragmented from cancer care. Oncology social workers urgently need new care-delivery models to increase access to cancer care and decrease the suffering adults with SMI experience.

To address the disparity in cancer outcomes for people with SMI, this chapter discusses the key components of person-centered collaborative care across the cancer continuum. It highlights different team members (social work, psychiatry, navigator) and focuses on the social work role from cancer diagnosis through end of life. Finally, this chapter provides guidance on how to tailor the model to the needs of patients, caregivers, clinicians, and health care systems.

What We Have Learned So Far

Serious Mental Illness

Serious mental illness (SMI) commonly includes schizophrenia spectrum disorders, bipolar disorder, and severe major depressive disorder. People with SMI may be coping with untreated psychiatric symptoms, which can impact their understanding of a cancer diagnosis and treatment options. These symptoms can also make it difficult to build rapport and trust. Social workers are often the first line of treatment for people affected by SMI in the health care system. At the state and community agency level, social workers provide therapy, case management, and home-based services to people with SMI. They are also on the front lines in emergency departments and guide discharges from inpatient hospitalizations. The public mental health system is complex and underfunded, which leads to challenges accessing care and support.

Inequities in Cancer Care

People with SMI face inequities in the health care system that lead to poorer care and to patients being late to diagnosis, treatment, and palliative care. People with SMI have lower rates of cancer prevention, cancer screening, and receiving guideline-concordant cancer care. Untreated psychiatric symptoms (e.g., disorganization, paranoia, depression) and mental health stigma from the patient and the clinician are contributors to these low rates. Mental health care and cancer care are fragmented and delivered in separate health care systems with separate medical records, leading to challenges with clinician communication about patient care. Mental health treatment is difficult to access, and these barriers may be compounded by the limitations of public insurance, leading to long wait times to initiate care. Financial instability adds to the challenge of cancer care. Studies show that patients with SMI face challenges to retain gainful employment, housing, and insurance and meet basic living needs (Evans et al., 2016). Caregivers are tasked with taking care of the patient's financial needs, which adds a burden to both patient and caregiver.

Collaborative Care in Cancer Care

Current systems in cancer care are not especially helpful to people with both cancer and SMI, and new models need to be implemented. Collaborative care is a population-based model that employs an interdisciplinary team (e.g., a nurse or case manager embedded within the medical team) to identify patient goals, engage the patient and caregiver, and facilitate access to psychiatric expertise. The social worker on the team coordinates care, facilitates communication within the patient's team, and tracks patient outcomes with validated measures. Collaborative care models studied in cancer patients with depression have shown positive outcomes (Sharpe et al., 2014). Adults with SMI and cancer need rapid access to specialty care and a person-centered approach to decrease burden and build trust. Adapting the collaborative care model for the patient with SMI and cancer is the next step in cancer care for this population.

The Bridge Model: Adapting Collaborative Care for People With SMI and Cancer

Informed by qualitative interviews and retrospective research, we adapted the collaborative care model for people with SMI and cancer (Irwin et al.,

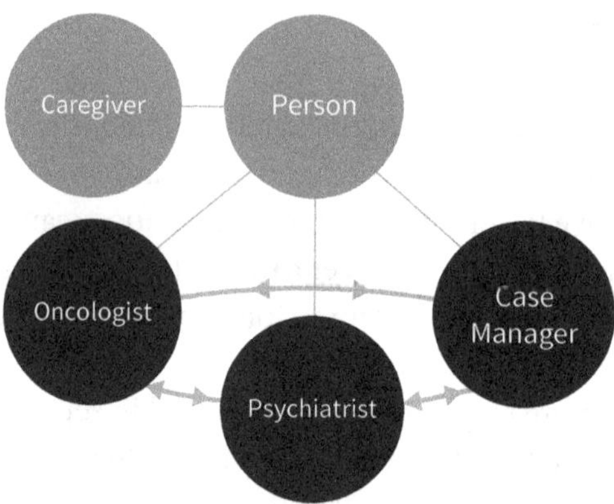

Figure 11.1 Bridge: Person-centered collaborative care for serious mental illness and cancer.

2019). The Bridge model ensures that patients with SMI and cancer have access to a social worker, psychiatrist, and community health navigator as part of their cancer care team (Figure 11.1). Based on a standardized assessment at the time of cancer diagnosis and collaboration with the oncology team, the team develops a plan for the patient's mental health and cancer treatment. Patient-reported outcomes and progress in cancer care are then reviewed in a team clinical meeting weekly led by the social worker. The clinical meeting includes care coordination, identification of barriers to care, and treatment planning.

A single-arm pilot trial demonstrated that the Bridge model was feasible and acceptable to patients, caregivers, and clinicians and showed promise for increasing access to cancer care for people with SMI (Irwin et al., 2019). Currently, a randomized trial is investigating the Bridge model (Harvard Risk Management Foundation & National Cancer Institute NCT03360695). Caregivers are enrolled to the same arm as the patient, which allows for study of this underresearched caregiver population as well.

Importance of Building a Team

Patients with SMI need a tailored approach to cancer care with a team that collaborates directly with the patient, their caregiver, and the cancer care and mental health teams. This approach offers diverse perspectives, combines expertise, and reduces burnout within the team. Key staff within the team are the social worker, psychiatrist, and community health navigator.

Social Worker

The social worker is a fundamental part of the collaborative care team and engagement of the patient in care. The social worker engages the patient, caregiver, and community supports, works to build trust/rapport, conducts a clinical assessment, refers to resources and evidence-based therapies, and bridges the oncology and mental health teams. The role is flexible, based on patient and caregiver needs and strengths, as well as the urgency and severity of both the patient's cancer and their mental illness. To decrease burden and build trust within this complex medical and mental health context, the social worker can connect with patients and their caregivers in a variety of settings, including inpatient and outpatient facilities, patients' homes, skilled nursing facilities, shelters, group homes, or mental health clinics. Additionally, social workers must adapt use of technology flexibly to promote engagement in care while maintaining safety.

Social Worker's Roles

- Build alliances with patient and caregivers and cultivate trust with ongoing check-ins and outreach.
- Increase illness understanding through joint visits with the patient's team (oncology or psychiatry) and individual meetings with patient and caregivers.
- Bridge communication between the oncology, psychiatry, and outpatient teams through e-mail, phone, text, or in-person visits.
- Address barriers to cancer care (e.g., access to transportation) with a thorough assessment of the patient and their caregiver.
- Incorporate brief, evidence-based treatments and referrals with the patient or their caregiver. such as motivational interviewing, problem-solving therapy, mindfulness, and cognitive behavioral strategies (e.g., diaphragmatic breathing to decrease anxiety prior to start of radiation).
- Support the patient's and caregiver's self-management and engagement in oncology care.

Psychiatrist

The psychiatrist (who has expertise in psycho-oncology and serious mental illness) assesses the patient's psychiatric history and current symptoms and collaborates with the oncology and mental health teams to develop a plan for cancer and mental health treatment. Common issues include assessing a patient's capacity to consent to treatment or clinical trials, considering medication interactions, and creating guidelines to prevent worsening of mental health symptoms. The collaborative care psychiatrist collaborates with the outpatient mental health team (particularly the psychiatrist or psychiatric nurse practitioner when present), oncology team, or primary care team to offer psychiatric care and consultation throughout treatment planning. When feasible, it is important to have proactive consultation or case review by the psychiatrist at the time of cancer diagnosis. Given limited access to psychiatry, a psychiatric consultation can be initiated at other phases in cancer care. The psychiatrist is available for consultation across care settings (inpatient, outpatient, group living environments, skilled nursing) to promote continuity.

When to Consult a Psychiatrist?

- Patient has no psychiatrist in the community and is having symptoms that are a barrier to treatment.
- Oncology team has concerns about the patient's cancer treatment interfering with their psychiatric medications.
- Oncology team shares worries that the patient does not understand the risks and benefits of cancer treatment or has declined treatment without clear understanding.

What If a Psychiatrist Is Not Accessible?

- Social worker could add the primary care physician or nurse practitioner as a team member during cancer care to advise on psychiatric medications.
- Team could explore community mental health options and availability given the patient's urgent needs due to new cancer diagnosis.
- Social worker can collaborate with the caregiver and team to ensure that a shared decision is obtained and a plan is agreed upon to make the patient feel more in control and open to seeking services.

What If the Patient Does Not Want to Meet With a Psychiatrist?

- Oncology team members can talk to the patient about their fears and concerns with involving a psychiatrist in the team.

- Normalize the presence of psychiatry on the oncology team by letting the patient know that the team will also be reaching out to different specialties like cardiology or orthopedics to give them comprehensive care (i.e., to reassure them that bringing in specialists to the team is not entirely due to their SMI).
- Ask the oncologist to meet with both patient and psychiatrist to introduce the patient to the importance of the role of psychiatry in their cancer care.
- Psychiatrist can provide guidance for the oncology team, which can choose to prescribe psychiatric medications with ongoing access to consultation.

Community Health Navigator

The community health navigator strengthens the team's capacity to deliver person-centered care. The navigator can meet the patient where they are—whether at home or in a hospital, cancer center, or skilled nursing facility. The navigator arranges for resources crucial to the patient's treatment plan, which may include anything from transportation, medication delivery, pet care, or accompaniment to appointments. Having expertise in community mental health facilities fosters strong collaboration with frontline community mental health staff. Navigators with a common background or sense of shared community with the patient may also be able to address language barriers or explain processes in a way that increases the patient's trust in the health care system.

Community Health Navigator's Role

- Track patients to assess whether they are facing urgent issues, have been hospitalized, or have missed appointments or treatments.
- Schedule appointments and follow up with patients to assess whether they have questions about premedication or appointment timing or are facing barriers to the cancer care.
- Accompany patients to and facilitate dialogue during visits.

Caregivers for People With SMI and Cancer

Caregivers for people with SMI and cancer can include spouses, siblings, adult children, and community-based caregivers (Irwin et al., 2019). It is important for social workers to identify caregivers early in treatment planning. This allows not only for the caregiver to be a part of the process but also for the social worker to assess the caregiver's needs. Including the caregiver will hopefully lead to better cancer care outcomes for the patient and less burden on the caregiver. When working with caregivers, it is important to seek collateral information from the caregiver to fill in questions, such as Who will manage the patient's medication? What services already exist in the home? Is there a guardian? If so, what is their relationship to the patient?

Assessing the Patient With SMI and Cancer: Values, Needs, and Strengths

A key component to assessing a patient with SMI and cancer is building trust. Patients with SMI have experienced stigma and discrimination throughout their experience in the health care system. Providers make assumptions when they open a patient's chart and see diagnoses of schizophrenia or bipolar disorder. Trust is crucial with patients who have had medical trauma and are accustomed to being invalidated or mistreated in the health care system. To build trust, a social worker can:

- Meet the patient where they are in terms of location, cognition, and emotion.
- Avoid arguing with the patient about beliefs regarding cancer or mental illness.
- Help the patient find an ally. Ask, Who is important to this person? Who do they call if they need help?
- Communicate with the oncology team and the community mental health team to show the patient that everyone is working together.
- Remember and honor the patient's autonomy.

Approach patients with SMI and their caregivers with curiosity and openness. You may need to tailor the language you use or questions you ask based on how the patient is feeling that day or what kind of information they are processing about their cancer care. Helpful questions to ask are:

- What are your goals? What matters most to you?
- What do you know about your cancer currently?
- Who are your current providers?
- What are the barriers you face to treatment?

- What are the best ways to reach you? E-mail? Text? Phone?
- How can our team be helpful to you?
- What/Who means the most to you? (Who are you closest to?)
- What are your strengths?
- What brings you joy/keeps you going each day?
- What questions do you have for the team?

Jane is a 74-year-old woman with a new lung cancer and a diagnosis of schizophrenia. Her treatment plan is daily radiation, and she has a good prognosis with curative intent. When you meet with Jane, you learn that she lives alone with her cat. Her family is supportive, but she often feels that they do not understand her mental illness. Her sister, Lynn, helps with appointments and overall management of Jane's medical needs.

During this first assessment, you learn that Jane mistrusts the health care system. She spent many years in a state hospital, where she saw fellow patients being abused and was mistreated herself. She tells you that she is extremely proud of being able to leave the hospital and work as a peer specialist to help guide other people with mental illness through the process.

Jane struggles to answer direct questions, and your time with her is best spent validating her worries and listening to her story. Active listening leads her to trust you and your team. The psychiatrist on the team builds trust with Jane by being in contact with her primary care physician and collaborating with Jane about medication changes. She meets with Jane in person, which helps reduce her paranoia. The social worker and community health navigator meet with Jane; they listen to and validate her personal experience of having a mental illness.

After Jane receives her cancer treatment, her scans are initially clear. However, her disease returns, and during her second round of treatment, she begins to struggle more with her memory and self-care. Her sister Lynn communicates to the team her concern that Jane is feeling worse and having more symptoms. Jane has been falling at home, and it becomes clear that she cannot live alone anymore. Palliative care becomes more involved in the management of both pain and overall symptoms. The psychiatrist simplifies her medications and provides guidance to prevent delirium. Lynn offers for Jane to live with her, and hospice joins the care team.

You speak with Lynn often, and she lets you know that Jane is sleeping more and reaching the end of her life. She is not in pain, and family have come from all over the state and country to stay with her. Jane can die a death with dignity and without pain surrounded by loved ones. The collaborative care approach helped make it possible for Jane to receive treatment, build trust in her oncology team, and have end-of-life care that honored her wishes.

Palliative Care for Patients With SMI and Cancer

Early, integrated palliative care improves quality of life and is recognized by oncologists as a standard of cancer care for all patients. However, not all patients have the same access to palliative care, particularly outside the hospital setting. Research on patients with SMI and their end-of-life care needs is scant. But what is known is that people with schizophrenia are less likely to receive palliative care consultation at the end of life and more likely to die in a nursing home (Chochinov et al., 2012). Patients with SMI may have less access to pain management and may not be receiving appropriate care as they reach the end of life (Martens et al., 2013). Social workers must consider where patients with SMI and cancer can live as they approach the end of life, as it may not be possible for them to live independently. Many group living environments are not designed to care for residents with advanced cancer. This can lead patients to be transferred to skilled nursing facilities, where they can become cut off from their psychiatric care and social supports. During the COVID-19 pandemic, social supports were further limited with facilities closed to outside visitors. We need new models with embedded services, such as integrated training for oncology, mental health, and palliative care clinicians and community supports, to help patients stay where they are for as long as possible. This training should include how to transition patients to hospice care so their goals of care can be fully realized while also maintaining autonomy and dignity as priorities.

People with SMI already face inequities in both mental health services and general health care that can lead to mistrust and make it harder to initiate or complete cancer care. Maximizing these patients' chances for receiving quality cancer care requires a tailored, person-centered approach to treatment (Irwin & Loscalzo, 2020). A collaborative care model like the Bridge has been shown to be feasible and acceptable to patients, caregivers, and clinicians (Irwin et al., 2019). This model allows for a social worker, psychiatrist, and community health navigator to provide clinical and community-based care that treats the patient, caregiver, and clinical team. Palliative care research in this population shows that people with SMI are less likely to receive palliative care and more likely to transition to nursing homes (Shalev et al., 2020). Members of the team must acknowledge the discrimination that patients with SMI have experienced and work to create a collaborative care experience that prioritizes the patient's autonomy and dignity. Social workers are often the first provider that patients meet, and adjusting the assessment process can support a higher quality of overall cancer care. In addressing this equity gap faced by patients with cancer and SMI, it is important to acknowledge the role of cultural humility in building trust and improving care outcomes. As such, working on cultural humility can help expand the collaborative care model and ensure that this approach also works for those intersectional identities that have been overlooked in the health care system.

Guiding Best Practices for the Future

To decrease the inequities people with SMI face in cancer care, we need to meet people where they are. This means meeting people physically and cognitively where they are in their cancer care experience, including talking to people about the goals they have for care, being inclusive of people with SMI in cancer research, and being aware of the bias that may exist among clinicians about this population. Early research on the collaborative care model is promising, but more studies are needed, especially regarding how best to tailor care for patients with metastatic disease and how to help patients in group-home living environments transition to end-of-life care. Social workers will continue to be at the forefront of the clinical care needed to improve cancer care and mental health outcomes and decrease suffering for patients with SMI.

Pearls

- A tailored, collaborative approach to cancer care for patients with SMI can benefit the patient, caregiver, and cancer care team.
- Early psychiatry involvement with patients who are diagnosed with cancer can include collaborating with oncology to inform treatment planning, establishing communication with the outpatient mental health team, and assessing the need to adjust psychiatric medications.
- The social worker builds trust, provides supportive, evidence-based therapies to patients and their caregivers, bridges communication between cancer care and psychiatry, and addresses barriers to care that may impact cancer treatment.
- Talk to the patient and their caregiver: find out what brings them to treatment, their goals for treatment, and what their questions are regarding care and treatment.
- When we consider a person's strengths, we can think creatively (Irwin & Loscalzo, 2020).
- Use person-centered language when talking to patients (i.e., *a person with schizophrenia* not *a schizophrenic*).

Pitfalls

- The team does not ask about the patient's mental health team and does not connect with them to establish communication.
- Lack of collaboration with the caregiver (whether that person is family or a community member) can cause the caregiver to feel alienated from the team and confused about who to call for help.
- The team fails to consult psychiatry and social work from the time of diagnosis.
- The team assumes that the patient is not interested in research or able to consent without a full assessment.

Additional Resources

The Engage Initiative (Cancer and Mental Health Collaborative): www.engageinitiative.org.

A coalition that seeks to make sure that mental illness is never a barrier to cancer care. This stakeholder-led collaborative hosts virtual events that focus on cancer care for individuals with serious mental illness and their caregivers. The website also contains links to research, resources for advocacy, and a tool kit that highlights how to design research studies for patients with SMI. Clinicians, patients, caregivers, researchers, and advocates are welcome to join.

SAMHSA's National Helpline: https://www.samhsa.gov/find-help/national-helpline

SAMHSA's National Helpline, 1-800-662-HELP (4357), (also known as the treatment referral routing service) or TTY 1-800-487-4889 is a confidential, free, 24-hour-a-day, 365-day-a-year, information service provided in English and Spanish for individuals and family members facing mental health and/or substance use disorders. This service provides referrals to local treatment facilities, support groups, and community-based organizations. Callers can also order free publications and other information.

NAMI—National Alliance on Mental Illness: https://www.nami.org/Home

NAMI is a nonprofit, grassroots, support and advocacy organization of individuals with mental disorders and their families. The website provides numerous resources, including support groups, education, and training.

References

Applebaum, A. J., & Breitbart, W. (2013). Care for the cancer caregiver: A systematic review. *Palliative & Supportive Care*, *11*(3), 231–252. https://doi.org/10.1017/S1478951512000594

Awad, A. G., & Voruganti, L. N. (2008). The burden of schizophrenia on caregivers: A review. *PharmacoEconomics*, *26*(2), 149–162. https://doi.org/10.2165/00019053-200826020-00005

Chochinov, H. M., Martens, P. J., Prior, H. J., & Kredentser, M. S. (2012). Comparative health care use patterns of people with schizophrenia near the end of life: A population-based study in Manitoba, Canada. *Schizophrenia Research*, *141*(2–3), 241–246. https://doi.org/10.1016/j.schres.2012.07.028

Evans, T. S., Berkman, N., Brown, C., Gaynes, B., & Weber, R. P. (2016). *Disparities within serious mental illness*. U.S. Agency for Healthcare Research and Quality.

Harvard Risk Management Foundation and National Cancer Institute. (2017, December 11–). Bridge: Proactive psychiatry consultation and case management for patients with cancer. Identifier NCT03360695. https://clinicaltrials.gov/study/NCT03360695?a=4

Haskins, C. B., McDowell, B. D., Carnahan, R. M., Fiedorowicz, J. G., Wallace, R. B., Smith, B. J., & Chrischilles, E. A. (2018) Prevalence of preexisting mental illness in SEER–Medicare breast cancer patients. *Journal of Clinical Oncology*, *36*(15, suppl.), e13564–e13564.

Humphreys, K., Blodgett, J. C., & Roberts, L. W. (2015). The exclusion of people with psychiatric disorders from medical research. *Journal of Psychiatric Research*, *70*, 28–32. https://doi.org/10.1016/j.jpsychires.2015.08.005

Irwin, K. E., & Loscalzo, M. L. (2020). Witnessing unnecessary suffering: A call for action and policy change to increase access to psycho-oncology care. *Psycho-Oncology*, *29*(12), 1977–1981. https://doi.org/10.1002/pon.5599

Irwin, K. E., Park, E. R., Fields, L. E., Corveleyn, A. E., Greer, J. A., Perez, G. K., Callaway, C. A., Jacobs, J. M., Nierenberg, A. A., Temel, J. S., Ryan, D. P., & Pirl, W. F. (2019). Bridge: Person-centered collaborative care for patients with serious mental illness and cancer. *Oncologist*, *24*(7), 901–910. https://doi.org/10.1634/theoncologist.2018-0488

Martens, P. J., Chochinov, H. M., & Prior, H. J. (2013). Where and how people with schizophrenia die: A population-based, matched cohort study in Manitoba, Canada. *Journal of Clinical Psychiatry*, *74*(6), e551–e557. https://doi.org/10.4088/JCP.12m08234

Murphy, K., Corveleyn, A., Park, E., & Irwin, K. E. (2022, March 9–11). *Rewards, challenges, and lessons learned from familial and community caregivers of individuals with serious mental illness and cancer* [Conference presentation]. American Psychosocial Oncology Society 2022 Convention, Portland, OR, United States.

Olfson, M., Gerhard, T., Huang, C., Crystal, S., & Stroup, T. S. (2015). Premature mortality among adults with schizophrenia in the United States. *JAMA Psychiatry*, *72*(12), 1172–1181. https://doi.org/10.1001/jamapsychiatry.2015.1737

Shalev, D., Fields, L., & Shapiro, P. A. (2020). End-of-life care in individuals with serious mental illness. *Psychosomatics*, *61*(5), 428–435. https://doi.org/10.1016/j.psym.2020.06.003

Sharpe, M., Walker, J., Holm Hansen, C., Martin, P., Symeonides, S., Gourley, C., Wall, L., Weller, D., Murray, G., & SMaRT (Symptom Management Research Trials) Oncology-2 Team. (2014). Integrated collaborative care for comorbid major depression in patients with cancer (SMaRT Oncology-2): A multicentre randomised controlled effectiveness trial. *Lancet*, *384*(9948), 1099–1108. https://doi.org/10.1016/S0140-6736(14)61231-9

12
Interprofessional Spiritual Care Along the Cancer Care Trajectory

Debra Mattison, Sandra Blackburn, and Christopher Brady

Key Concepts

- Biopsychosocial-spiritual assessment is a foundational component of oncology and palliative care social work practice, yet social workers often neglect spirituality in this assessment process.
- Religion and spirituality may be sources of strength-based coping and emotional comfort and hope for some; for others, they may cause hurt, confusion, and conflict. Thus, the subject is critical for oncology social workers to explore.
- Social workers have an ethical and professional responsibility to explore their own religious and spiritual values, beliefs, and experiences to effectively engage and serve clients.

Keywords: biopsychosocial-spiritual assessment, religion, social work, spirituality, spiritual assessment

> We also know that many of the people we serve draw upon spirituality, by whatever names they call it, to help them thrive, to succeed at challenges and to infuse the resources and relationships we assist them with to have meaning beyond mere survival value.
>
> **(Canda & Furman, 2010, p. 3.)**

A cancer diagnosis is often a stunning, life-changing event that affects the wholeness of one's being. Despite many advances in cancer care and symptom management from diagnosis to the end of life, cancer remains a chronic illness that by nature can be prolonged and challenging emotionally, physically, and spiritually.

Social workers must develop a clinical skill set to provide competent biopsychosocial-spiritual care as collaborators with interprofessional teams

Debra Mattison, Sandra Blackburn, and Christopher Brady, *Interprofessional Spiritual Care Along the Cancer Care Trajectory*
In: *Oncology and Palliative Social Work*. Edited by: Susan Hedlund, Bryan Miller, Grace Christ, and Carolyn Messner,
Oxford University Press. © Oxford University Press 2024. DOI: 10.1093/oso/9780197607299.003.0012

addressing spiritual distress in oncology and palliative care. This holistic approach to care supports patients as they seek to maintain a sense of self, even in the face of the ever-present demands of their cancer experience. Social workers must also be aware of their own religious and spiritual beliefs and how they might impact their social work practice and patients.

This chapter provides a contextual review of literature related to religion and spirituality in social work practice; addresses foundational concepts and tools for spiritual assessments with consideration of diverse spiritual identities, beliefs, and expression; identifies general intervention approaches; and encourages social workers to explore their own spiritual beliefs as clinicians who companion and respond to human suffering with both skills and limitations.

Defining Religion and Spirituality

Definitions of religion and spirituality are complex and individualistic with diverse terminology used to refer to, understand, and express individual experiences of drawing on them in one's life. Spirituality encompasses a vast domain, and hundreds of definitions attempt to capture its meaning. While the words *religion* and *spirituality* are often used interchangeably, failure to consistently differentiate between them has led to lack of clarity in research, as well as disputes and hesitancy about inclusion of religion and/or spirituality in social work practice.

Both religion and spirituality affect how humans think, feel, and behave and have overlapping as well as distinctive qualities. Religion often involves organized and institutionalized sets of beliefs, creeds, and moral codes of conduct; potential affiliation with an organized community; and belief in a superhuman power. Spirituality is a concept often described as being related to meaning, purpose, connectedness, and transcendence beyond mind and body. Furthermore, spirituality is often differentiated in the literature as personal, inner, and individually defined, while religion often focuses on outward expression and observable actions through gatherings, rituals, and actions of worship. Spirituality can be viewed as an overarching concept of which religion is a subset; religion is one of many ways an individual may express their spirituality. There is no single, quantifiable definition of spirituality that can encompass the vastness of individual experience of the part of humanness that is not body and mind but spirit. Crisp (2010) provides a summarizing perspective, stating, "at the bottom line, spirituality is concerned with the things that matter to people, which may or may not include religion" (p. 28).

Spirituality in Social Work Practice

Relevance of Spirituality to Oncology and Palliative Care Social Work Practice

A growing body of evidence-informed literature attests to the value of spirituality in positively contributing to a range of health and mental health outcomes (Oxhandler & Pargament, 2014). Koenig (2012) notes that many patients have spiritual needs that intersect with health needs, and that religion and/or spirituality can influence health care decisions, affect a providers' interventions, and help patients cope.

Spirituality can play an even more prominent role in people's lives when they are facing hospice care and death and dying (Crisp, 2010). At the end of life, patients naturally ponder questions regarding the meaning of life, nature of suffering, and uncertainty of the future, all of which involve a spiritual component. Existential questions and concerns may result both in the challenging of long-held worldviews and a need to find sources of hope and comfort. While there is no quick "fix" for these concerns, social workers can provide a safe space and empathetic presence that welcomes patients to share both spiritual struggles and spiritual strengths and can facilitate comfort, peace, and hope, even as one faces the unknown and death.

Ethical Social Work Practice: Acknowledging and Addressing Spirituality

Social work is a value-based profession guided by a code of ethics that embraces a person-in-environment approach and considers the holistic domains of mind, body, and spirit. Spirituality is an essential element of a biopsychosocial-spiritual assessment of the wholeness of each unique person. Multiple professional guidelines attest to spirituality as key to diverse, inclusive, and culturally sensitive social work practice (e.g., NASW, 2021, 2015). Addressing spirituality is also congruent with valuing diversity and advocating against discrimination and bias based on any aspect of human diversity.

Clients' Desires and Experiences About Integration of Spirituality in Care

While there is a wide range among clients regarding whether or how they want their spiritual and religious needs to be addressed, many clients express both a need and a desire for discussions about these topics with their health care providers (Darrel & Rich, 2017). Despite clients' interest in spirituality, some social workers are reluctant to raise the subject. One in five social workers report waiting for the client to mention spirituality despite clients often stating a preference that clinicians initiate these discussions (Oxhandler & Giardina, 2017). Patients can perceive a social worker's lack of communication about spirituality as a barrier they must break through to have spirituality addressed in their care.

A discrepancy also exists between social workers' attitudes about and practices around spirituality. Oxhandler et al. (2015) notes that while many social workers express positive attitudes regarding the integration of spirituality into their practices, far fewer actually do so. Identified barriers to integration cluster more frequently around practitioner-related barriers (e.g., lack of training or provider discomfort and perception that spirituality is not relevant) than client- or agency-related barriers (Oxhandler & Giardina, 2017). This fact raises concerns about social workers' commitment to patient-centered care.

While a guiding principle of therapeutic relationships is to provide a nonjudgmental, accepting space, some clients perceive counselors as being likely to ignore, minimize, or pathologize their spiritual beliefs (Harris et al., 2016). Gotterer (2001) found it was common for clients to perceive their mental health providers as uncomfortable discussing spirituality, noting that the topic felt "taboo" in a counseling setting. Thus, social workers' lack of skills, as well as any discomfort they might have with discussing spirituality, may intensify clients' own fear and uncertainty about these topics as important and safe to discuss with the social worker (Oxhandler & Giardina, 2017).

Oncology and palliative care social workers need to be aware of the risks and impact of avoiding, distancing, and unintentionally invalidating a client's spirituality. Behavior that conveys a lack of interest or attention to spirituality can potentially harm clients by leading not only to incomplete assessments but also possibly negative or even harmful experiences and unmet spiritual needs (Oxhandler et al., 2015, 2017).

Spiritual Assessment

Assessment is a critical clinical skill in social work practice designed to gather and synthesize information to inform effective client-centered interventions. As research regarding the relationship between spirituality and health has grown over the last 20 years, so has the development of available spiritual assessment tools. A systematic literature review conducted by Monod et al.

(2011) identified over 60 spiritual assessment instruments used in clinical research. Blaber et al. (2015) reviewed four of the most widely used history-taking tools (FICA, FAITH, SPIRITual, and HOPE) and noted that spiritual history-taking tools have an important role in identifying spiritual needs of health care patients, particularly those at end of life.

Social workers can also draw on spiritually focused assessment questions (Box 12.1), which use broad conceptual and inclusive terminology, to provide open invitations that clearly signal to the patient that the clinician is interested in and able to hear their spiritual beliefs and experiences. Asking these questions as part of a narrative framework with a genuinely conveyed "tell me more" attitude allows patients to use whatever diverse terms they choose to tell their stories and enhances mutual understanding of the patient's worldview.

Box 12.1 Selected Spirituality Focused Assessment Questions

- *Do you have any spiritual, religious, or philosophical beliefs that are important to you?*
- *Who or what comforts, encourages, or helps you have hope?*
- *What helps you when you are afraid or in pain?*
- *What are you still hoping to experience or get out of life?*
- *What do your beliefs say about trials, suffering, sickness, and hope?*
- *Tell me about any practices or rituals you do that are helpful right now.*

Stewart (2014) encourages oncology social workers to pay attention to spiritual language that indicates patients may be "standing on a threshold of a spiritual dialogue" (p. 68). Patients may not always use the word *spiritual* in expressing their thoughts, feelings, or needs, and yet spirituality is often embedded in statements that await the clinician's attention and invitation for exploratory dialogue, such as:

Patient: "I guess I deserve this."
Clinician: "Can you tell me more about your thoughts on what you think you deserve?"
Patient: "I don't know what to believe about life anymore."
Clinician: "It sounds like some of the beliefs you once held aren't so clear now. I'm interested in hearing more about this."

Box 12.2

A palliative care social worker conducts a biopsychosocial-spiritual assessment, indicating spiritual distress, at her initial meeting with a 63-year-old female with progressive, stage IV breast cancer. The patient shares that she and her son are both faithful members of a conservative religious denomination and recently argued about her decision to discontinue cancer-targeted treatment. Her son accused her of embracing euthanasia, which he states is expressly forbidden in their faith and would result in eternal separation from God. The patient is at peace with her decision.

After the session, the social worker recognizes her feelings of frustration and anger that the patient's son has introduced guilt into his mother's right to make her treatment decisions. She reflects on her attitude toward "conservative" religion and her strong feeling that the patient's son is just plain "wrong" in this situation. She discusses this encounter with her chaplain colleague, and they propose a care conference to the patient, which would include her son and others they trust—their pastor and her physician and nurse practitioner.

At the care conference, they could address what palliative care means in the context of both the family's deep and meaningful religious beliefs and center on mutual goals of honoring the patient's treatment decisions, while making space for her son's fears to be included and addressed. The social worker plans to continue to meet with this patient to provide end-of-life spiritual support and to explore her legacy and hopes and fears at the end of life.

Clinical Interventions

Spiritual interventions with patients across the cancer care continuum may focus on broad themes such as questioning fulfillment of one's purpose, existential contemplation of death, guilt and regret over things done (or not done), the need to forgive others or be forgiven, and end-of-life planning. Conversations using a strengths-based model and compassionate presence invite and make space for patients, families, and team members to share their strengths, hopes, and fears, and can be organic, naturally occurring interventions. Puchalski et al. (2019) offers a centering framework for spiritual interventions, noting that their purpose is to create "a connection with the patient that enables them to express their deepest concerns" while the clinician's ability to offer a "deep non-judgmental listening helps the patient give voice to their suffering" (p. 9) (Boxes 12.2 & 12.3).

Some interventions may be more structured, such as spiritually modified cognitive behavioral therapy (CBT), which has been found effective in targeting depression (Rosmarin, 2018), or manualized, structured therapy approaches, such as meaning-centered psychotherapy (MCP), which has demonstrated therapeutic outcomes related to anxiety, spiritual well-being, and sense of meaning (Breitbart et al., 2018).

When considering spiritual interventions, key recommendations emerge in the literature centering on using interventions that respect and are congruent with patients' values and cultural beliefs, assessing patient interest and readiness for such interventions, and ensuring that practitioners have adequate training and expertise regarding specific intervention techniques (Francoeur et al., 2016; Hodge, 2011).

Box 12.3

A hospice patient was expressing existential distress, wondering if his life has mattered, and if there is anything beyond. He was concerned that his life has passed so quickly and has been perhaps wasted, stating, "All I ever did was focus on my career." Over several interactions, his social worker explored his beliefs about life, death, and afterlife, and what he hoped for as he sat with the "not knowing."

The social worker, trained in MCP, engaged in life review, focusing on the patient's strengths, listening to his "mountain-top experiences," and allowing space for regret and loss for the things he wished he had done. The social worker explored the patient's legacy and was able to help him claim the value and impact of his mentorship of younger colleagues and importance of his love of animals and volunteer work at an animal rescue agency.

The social worker's ability to identify spiritual concerns, be present, make space for spirituality to be discussed, and use of specific spiritually focused interventions resulted in mitigation of the patient's distress and supported a sense of meaning and purpose as he explored his self-identified hopes at the end of life.

Clinician Self-Exploration of One's Own Spirituality

The revised National Association of Social Workers *Code of Ethics* (2021) reaffirmed that critical self-reflection and cultural humility are cornerstones of social work practice. Introspection about one's own religious and spiritual beliefs, biases, stereotypes, prejudices, attitudes, and experiences is essential to ethical, competent practice and how one sees, understands, interacts with, and responds to clients while attending to their spiritual needs (Canda & Furman, 2010).

Significant differences have been noted between licensed social workers and the general population regarding beliefs, practices, and the perceived degree of importance of religion and spirituality in one's life (Oxhandler et al., 2018). Social workers commonly find themselves working with clients whose beliefs are different from their own. Discussions of religion and spirituality may evoke powerful personal, social, emotional, and political reactions.

Clinicians need to be alert to implicit bias, countertransference, and microaggressions, such as pathologizing or exoticizing spirituality, that could impede effective relationships with patients of diverse religious backgrounds or spiritual perspectives (Hodge, 2020). Appropriately and openly acknowledging a fear of imposing one's beliefs on clients and possible resulting harm is simply good practice. However, avoiding, neglecting, or discounting religion and spirituality have less often been acknowledged as potentially "imposing" one's values. Both addressing and failing to address spiritual needs have potentially significant consequences for patients.

Interprofessional Practice

Some social workers may view spirituality as outside the scope of social work practice and an area that only clergy, chaplains, or other spiritual advisors should address. Relegating the responsibility for assessing and addressing spirituality to individual disciplines or health care provider roles is incongruent with the more holistic, interprofessional approach used in addressing other core issues such pain, symptom management, or depression in which multiple members of the interprofessional team may effectively work to meet a client's needs.

In the last decade, interprofessional practice (IPP) has become a standard in health care. IPP focuses on the goal of interprofessional health care team members collaborating across the care-delivery spectrum (Morgan et al., 2015; Schot et al., 2020). This collaboration is ideally patient-family centered and team based with shared goals, decision-making, and responsibility for outcomes. IPP demonstrates understanding, valuing, and using the roles of other disciplines in optimal service to the patient.

In IPP, every interprofessional team member plays a valuable role in addressing spirituality. It is common in collaborative environments for multiple team members to interdependently address a specific patient need based on their discipline-specific training and skill competencies (Francoeur et al., 2016). Various team members can facilitate integration of spirituality into holistic patient care whether it be recognizing and validating a patient's spirituality as a coping strength or concern; referring patients to other team members for further assessment; or providing clinical assessment and interventions regarding spiritual concerns ranging from a need for prayer or ritual to counseling regarding long-held resentments and anger. Effective IPP involves much more than a series of individual contacts with the patient by a team of experts. Rather, it demands an expert team regularly communicating and consulting with each other to effectively marshal their individual and collective expertise in providing holistic care.

Collaborative teamwork is also mutually beneficial to IPP team members themselves. Professionals who are a part of interprofessional teams more often report a sense of work-related empowerment to conduct their roles and that their work is meaningful compared to those who work outside of teams (Siekkinen et al., 2021).

Social workers are critical members of the overall oncology team when it comes to helping patients navigate the multidimensional challenges a cancer diagnosis presents. Social workers who embody openness in seeking to understand a patient's diverse spiritual worldview, as well as their own, bring valuable information regarding coping strengths and spiritual distress to the team's holistic understanding of the patients we collectively serve. We must be prepared to initiate, engage, and respond to spirituality as an essential component of daily practice in holistic patient care skillfully and actively. This requires us to actively engage in ensuring proper training in this area to intentionally address discomfort, passivity, or worse, neglect in exploring patients' spirituality.

Spirituality is a coping mechanism for many experiencing the frailty of life, as well as adapting to the new and ongoing pandemic-related challenges that have resulted in additional layers of loss, isolation, and complexity to their cancer experience. When social workers walk alongside patients and honor their spiritual worldviews, our capacity to truly see, hear, engage, and empathetically practice expands. In this space, the trust needed to serve and companion our clients as they face the challenges of cancer is strengthened.

Guiding Best Practices for the Future

Every patient embodies unique intersections of identity, values, beliefs, and personal histories of "-ism" discrimination, oppression, and/or privilege that social workers must acknowledge as having an influence on an individual's experience of their cancer care trajectory. Religious affiliations and spirituality may be a source of comfort and strength for some patients. Conversely, for others, they may be a source of harm and oppression that also warrants clinician assessment. Religious practices and spiritual beliefs are not static, and a patient's practices or beliefs may currently be different from those of one's family of origin, which may cause discomfort or ambiguity; some experience having different practices or beliefs as a loss and alienation. Because practices and beliefs are often evolving during one's cancer experience, they require ongoing attention and assessment.

While religion and spirituality are often associated with specific beliefs, systems, and practices, social workers must be cautious to neither universalize nor assume homogeneity in their understandings of these systems but rather recognize the vast spectrum of diversity that exists both within and among various groups (Canda & Furman, 2010). For example, an atheist may have a belief system that is not defined by a relationship to a deity while still self-identifying as a highly spiritual person who regularly draws on spiritual meaning-making practices. Practicing from a posture of cultural awareness and humility, which focuses on the client as an "expert" in their own experience, fosters a sense of welcoming, engagement, and affirmation of diverse worldviews (Pandya, 2016) (Box 12.4).

Box 12.4

"The potential of spirituality for both clients and social workers is great. Rather than trying to squeeze the non-quantifiable qualities of human nature into scientific parameters, it is better that social workers not forget the humane art of listening, hearing the mysteries it may reveal and the troubles it may resolve" (Gotterer, 2001, p. 192).

Pearls

- Spirituality matters to clients; is an essential, core part of a biopsychosocial-spiritual assessment; and is critical to a holistic understanding and effective interventions in service to patients across their cancer trajectory.
- Spirituality is a multifaceted, diverse concept that requires intentional attention and exploration of patients' beliefs, values, culture, and

lived experience, which may affect their coping, decision-making, and well-being.
- Social workers need to critically reflect on their own spirituality and their effects on one's social work practice and ability to effectively engage and address spiritual aspects of patient care.
- It takes an engaged, collaborative interprofessional team to effectively meet the holistic spiritual needs of individual, unique patients.

Pitfalls

- Assuming that religion and spirituality are the same thing while ignoring the complexity of the differences, similarities, and intersectionality of these individual concepts.
- Believing that spirituality is the professional domain of only one discipline (e.g., a chaplain or religious leader) has led to neglect of spirituality in social work training and practice.
- Lack of attention and failure to actively engage in valuing and validating spirituality in social work practice may result in inadequate assessment, missed intervention opportunities, and unmet patient needs.
- Failure to self-reflect on one's own spiritual beliefs, values, and practices can result in implicit bias and neglect of spirituality as an area of importance and meaning for our clients.

Additional Resources

Society for Spirituality and Social Work: https://spiritualityandsocialwork.org/
George Washington Institute for Spirituality and Health: https://smhs.gwu.edu/spirituality-health/
Council on Spiritual Practices: http://csp.org/
Conference on Medicine and Religion: http://www.medicineandreligion.com/about-us.html
Spiritual Competency Academy: https://www.spiritualcompetencyacademy.com/
Center for Spirituality, Theology and Health Duke University: https://spiritualityandhealth.duke.edu/
John Templeton Foundation: http://www.templeton.org/

References

Blaber, M., Jone, J., & Willis, D. (2015). Spiritual care: Which is the best assessment tool for palliative settings? *International Journal of Palliative Nursing, 21*(9), 430–438. https://doi.org/10.12968/ijpn.2015.21.9.430

Breitbart, W., Pessin, H., Rosenfeld, B., Applebaum, A. J., Lichtenthal, W. G., Li, Y., Saracino, R. M., Marziliano, A. M., Masterson, M., Tobias, K., & Fenn, N. (2018). Individual meaning-centered psychotherapy for the treatment of psychological and existential distress: A randomized controlled trial in patients with advanced cancer. *Cancer, 124*(15), 3231–3239. https://doi.org/10.1002/cncr.31539

Canda, E. R., & Furman, L. D. (2010). *Spiritual diversity in social work practice: The heart of helping* (2nd ed.). Oxford University Press.

Crisp, B. R. (2010). *Spirituality and social work*. Routledge. https://doi.org/10.4324/9781315610399

Darrell, L., & Rich, T. (2017). Faith and field: The ethical inclusion of spirituality within the pedagogy of social work. *Field Educator, 7*(1), 1–10.

Francoeur, R. B., Burke, N., & Wilson, A. M. (2016). The role of social workers in spiritual care to facilitate coping with chronic illness and self-determination in advance care planning. *Social Work in Public Health, 31*(5), 453–466. https://doi.org/10.1080/19371918.2016.1146199

Gotterer, R. (2001). The spiritual dimension in clinical social work practice: A client perspective. *Families in Society, 82*(20), 187–193. https://doi.org/10.1606/1044-3894.209

Harris, K. A., Randolph, B. E., & Gordon, T. D. (2016). What do clients want? Assessing spiritual needs in counseling: A literature review. *Spirituality in Clinical Practice, 3*(4), 250–275. https://doi.org/10.1037/scp0000108

Hodge, D. R. (2011). Using spiritual interventions in practice: Developing some guidelines from evidence-based practice. *Social Work, 56*, 149–158. https://doi.org/10.1093/sw/56.2.149

Hodge, D. R. (2020). Spiritual microaggressions: Understanding the subtle messages that foster religious discrimination. *Journal of Ethnic & Cultural Diversity in Social Work, 29*(6), 473–489. https://doi.org/10.1080/15313204.2018.1555501

Koenig, H. G. (2012). Religion, spirituality, and health: The research and clinical implications. *International Scholarly Research Notices, 2012*. https://doi.org/10.5402/2012/278730

Monod, S., Brennan, M., Rochat, E., Martin, E., Rochat, S., & Büla, C. J. (2011). Instruments measuring spirituality in clinical research: A systematic review. *Journal of General Internal Medicine, 26*(11), 1345–1357. https://doi.org/10.1007/s11606-011-1769-7

Morgan, S., Pullon, S., & McKinlay, E. (2015). Observation of interprofessional collaborative practice in primary care teams: An integrative literature review. *International Journal of Nursing Studies, 52*(7), 1217–1230. https://doi.org/10.1016/j.ijnurstu.2015.03.008

National Association of Social Workers. (2015). Standards and indicators for cultural competence in social work practice. https://www.socialworkers.org/LinkClick.aspx?fileticket=7dVckZAYUmk%3D&portalid=0

National Association of Social Workers. (2021). *Code of ethics of the National Association of Social Workers*. Retrieved from https://www.socialworkers.org/About/Ethics/Code-of-Ethics

Oxhandler, H. K., & Giardina, T. D. (2017). Social worker's perceived barriers to and sources of support for integrating clients' religion and spirituality in practice. *Social Work, 62*(4), 323–332. https://doi.org/10.1093/sw/swx036

Oxhandler, H. K., & Pargament, K. I. (2014). Social work practitioners' integration of clients' religion and spirituality in practice: A literature review. *Social Work, 59*(3), 271–279. https://doi.org/10.1093/sw/swu018

Oxhandler, H. K., Parrish, D. E., Torres, L. R., & Achenbaum, W. A. (2015). The integration of clients' religion and spirituality in social work practice: A national survey. *Social Work, 60*(3), 228–237. https://doi.org/10.1093/sw/swv018

Oxhandler, H. K., Polson, E. C., & Achenbaum, W. A. (2018). The religiosity and spiritual beliefs and practices of clinical social workers: A national survey. *Social Work, 63*(1), 47–56. https://doi.org/10.1093/SW/SWX055

Pandya, S. P. (2016). Hospital social work and spirituality: Views of medical social workers. *Social Work in Public Health, 31*(7), 700–710. https://doi.org/10.1080/19371918.2016.1188740

Puchalski, C. M., Sbrana, A., Ferrell, B., Jafari, N., King, S., Balboni, T., Miccinesi, G., Vandenhoeck, A., Silbermann, M., Balducci, L., Yong, J., Antonuzzo, A., Falcone, A., & Ripamonti, C. I. (2019). Interprofessional spiritual care in oncology: A literature review. *ESMO Open*, *4*(1), e000465. https://doi.org/10.1136/esmoopen-2018-000465

Rosmarin, D. H. (2018). *Spirituality, religion, and cognitive-behavioral therapy: A guide for clinicians*. Guilford.

Schot, E., Tummers, L., & Noordegraaf, M. (2020). Working on working together: A systematic review on how healthcare professionals contribute to interprofessional collaboration. *Journal of Interprofessional Care*, *34*(3), 332–342. https://doi.org/10.1080/13561820.2019.1636007

Siekkinen, M., Kuokkanen, L., Kuusisto, H., Leino-Kilpi, H., Rautava, P., Rekunen, M., Seppänen, L., Stolt, M., Walta, L., & Sulosaari, V. (2021). Work empowerment among cancer care professionals: A cross-sectional study. *BMC Health Services Research*, *21*(1), 1–11. https://doi.org/10.1186/s12913-021-06528-8

Stewart, M. (2014). Spiritual assessment: A patient-centered approach to oncology social work practice. *Social Work in Health Care*, *53*(1), 59–73. https://doi.org/10.1080/00981389.2013.834033

13 The Burdens and Rewards of Informal Cancer Caregivers

Issues and Interventions

Kelly R. Tan, Tamryn F. Gray, Alyson Erardy, and Erin E. Kent

Key Concepts

- Social workers in oncology palliative care seek to understand the diverse needs of family caregivers across the life span, various inpatient and community-based settings, and spanning the illness trajectory from prevention and diagnosis to survivorship or end of life.
- Social workers are equipped to assist patients and their caregivers using a strengths-based, person-in-environment perspective.
- Cancer caregivers are at risk for stress and stress-related health problems (e.g., anxiety, depression, financial burden). They may also experience positive aspects of caregiving (e.g., finding benefits and strengthening relationships with care recipients).
- Social workers are instrumental in the assessment and management of palliative and end-of-life care needs of patients and their caregivers.

Keywords: assessment, caregiver, family, quality of life, supportive-care interventions

This chapter provides an overview of cancer caregiving and the role of social work in this context. While oncology care is often patient-centered, clinicians may overlook other individuals impacted by cancer, such as caregivers—family and friends "provide care that is typically uncompensated and usually at home" (Kent et al., 2016, p. 1987). The *Caregiving in the U.S.* (2020) report estimated there were 53 million Americans (approximately 1 in 5) caring for a loved one, representing a 3% increase from 2015. Despite their prominent presence, caregivers are often overlooked in serious illness discussions

Kelly R. Tan, Tamryn F. Gray, Alyson Erardy, and Erin E. Kent, *The Burdens and Rewards of Informal Cancer Caregivers*
In: *Oncology and Palliative Social Work*. Edited by: Susan Hedlund, Bryan Miller, Grace Christ, and Carolyn Messner,
Oxford University Press. © Oxford University Press 2024. DOI: 10.1093/oso/9780197607299.003.0013

(National Alliance for Caregiving [NAC] and the American Association of Retired Persons [AARP], 2020).

In 2016, the authors of *Cancer Caregiving in the U.S.* estimated that caregivers provided an average of 33 hours of care for a loved one each week; however, services to support caregivers are limited. Social workers in oncology and palliative care settings can address this gap by delivering interventions directly to caregivers, including case management, emotional support, advocacy, and coordination of services and benefit programs. The supports social workers offer can improve caregiver well-being and enable caregivers to continue providing care.

The following vignette demonstrates how social workers are equipped with the necessary skills to support cancer caregivers and provides guided questions social workers may ask during conversations (Box 13.1).

Box 13.1

Michael is a 50-year-old Black man who is caring for his 48-year-old wife, Dina. Dina will start chemotherapy for stage II triple negative breast cancer next month. Michael and Dina have two school-aged children who do not know about their mother's diagnosis. Dina is taking a leave of absence from her job to pursue treatment, so Michael must continue working, care for his children, and manage the home in addition to his caregiving role. An oncology nurse suggests Michael and Dina connect with the social worker, Morgan, for support.

When Michael and Dina sit down in the social worker's office, Morgan observes their body language. Dina appears closed off, her arms and legs are crossed and her eyes are down; Michael appears anxious, his body upright and tense. Morgan smiles in an effort to ease their discomfort, offering them each a cup of water. They each take a few moments to drink some water and breathe. Dina's gaze shifts upward, and Michael noticeably relaxes in his chair.

Morgan introduces herself, describes her role within the health care team and offers to meet with Michael in addition to Dina during her visits. Morgan informs the couple that she has community connections and can refer them to organizations and supportive services. Morgan shares that she wants to prioritize the children and help the couple create a plan to discuss Dina's diagnosis effectively and age-appropriately. Morgan helps the couple identify individuals they trust to assist with childcare and provides them with information about another social worker, who works with children affected by cancer.

At the end of the meeting, Morgan checks in with Michael and Dina and acknowledges the overwhelming amount of information they received. Michael expresses gratitude to Morgan for informing them about available services, especially for himself and the children. Dina shares that she is scared about chemotherapy but thanks Morgan for the help. Morgan and Michael schedule a meeting for the following week to complete some resource applications.

Below are questions Morgan would have asked during her conversation with Michael and Dina to better understand their circumstances.

- *Does the family have a plan to pay for medical bills and delegate household and childcare tasks to family and friends?*
- *In what ways can school administrators and teachers support the family, particularly the children, during this time?*
- *What are the parents' main concerns about discussing the cancer diagnosis with their children?*
- *Has Michael notified his employer about Dina's diagnosis? Does Michael know his options regarding paid family leave?*

Cancer Caregiving: What Do We Know Now?

In 2020, a reported 3.2 million Americans were providing care to someone with cancer (NAC and AARP, 2020, p. 30). Most caregivers of people with cancer identify as female (58%), are age 35 to 64 (67%), identify as non-Hispanic White (65%), and are caring for a family member (90%). Most care recipients are women (70%) and in late adulthood (62%) (NAC et al., 2016).

Compared to caregiving for other chronic health conditions, such as old age or Alzheimer's, cancer caregiving is often shorter in number of years but requires more intensive care. On average, cancer caregivers provide care for approximately 2 years compared to noncancer caregivers, who typically provide care for over 4 years. Cancer caregivers provide an average of 33 hours of care per week versus 25 hours for noncancer caregivers. Cancer caregivers assist with activities of daily living and perform medical and nursing tasks, with nearly half reporting feeling unprepared to do so (NAC et al., 2016).

General Principles in Palliative and Oncology Social Work Related to Cancer Caregiving

A cancer diagnosis often comes as a shock to patients and caregivers. Social workers can assess family history, functioning, and communication patterns between the patient and caregiver to obtain a better understanding of their dynamics. Social workers also assess family culture and beliefs that may influence their response to illness (Hedlund, 2015). Information from assessments provides essential guidance for the health care team to provide high-quality family-centered care.

The Role of Social Work in the Psychosocial Support of Caregivers

Cancer caregivers may have a variety of concerns and not be aware of the services offered by social workers. Shortly after receiving a cancer diagnosis, social workers should inform caregivers of the role the social worker can play in linking up the caregiver with available support services, such as community organizations (e.g., local health departments, chapters of cancer advocacy groups, volunteer corps) and support groups. After initial contact, social workers can provide targeted psychosocial support to patients and caregivers to meet specific needs (Varner, 2015).

Social workers should use a strengths-based approach with caregivers to remind them of their resources, encourage them to build their support network, and discuss ways to engage in self-care. Caregivers can also receive psychoeducation from social workers on what to expect depending on the phase of cancer their loved one is in. Social workers can introduce new coping skills, connect caregivers to support, coordinate services, and offer emotional support by creating a safe space for caregivers to process their feelings. Notably, sometimes the best clinical intervention a social worker can provide is listening and validating personal experiences (Varner, 2015).

Social workers rely on the National Association of Social Workers (NASW) *Code of Ethics*, a set of standards that guide the professional conduct of social workers. There are six core values of social work: service, social justice, dignity and worth of the person, importance of human relationships, integrity, and competence (NASW, 2021). These values illustrate why social workers hold a vital role in the psychosocial support for cancer caregivers.

Core Values of Social Work

The primary goal for social workers in palliative care and oncology is to help those affected by cancer, including caregivers. Social workers use their knowledge and skills to support a person through times of hardship; they may be called on to challenge injustice if they find a caregiver and/or patient are being treated unfairly by their health care team. Social workers are trained to respect all persons, with awareness of differences among individual patients and caregivers. To maintain individual autonomy, social workers promote self-determination, which is a person's ability to make their own decisions and be recognized as the expert of their own experience. Social workers help caregivers find ways to cope with their care recipient's decisions, even if the caregiver disagrees with those decisions. Finally, social workers are expected to practice with integrity within their scope of practice (NASW, 2021).

Competencies in Caregiving for Clinicians

Experts in the field of family caregiving have created two documents that provide guidance on key competencies and best practices in assessment of family caregivers (Betty Irene Moore School of Nursing [BIMSN], 2021). The first document, "Interprofessional Caregiving Competencies," describes four competency domains: the nature of family caregiving, family caregiving identification and assessment, providing family-centered care, and the context of family caregiving (BIMSN, 2021). These competencies outline key knowledge for social workers to create a family-centered approach to oncology care. The second document, "Family Caregiver Domains of Preparedness," describes how health professionals can assess the preparedness of family caregivers to take on care-related tasks. The nine domains include household tasks, personal care, mobility, health monitoring, emotional and social support, care coordination, medical/nursing tasks, shared decision-making, and caregiver self-care (BIMSN, 2021). A social worker's assessment and referrals to appropriate services can help fill identified support gaps and are likely to improve the caregiver's and patient's well-being by reducing stress and anxiety.

Principles and Foundations in the Science of Caregiving

New conceptual frameworks have emerged in caregiving research, including ways to both understand and address the needs of cancer caregivers. Many of these frameworks fit well with social work perspectives that understand humans in the context of their family system and broader social environment. New frameworks highlight key contextual factors that affect the caregiving experience, including stress and coping, relationship building, and

Table 13.1 Examples of Conceptual Frameworks Related to Caregiving

Author, Year	Conceptual Framework	Summary
Marshall et al., 2011	Model of Culture and Social Class for Families Facing Cancer	Facilitates health promotion and strengths-based psychosocial interventions among families that are diverse in culture and social class by depicting the person with cancer as embedded their social context that includes the family, caregiver(s), and broader social network.
Fletcher et al., 2012	Cancer Family Caregiving Experience	Illustrates a comprehensive model of cancer family caregiving experience to emphasize stress processing, contextual factors, and cancer trajectory.
Laidsaar-Powell et al., 2017	TRiadic Interactions in Oncology (TRIO) Framework	Depicts family caregivers in the existing conceptualization of clinician–patient decision-making and variability of family caregiver involvement in decision-making.
Manne & Badr, 2018	Intimacy and Relationship Process Model	Proposes that patients and their partners engage in behaviors that either promote or undermine relationship intimacy.
Lyons & Lee, 2018	Theory of Dyadic Illness Management	Posits that illness management is a dyadic phenomenon and highlights how dyads appraise illness as a unit and engage in behaviors to manage illness together.
Young et al., 2020	Heterogeneity of Caregiving Model	Recognizes that family caregivers are diverse and have unique needs that requires context-specific interventions.
Thompson et al., 2021	Dyadic Cancer Outcomes Framework:	Highlights individual- and dyad-level predictors and outcomes while incorporating disease trajectory and social context.

decision-making. Table 13.1 describes examples of conceptual frameworks related to family caregiving.

Psychosocial Challenges in Caregiving for a Person With Cancer

Cancer caregivers are more likely to report emotional distress than noncancer caregivers, and approximately 1 in 5 indicate that cancer caregiving has had a negative impact on their own health (NAC et al., 2016). Cancer is often characterized by a rapid deterioration in health, the need to manage illness with complicated medication regimens, and complex treatment decision-making. In particular, during times of high patient need, caregivers take on greater responsibility, which can result in neglecting their own health needs (Northouse et al., 2012). When faced with increased demands, caregivers may struggle to perform caregiving duties, and the resulting strain can have deleterious effects, such as caregiver anxiety or depression (Hodges et al., 2005), fear of cancer recurrence (Northouse et al., 2012), and reduced quality of life (Geng et al., 2018).

Cancer caregivers report more financial strain (25% versus 17%) than noncancer caregivers (NAC et al., 2016). This financial burden is associated with increased risk of poorer health outcomes, including distress and higher mortality, among both patients and caregivers (Bradley, 2019). About half of cancer caregivers report working while caregiving; most of those work full-time. Some caregivers may experience tension between reducing work hours to care for recipients and maintaining health insurance. A third of cancer patients and their partners report having to stay employed to maintain health insurance for themselves or their partners (Kent et al., 2016).

Positive Aspects of Providing Care for a Person With Cancer

Beyond these challenges, some caregivers have also reported experiencing positive aspects of caregiving, such as an increased meaning in life, benefit finding, a sense of achievement, self-efficacy, personal growth, and pride in one's ability to provide care (Li & Loke 2013). Young and Snowden (2017) note creating meaning in life from caregiving experiences stems from having a positive appraisal of caregiving (e.g., having a choice, providing care out of a sense of love, acceptance of the situation) instead of a negative appraisal (e.g., seeing caregiving as an obligation, having no choice). In addition, personal positive aspects may both have protective functions and be outcomes (Young & Snowden, 2017). When addressing psychosocial challenges, social workers can identify positive aspects and intervene to increase a caregiver's ability to be more aware, build more capacity to experience positive aspects of caregiving, and develop a greater sense of meaning while caregiving.

Patient–caregiver dyads often report strengthened relationships as a result of cancer caregiving experiences (Li & Loke, 2013). Some proposed mechanisms for how relationships become strengthened during caregiving include expressions of gratitude to the caregiver, improved communication skills, and increased time spent with each other. Research on the positive psychosocial processes of caregiving is still developing, however, caregivers may benefit from being assessed for these aspects to enable caregivers to be more aware of the good in caregiving and identify aspects that are not being experienced so that a social worker can provide coping skills training to increase opportunities to experience these positive aspects.

Assessments of Caregiving Psychosocial Issues

Caregiver assessment refers to the systematic process of identifying specific problems, experiences, resources, and needs; pinpointing positive aspects of caregiving; and assessing the caregiver's ability to provide care (Varner, 2015). Social workers assessing caregivers should take into consideration the appropriateness, length, and utility of measurement instruments. Social workers may benefit from asking themselves the following prior to conducting a needs assessment: What is the caregiver's current personal context? What will I do with the results of the assessment? How long is the assessment? When will the caregiver take the assessment? Has the caregiver completed the assessment for another health care provider? When do I need to reassess the caregiver?

Social workers should complete assessments during their initial contact with both the person with cancer and the caregiver. For a comprehensive list of available psychosocial instruments as well as several short-form instruments using item-response theory, refer to the websites listed in the Additional Resources section.

Interventions to Treat Caregiving-Related Psychosocial Issues

Social workers should offer caregivers who currently have or are identified as at risk for psychosocial challenges appropriate interventions to address these issues. Applebaum and Breitbart's (2013) systematic review of interventions for cancer caregivers published between 1980 and 2011 categorized these interventions into eight categories: psychoeducation, problem-solving/skill-building interventions, supportive therapy, family/couples therapy, cognitive behavioral therapy, interpersonal therapy, complementary and alternative medicine interventions, and existential therapy.

Several systematic reviews have evaluated the effectiveness of psychosocial interventions among cancer caregivers, focusing on addressing and improving anxiety, depression, quality of life, and self-care, as well as enhance coping abilities and skills training (e.g., Applebaum & Breitbart, 2013; Ferrell

& Wittenberg, 2017; Lee et al., 2021). Interventions aimed at improving cancer caregiving generally focus on one of three sets of outcomes—patient outcomes, caregiver outcomes, or combined patient–caregiver (dyad) outcomes—and target either caregivers only or both patients and caregivers (dyadic interventions).

Dyadic Interventions

Research on family caregiving continues to shift from the individual to the dyadic level because of the growing evidence that caregiver and patient health are intertwined. Findings from a review of spousal couple-based intervention studies highlight beneficial outcomes of couple-based interventions, including improvements in communication, dyadic coping, psychosocial distress, sexual functioning, and marital satisfaction (Li & Loke, 2014). Using a combination of face-to-face, web-based, app-based, and telephone contacts, specially trained counselors, psychologists, nurses, and social workers deliver interventions and focus on skills training, therapeutic and marital counseling, self-care, coping, communication, and psychoeducation (Li & Loke, 2014). Table 13.2 provides exemplar individual and dyadic interventions for patients with cancer and their family caregivers.

Caregivers are essential to the support of people with cancer, particularly as cancer care is increasingly shifting to the outpatient setting, thus increasing the burden of care responsibilities on caregivers. They face many challenges as their care recipients transition through cancer care from diagnosis to end of life or survivorship. Social workers are uniquely prepared to assess caregiver well-being, connect them with supportive care and community-based resources, and deliver interventions to improve their overall quality of life.

Guiding Best Practices for the Future

The development and implementation of several policies may affect cancer caregiving in the future. The RAISE (Recognize, Assist, Include, Support, and Engage) Family Caregivers Act (S.1028/H.R.3759) was passed in 2018 to develop a national strategy to support family caregivers. In September 2021, a report to Congress detailed 26 recommendations that fell under 5 major areas: increased awareness of family caregiving, increased emphasis on caregiver integration, increased access to services and supports for family caregivers, increased financial and workplace protection for caregivers, and better and more consistent

Table 13.2 Selected Exemplar Interventions

Author, year, intervention	Pilot/ RCT*	Components	Cancer Site(s)	Individual/ Dyad	Primary Outcome
Northouse et al., 2013 Brief FOCUS Program	RCT	Three contacts (two 90-minute home visits and one 30-minute phone session) addressing five content areas (family involvement, optimistic attitude, coping effectiveness, uncertainty reduction, and symptom management)	Advanced breast, colorectal, lung, or prostate cancer	Dyad	Quality of life
Sahler et al., 2013 Bright IDEAS: Problem-Solving Skills Training	RCT	Eight-session intervention covering the five steps of problem-solving skills training (*I*dentify the problem; *D*etermine options; *E*valuate options and choose the best; *A*ct; and *S*ee if it worked)	Various cancers	Individual	Coping and emotional distress
Rolbiecki et al., 2020 Caregiver Speaks	Pilot single-arm feasibility study	Six-week online intervention using photo-elicitation as a tool to facilitate the exchange of personal stories among bereaved cancer caregivers.	Various cancers	Individual	Meaning making
Applebaum et al., 2020 ERT-C	RCT	Emotion regulation therapy adapted for caregivers of people with cancer. Eight 60-minute session with a trained therapist (sessions focus on psychoeducation, emotion regulation training, attention skills, detection of problematic emotion responses)	Various cancers	Individual	Emotional well-being
Watabayashi et al., 2020 Financial navigation program	Pilot single-arm feasibility study	Comprehensive financial navigation program consisting of a financial education video, monthly contact with a financial counselor and case manager for 6 months.	Various- solid tumors	Dyad	Financial burden

*RCT (randomized controlled trial)

Refer to the Additional Resources section for recommended articles for these selected interventions.

research and data collection. Another important recent legislative action is the CARE (Caregiver Advise Record Enable) Act, designed to ensure that for hospitalized patients, a caregiver is documented, notified prior to discharge, and involved in discharge planning (Mason, 2017). Currently, federal programs are in place to protect employees if they need to care for a close relative with a health problem. For example, the Family Medical Leave Act offers employment protection for up to 12 weeks but no wage benefits and does not cover employees who are self-employed or work for small businesses. Though these benefits are not specific to cancer caregivers, there are real implications for the oncology context in terms of alleviating burden and providing more supports.

Pearls

- Psychosocial interventions should be tailored to caregiver's individual needs, assessed using validated and reliable measures, and addressed using evidence-based interventions.
- Using a strength-based approach when working with caregivers may help them identify existing resources and assets to help them cope with cancer.
- Connecting caregivers to resources and practical and emotional support may benefit their overall health and quality of life.

Pitfalls

- Cancer care is often patient focused; however, the negative impact of cancer extends beyond the patient, warranting the need to support the whole family.
- A cancer diagnosis is often sudden and disruptive to both patients and caregivers, which may result in the need to adopt new coping strategies.
- There is insufficient evidence of the effectiveness of family and caregiver interventions over usual care, though intervention research has grown significantly in the past decade.

Additional Resources

National Cancer Institute, Evidence-Based Cancer Control Programs. https://ebccp.cancercontrol.cancer.gov/searchResults.do

Northouse, L. L., Mood, D. W., Schafenacker, A., Kalemkerian, G., Zalupski, M., LoRusso, P., Hayes, D. F., Hussain, M., Ruckdeschel, J., Fendrick, A. M., Trask, P. C., Ronis, D. L., & Kershaw, T. (2013). Randomized clinical trial of a brief and extensive dyadic intervention for advanced cancer patients and their family caregivers. *Psycho-Oncology*, *22*(3), 555–563. https://doi.org/10.1002/pon.3036

Palliative Care Research Cooperative Group Caregiver Core. https://palliativecareresearch.org/corescenters/caregiver-core

Patient Reported Outcomes Measurement Information System (PROMIS). http://healthmeasures.net/

Rolbiecki, A. J., Oliver, D. P., Washington, K., Benson, J. J., & Jorgensen, L. (2020). Preliminary results of Caregiver Speaks: A storytelling intervention for bereaved family caregivers. *Journal of Loss and Trauma*, *25*(5), 438–453. https://doi.org/10.1080/15325024.2019.1707985

Sahler, O. J., Dolgin, M. J., Phipps, S., Fairclough, D. L., Askins, M. A., Katz, E. R., Noll, R. B., & Butler, R. W. (2013). Specificity of problem-solving skills training in mothers of children newly diagnosed with cancer: Results of a multisite randomized clinical trial. *Journal of Clinical Oncology*, *31*(10), 1329–1335. https://doi.org/10.1200/JCO.2011.39.1870

Watabayashi, K., Steelquist, J., Overstreet, K. A., Leahy, A., Bradshaw, E., Gallagher, K. D., Balch, A. J., Lobb, R., Lavell, L., Linden, H., Ramsey, S. D., & Shankaran, V. (2020). A pilot study of a comprehensive financial navigation program in patients with cancer and caregivers. *Journal of the National Comprehensive Cancer Network*, *18*(10), 1366–1373. https://doi.org/10.6004/jnccn.2020.7581

References

Applebaum, A. J., & Breitbart, W. (2013). Care for the cancer caregiver: A systematic review. *Palliative and Supportive Care*, *11*(3), 231–252. https://doi.org/10.1017/S1478951512000594

Applebaum, A. J., Panjwani, A. A., Buda, K., O'Toole, M. S., Hoyt, M. A., Garcia, A., Fresco, D. M., & Mennin, D. S. (2020). Emotion regulation therapy for cancer caregivers: An open trial of a mechanism-targeted approach to addressing caregiver distress. *Translational Behavioral Medicine*, *10*(2), 413–422. https://doi.org/10.1093/tbm/iby104

Betty Irene Moore School of Nursing at UC Davis. (2021). *Interprofessional family caregiving competencies and family caregiver domains of preparedness*. https://health.ucdavis.edu/family-caregiving/education/caregiving-competencies-and-domains

Bradley, C. J. (2019). Economic burden associated with cancer caregiving. *Seminars in Oncology Nursing*, *35*(4), 333–336.

Ferrell, B., & Wittenberg, E. (2017, July 8). A review of family caregiving intervention trials in oncology. *CA: Cancer Journal for Clinicians*, *67*(4), 318–325. https://doi.org/10.3322/caac.21396

Fletcher, B. S., Miaskowski, C., Given, B., & Schumacher, K. (2012). The cancer family caregiving experience: An updated and expanded conceptual model. *European Journal of Oncology Nursing*, *16*(4), 387–398. https://doi.org/10.1016/j.ejon.2011.09.001

Geng, H. M., Chuang, D. M., Yang, F., Yang, Y., Liu, W. M., Liu, L. H., & Tian, H. M. (2018). Prevalence and determinants of depression in caregivers of cancer patients: A systematic review and meta-analysis. *Medicine*, *97*(39), e11863. https://doi.org/10.1097/MD.0000000000011863

Hedlund, S. (2015). Introduction to working with families in oncology. In G. Christ, C. Messner, & L. Behar (Eds.), *Handbook of oncology social work: Psychosocial care for people with cancer* (pp. 380–382). Oxford University Press.

Hodges, L. J., Humphris, G. M., & Macfarlane, G. (2005). A meta-analytic investigation of the relationship between the psychological distress of cancer patients and their careers. *Social Science and Medicine*, *60*(1), 1–12. https://doi.org/10.1016/j.socscimed.2004.04.018

Kent, E. E., Rowland, J. H., Northouse, L., Litzelman, K., Chou, W. Y., Shelburne, N., Timura, C., O'Mara, A., & Huss, K. (2016). Caring for caregivers and patients: Research and clinical priorities for informal cancer caregiving. *Cancer, 122*(13), 1987–1995. https://doi.org/10.1002/cncr.29939

Laidsaar-Powell, R., Butow, P., Charles, C., Gafni, A., Entwistle, V., Epstein, R., & Juraskova, I. (2017). The TRIO Framework: Conceptual insights into family caregiver involvement and influence throughout cancer treatment decision-making. *Patient Education and Counseling, 100*(11), 2035–2046. https://doi.org/10.1016/j.pec.2017.05.014

Lee, J., Chen, H. C., Lee, J. X., & Klainin-Yobas, P. (2021). Effects of psychosocial interventions on psychological outcomes among caregivers of advanced cancer patients: A systematic review and meta-analysis. *Supportive Care in Cancer, 29*(12), 7237–7248. https://doi.org/10.1007/s00520-021-06102-2

Li, Q., & Loke, A. Y. (2013). The positive aspects of caregiving for cancer patients: A critical review of the literature and directions for future research. *Psycho-Oncology, 22*(11), 2399–2407. https://doi.org/10.1002/pon.3311

Li, Q., & Loke, A. Y. (2014). A systematic review of spousal couple-based intervention studies for couples coping with cancer: Direction for the development of interventions. *Psycho-Oncology, 23*(7), 731–739. https://doi.org/10.1002/pon.3535

Lyons, K. S., & Lee, C. S. (2018). The theory of dyadic illness management. *Journal of Family Nursing, 24*(1), 8–28. https://doi.org/10.1177/1074840717745669

Manne, S., & Badr, H. (2008). Intimacy and relationship processes in couples' psychosocial adaptation to cancer. *Cancer, 112*(11 Suppl), 2541–2555. https://doi.org/10.1002/cncr.23450

Marshall, C. A., Larkey, L. K., Curran, M. A., Weihs, K. L., Badger, T. A., Armin, J., & García, F. (2011). Considerations of culture and social class for families facing cancer: The need for a new model for health promotion and psychosocial intervention. *Families, Systems & Health: The Journal of Collaborative Family Healthcare, 29*(2), 81–94. https://doi.org/10.1037/a0023975

Mason, D. (2017). Supporting family caregivers, one state at a time: The CARE Act. *JAMA Forum Archive.* https://doi.org/10.1001/jamahealthforum.2017.0055

National Alliance for Caregiving and American Association of Retired Persons. (2020). *Caregiving in the U.S. 2020.* https://www.caregiving.org/wp-content/uploads/2021/01/full-report-caregiving-in-the-united-states-01-21.pdf

National Alliance for Caregiving, National Cancer Institute, and Cancer Support Community. (2016). *Cancer caregiving in the U.S.: An intense, episodic, and challenging care experience.* https://www.caregiving.org/wpcontent/uploads/2020/05/CancerCaregivingReport_FINAL_June-17-2016.pdf

National Association of Social Workers. (2021). *Code of ethics of the National Association of Social Workers.* https://Socialworkers.org/About/Ethics/Code-of-Ethics/Code-of-Ethics-English

Northouse, L. L., Katapodi, M. C., Schafenacker, A. M., & Weiss, D. (2013). The impact of caregiving on the psychological well-being of family caregivers and cancer patients. *Seminars in Oncology Nursing, 28*(4), 236–245. https://doi.org/10.1016/j.soncn.2012.09.006

RAISE Family Caregivers Act of 2018, S.1028, 115th Congress (2017–2018). https://www.congress.gov/bill/115th-congress/senate-bill/1028/text

Rolbiecki, A. J., Oliver, D. P., Washington, K., Benson, J. J., & Jorgensen, L. (2020). Preliminary results of Caregiver Speaks: A storytelling intervention for bereaved family caregivers. *Journal of Loss and Trauma, 25*(5), 438–453. https://doi.org/10.1080/15325024.2019.17079

Sahler, O. J., Dolgin, M. J., Phipps, S., Fairclough, D. L., Askins, M. A., Katz, E. R., Noll, R. B., & Butler, R. W. (2013). Specificity of problem-solving skills training in mothers of children newly diagnosed with cancer: Results of a multisite randomized clinical trial. *Journal of Clinical Oncology, 31*(10), 1329–1335. https://doi.org/10.1200/JCO.2011.39.1870

Thompson, T., Ketcher, D., Gray, T. F., & Kent, E. E. (2021). The Dyadic Cancer Outcomes Framework: A general framework of the effects of cancer on patients and informal caregivers. *Social Science and Medicine*, *287*, 114357. https://doi.org/10.1016/j.socscimed.2021.114357

Varner, A. (2015). Caregivers of cancer patients. In G. Christ, C. Messner, & L. Behar (Eds.), *Handbook of oncology social work: Psychosocial care for people with cancer* (pp. 385–390). Oxford University Press.

Young, H. M., Bell, J. F., Whitney, R. L., Ridberg, R. A., Reed, S. C., & Vitaliano, P. P. (2020). Social determinants of health: Underreported heterogeneity in systematic reviews of caregiver interventions. *Gerontologist*, *60*(Suppl. 1), S14–S28. https://doi.org/10.1093/geront/gnz148

Young, J., & Snowden, A. (2017). A systematic review on the factors associated with positive experiences in careers of someone with cancer. *European Journal of Cancer Care*, *26*(3). https://doi.org/10.1111/ecc.12544

Watabayashi, K., Steelquist, J., Overstreet, K. A., Leahy, A., Bradshaw, E., Gallagher, K. D., Balch, A. J., Lobb, R., Lavell, L., Linden, H., Ramsey, S. D., & Shankaran, V. (2020). A pilot study of a comprehensive financial navigation program in patients with cancer and caregivers. *Journal of the National Comprehensive Cancer Network*, *18*(10), 1366–1373. https://doi.org/10.6004/jnccn.2020.7581

14

Palliative and Hospice Care at the End of Life

Walking Alongside Patients and Families

Jamie Newell and Stephanie B. Broussard

Key Concepts

- Several models of palliative care exist for services within inpatient, outpatient, and home-based settings.
- Cultural humility and accountability are integral to providing quality palliative care for all populations.
- Oncology and palliative care clinicians must continually strive to better engage underserved populations to provide trauma-informed, comprehensive care.
- Comprehensive palliative care includes the treatment of total pain—attending to physical, emotional, spiritual, and existential pain.
- Cultivating prognostic awareness for patients and families allows them to engage in shared decision-making and better determine goals of care.
- Advance care planning is most valuable when the care team can engage in multiple conversations around the patient's illness to clarify goals of care and prioritize values.
- Meaning-making is an important part of coping with serious illness and end of life.

Keywords: biopsychosocial, disparities, hospice, meaning-making, palliative, underserved

Oncology teams strive to provide quality, compassionate care across the entire trajectory of treatment. For patients who grapple with incurable disease, the oncology team has the opportunity not only to treat their cancer but also to support preparation and meaning making as end of life approaches. Palliative

Jamie Newell and Stephanie B. Broussard, *Palliative and Hospice Care at the End of Life* In: *Oncology and Palliative Social Work*. Edited by: Susan Hedlund, Bryan Miller, Grace Christ, and Carolyn Messner, Oxford University Press.
 DOI: 10.1093/oso/9780197607299.003.0014

care is integral to this process. Embedding palliative care concurrently into oncologic care adheres to best practices in addressing symptom management, providing greater support for patients and families, and launching earlier discussions of advance care planning and goals of care.

What Is Palliative Care?

Palliative care originated in the pursuit of quality care for the dying in the early 1960s and grew throughout the 1970s into a wide network of hospice services (National Hospice and Palliative Care Organization [NHPCO], 2020). As modern medicine and technology have advanced, people with serious illnesses are living longer and the complexity of their needs are increasing. As a result, palliative care has evolved beyond solely end-of-life care into critical longer-term support for those with cancer and other life-limiting illnesses.

"Palliative care is provided by a specially trained team of doctors, nurses, social workers, and other specialists who work together with other members of the patient's care team to provide an extra layer of support. Palliative care is specialized care based on the needs of the patient, not on the patient's prognosis. It is appropriate at any age and at any stage in a serious illness, and it can be provided along with curative treatment" (Center to Advance Palliative Care [CAPC], n.d.). Palliative care attends to physical, intellectual, emotional, social, and spiritual distress to enhance quality of life, autonomy, and goal-concordant care (NHPCO, 2018).

Models of Palliative Care

The five major models of specialty palliative care delivery—outpatient clinics, inpatient consultation teams, acute palliative care units, community-based palliative care, and hospice care—create a continuum of care that comprehensively addresses patients' needs throughout the disease trajectory. Services can vary in team structures, approach, population served, location of care, and insurance coverage, each with their own benefits and challenges (Hui & Bruera, 2020).

Although evidence clearly shows that palliative care models improve the quality and reduce the cost of care as a patient nears the end of life, reimbursement models have not evolved commensurately. Physicians and advanced practice providers are reimbursed for individual services provided, like other specialists (Ferrell et al., 2017). The Medicare fee-for-service model and lack of reimbursement for comprehensive care can be a barrier to the provision of palliative care provided by a full interdisciplinary team as recommended. However, there are insurances and value-based payment models that reimburse for comprehensive palliative care services. (CAPC, n.d.).

Palliative care teams both provide specialized services to oncology patients and serve as teachers and consultants, helping oncologists practice primary palliative care. As most palliative care teams do not have the capacity to see all oncology patients, particularly in the outpatient setting, oncologists must have palliative care skills to address symptoms, distress, and important goals-of-care discussions. Palliative care specialists, when available in the outpatient setting, can provide secondary palliative care, offering specialized support in symptom management and advance care planning. Inpatient palliative care teams provide tertiary palliative care support, with more ability to provide enhanced pain interventions in a monitored environment. In recent years, more agencies provide in-home palliative care services, though they vary widely, and insurance coverage can be limited.

Access to palliative care services in rural settings often lags behind urban areas. Traditional barriers such as staffing shortages, lack of financial reimbursement and resources, and community misconceptions of palliative care are exacerbated in rural communities; having to travel greater distances to access or provide care poses an additional challenge. As a result, most successful rural models result from community collaboration and ingenuity. Telehealth services have also proven to improve access to specialty palliative care (Weng et al., 2022).

Due to limited access to palliative care specialists, many oncology patients are referred to clinics that manage and treat chronic pain. Patients may receive interventional procedures that are effective for some of their physical pain. These clinics specialize more in chronic pain, which is often intertwined with complex behavioral concerns, and do not necessarily provide specialized support around oncologic pain and existential pain related to serious illness and end of life.

Best Practices

Informed by multiple randomized trials, current American Society for Clinical Oncology (ASCO) guidelines stipulate that best practice oncology care for patients with advanced cancer includes concurrent palliative care. Concurrent palliative care demonstrably improves patients' quality of life and reduces symptoms, lessens caregiver distress, and makes care more congruent with a patient's stated goals and less aggressive at end of life (Smith et al., 2018).

In 2016, ASCO formally adopted clinical guidelines establishing that every patient with advanced cancer should be treated by a multidisciplinary palliative care team in addition to their oncologist within 8 weeks of diagnosis, with access to inpatient and outpatient services (Ferrell et al., 2017). The guidelines also recommend:

- Rapport and relationship building with patient and family caregiver(s).
- Symptom, distress, and functional status management (e.g., pain, dyspnea, fatigue, sleep disturbance, mood, nausea, or constipation).
- Education about illness and prognosis.
- Clarification of treatment goals.
- Assessment and support of coping needs.
- Assistance with medical decision-making.
- Coordination with other care providers.
- Provision of referrals to other care providers.

Early palliative care integration demonstrates improved quality of life and can prolong survival. Evidence indicates that early integration improves patient outcomes by reducing chemotherapy use at end of life, increasing length of stay on hospice, and reducing overall health spending (CAPC, n.d.). Many oncology practices rely on standardized criteria and/or triggers to identify patients for palliative care referrals. Pain scales and scores on validated tools like the Edmonton Symptom Assessment Scale also aid in identifying patients whose symptoms may require specialized services and help determine effectiveness of the symptom management provided (Halpern, 2020). Though best practice considers patients and loved ones as a unit of care, caregiver needs can get lost in the shuffle as patients are treated for their cancer. This has been particularly true during the COVID-19 pandemic, when many clinics have restricted visitors and not allowed loved ones to be physically present at crucial times in the patient's care and at end of life. Palliative care teams spend additional time with caregivers to attend to their distress and psychosocial needs. Often, palliative care clinicians facilitate family meetings to increase understanding of illness, attend to support needs, and engage in advance care planning.

Total Pain

Cicely Saunders, the founder of modern hospice, conceptualized the physical, social, psychological, and spiritual suffering of seriously ill patients as total pain (Krawczyk et al., 2018). Treatment of total pain is a key tenet of palliative care, and optimal relief cannot be attained if all domains are not addressed.

Social workers' education and training uniquely equip them with the skills to address the psychosocial and spiritual aspects of disease (Halpern, 2020). Social workers provide clinical assessments and nonpharmacological therapeutic interventions for emotional distress, depression, anxiety, trauma, and end-of-life concerns, along with stressors related to social determinants of health (Altilio et al., 2011). Screening tools include the National Comprehensive Cancer Network distress thermometer, in addition to clinical assessment tools such as comprehensive biopsychosocial assessments that reflect evidence-based literature and standards of clinical practice. Social workers can use such validated tools as quality-of-life, depression, and anxiety scales. Interventions will vary based on acuity, level of distress, biopsychosocial needs, and practice setting. They may include crisis intervention, motivational interviewing, cognitive behavioral therapy, psychoeducation, narrative therapy, grief work, and community referrals (Halpern, 2020).

Oncology Treatments for Advanced Cancer

Oncologists offer patients with advanced, incurable cancer palliative treatments, which can include chemotherapy, immunotherapy, targeted therapies, and radiation. The goal of these treatments is usually to extend survival time as well as reduce symptoms. However, many patients can experience adverse effects and must weigh how much time they spend in treatment versus spending valuable time elsewhere. Furthermore, studies demonstrate that palliative chemotherapy is associated with more aggressive end-of-life interventions, including more frequent hospital visits, intensive care, and intubation. It also results in decreased hospice use (Wu et al., 2016).

Prognostic Awareness, Advance Care Planning, and Meaning-Making

Oncologists tend to not readily discuss a patient's prognosis and are often overly optimistic when they do. Studies suggest this is frequently correlated with the length and depth of their relationships with patients; oncologists forge strong relationships with their patients and care deeply for them. These significant relationships can increase the drive to maintain hope and engage in wishful thinking, which makes it harder to have prognostic discussions in a timely and purposeful way (Abernethy et al., 2019). Although the motivation is understandable, a lack of clear statements regarding a poor prognosis can result in missed opportunities for patients and families to prepare for end of life and engage in meaning-making, including legacy work, and to prioritize how they want to spend the time they have left.

Palliative care teams can provide additional opportunities to enhance the prognostic awareness of patients and families in order to allow them to explore their values and goals of care. Honest and timely discussions can help patients as well as oncologists determine whether goals of care are congruent with patients' treatment plans. They also allow patients and families to prepare for the future, prioritize their values and goals, and engage in advance care planning.

Advance care planning has been a consistent part of palliative care work. Recent studies have suggested that the push to engage patients and families in advance care planning does not greatly affect quality of life, reduction in hospital care, or goal-concordant care at end of life. Nevertheless, the role of advance care planning arguably remains important in identifying health care surrogates as well as engaging in shared medical decision-making throughout the treatment process (Morrison et al., 2021). High-value advance care planning includes in-depth discussion of prognosis, thorough elicitation of understanding of illness and goals of care, and fostering multiple touch points at which clinicians and patients can engage in shared decision-making.

Oncologists and even palliative care clinicians sometimes worry that engaging in discussions about prognosis will negatively impact patients' capacity for hope, which has been shown to be associated with improved coping, better quality of life, and less pain and anxiety. While it is true that the timing of these discussions requires clinical insight and nuance, clinicians can balance hope with important truths about disease trajectory. A recent study demonstrated that hope was not decreased by discussions of advance care planning and end of life (Dillon et al., 2021).

A systematic review of 67 studies showed that legacy work for patients with advanced cancer improved well-being in multiple domains, including reduced symptoms of depression (Boles & Jones, 2021). Palliative care providers are uniquely trained and positioned to facilitate this work, helping patients engage in life review and create a written or video legacy for loved ones. This work can enhance quality of life, promote meaning-making, and assist with both anticipatory grief as well as postdeath grief.

Culture and Spirituality

The American Academy of Hospice and Palliative Medicine and ASCO issued a joint statement in 2016 targeting spiritual and cultural care as essential components of palliative care in oncology (Bickel et al., 2016). Spiritual care is a significant factor in quality of life, and spiritual distress is common for seriously ill patients. Spiritual beliefs, culture, values, and life experiences are often intertwined and impact patients' perceptions of illnesses, care, and death (Rego et al., 2020). Thus, oncology and palliative care teams must explore ways to assess and address patients' spiritual needs.

Cultural, religious, and spiritual beliefs may influence whether a patient elects to receive specific types of treatment or symptom relief. Conversely, when clinicians perceive spiritual and cultural beliefs as barriers, patients are less likely to be offered palliative and end-of-life care or symptom management. Clinicians who actively engage in cultural humility and learn the nuances of each patient's culture experience positive outcomes, including an improved patient/family perception of the care provided (Givler et al., 2022).

Underserved Populations

Disparities in care clearly exist in medicine, including oncology and palliative care. Just as structural racism is rooted in other institutions of our society, it is also entrenched in health care and is an important social determinant of health. Studies have demonstrated differences in care and outcomes for Black, Hispanic, and Native American patients, as well as for patients with lower socioeconomic status. Researchers have also noted incongruencies in patient reporting of symptom burden, as well as concern among treatment teams and patients for undertreated pain. Although less data is available to speak to the experiences of other marginalized populations—sexual and gender minorities, immigrants and people with language barriers, and people with disabilities—these groups can also face structural, social, and economic barriers as they navigate health care (Griggs, 2020).

A systematic review of 2,696 articles demonstrated significant differences in use of and beliefs around end-of-life care for people of color with cancer, factoring in considerations of socioeconomic status, access barriers (insurance, funding, navigating health care systems), and health literacy (LoPresti et al., 2016). Language barriers for non-English speakers contribute to a lack of thorough understanding of many aspects of the health care system, and scant resources exist to fund culturally appropriate and comprehensive written information in languages other than English (Watts et al., 2018). A scoping literature review indicated that low health literacy in homeless populations combined with a lack of understanding about the Importance of health literacy among health care professionals and organizations contributes to significant barriers in cancer care (Lawrie et al., 2020). Lack of discussions in oncology care about sexual orientation and gender identity negatively affect both quality of life and clinical outcomes (Cathcart-Rake et al., 2020).

Transitioning to Hospice

Palliative care teams help educate patients and families about options for care as they approach the end of life, including hospice care. The transition to hospice is often eased when a relationship has been established with palliative care and the patient's and family's values and goals of care have already been explored. Patients choose hospice when treatment options are no longer curative, when there is a six-month or less prognosis, and when they elect to focus on comfort, quality of life, and time at home rather than life-prolonging treatment. Hospice teams provide interdisciplinary care in homes as well as care facilities to provide symptom management, support, and guidance for caregivers. Hospice teams include physicians, nurses, social workers, chaplains, certified nursing assistants, physical therapists, occupational therapists, and other ancillary service workers such as volunteers who provide help around the house or opportunities for caregivers to take breaks. Focused visits provide expert symptom management as well as emotional and spiritual support for patients and families. Social workers can also assist with additional caregiving resources if there are unmet care needs, such as in-home caregiving shifts that are not covered by hospice.

Hospice benefits include durable medical equipment as well as medications related to the end-of-life diagnosis. Patients usually receive care in the home or a care facility. Occasionally, if symptom management is more complex than can be managed where the patient resides, patients go to an inpatient hospice or a specialized hospital under the hospice's general inpatient benefit. Hospice is covered by Medicare and Medicaid, and most commercial plans have similar coverage. However, some commercial plans present barriers to care, including high deductibles, paltry coverage, and unreasonable waiting periods. Hospice teams should assist patients in verifying coverage; occasionally, a higher level of advocacy will be needed with insurers to ensure that patients get the care they need.

Hospice is paid through a per diem rate that covers all care related to the admitting diagnosis, meaning that hospice can only cover care that is palliative focused. This can be a barrier to care if, for example, patients require frequent blood transfusions or IV fluids (which can be life prolonging but also palliative for some symptoms). Some hospices cover a limited number of these services and/or a brief period of palliative radiation but not chemotherapy due to both cost and focus of care. Even if patients would benefit from the services that hospice provides, forgoing other treatments can be a barrier to patients agreeing to hospice.

Misconceptions about what hospice is and what it provides—people often wrongly assume that hospice is only for the very final days of life or that hospice teams expedite death with focus on comfort medications—have led to underuse of hospice (Box 14.1). Additionally, new treatments such as immunotherapies and targeted therapies have presented additional options and changed illness trajectories (Patel et al., 2020).

Box 14.1

Mrs. M was a 29-year-old Chinese female with metastatic colon cancer. When first seen by palliative care, she was receiving third-line treatment. She had two young children and was very motivated to continue treatment as long as possible. Her functional status was changing rapidly, and she spent considerable time in clinic receiving fluids and other care as she continued chemotherapy. She understood that her illness was serious but was reluctant to discuss prognosis. Culturally, her family did not discuss illness and believed that talking about it could worsen someone's condition. Mrs. M's husband attended appointments infrequently and did not initially engage with the palliative care team. Although extended family provided tangible support (childcare, meals, etc.), Mrs. M felt uncomfortable discussing her fears and distress with them. She presented as significantly depressed and agreed to counseling sessions with the oncology palliative care social worker. During these sessions, Mrs. M was able to be more vulnerable and allowed herself to discuss the impacts of cancer. Eventually, she was able to engage in more serious illness conversations with the interdisciplinary palliative care team.

The oncology treatment team experienced moral distress over continuing treatment for Mrs. M and worried about the opportunity cost of time in the clinic rather than at home with family. The palliative care team provided staff support and additional context about Mrs. M's culture, values, and goals as a young parent. Over two months of continued clinical decline, palliative care interventions helped her identify and achieve prioritized family activities. She was also able to engage in limited legacy work, which was a huge shift given her initial reluctance to acknowledge her prognosis. Her husband became open to more support from the team, although he continued to believe that Mrs. M would stabilize. The palliative care team also supported her transition to hospice care. She was able to die at home with her family, a goal that advance care planning discussions identified. The palliative care team supported the oncology treatment team with this emotionally difficult case while providing education about cultural and developmental factors in the patient's decision-making.

Palliative care teams empower patients with the tools to enhance quality of life while living with serious illness and/or preparing for death with goal-concordant care. They also help teach primary palliative care skills to oncology providers. With additional expertise in symptom management and communication, as well as interdisciplinary teamwork, palliative care teams provide specialty care to patients and families.

Palliative care can help bridge gaps in care for patients of color; LGBTQ+ patients; patients with diverse backgrounds, cultures, and languages; patients experiencing poverty; and other underserved populations by acknowledging that structural racism and inequities exist, approaching patients and their families with cultural humility, and building relationships to offer emotional and spiritual support, better navigation of health care, and access to services (Box 14.1). Palliative care teams have unique opportunities to learn more about these inequities and spend additional time addressing barriers for underserved populations. Palliative care clinicians typically can spend more time with patients and families and, as a result, learn more about their values, cultural considerations, and access to resources. A trauma-informed approach and a concerted effort to learn about cultural perspectives, values, identity, and barriers to care can build rapport and lead to better care and outcomes.

Relationships with the palliative care team often result in earlier referrals to hospice care, as well as an easier transition to hospice. The interdisciplinary team provides important education and support around medical decision-making and facilitates the understanding of hospice as a service that supports quality of life and goals of care rather than hospice being a place to die. Palliative and hospice care explore hopes for end of life, focusing on values, rituals, cultural beliefs, and spiritual practices to enhance patients' quality of life and help them maintain dignity as they progress to end of life.

Box 14.2

Mr. B was a 76-year-old Black male with advanced lung cancer. Prior to diagnosis, Mr. B coached Little League baseball and was active in his church. After surgical resection, he experienced some relief in symptoms but did not return to his prior level of functioning. Mr. B denied discomfort despite visible symptoms, but his pain led him to seek emergency room treatment. Afterward, his oncologist discussed prognosis and explored goals of care with Mr. B and his wife. Mr. B became angry during the appointment, stating that he was not just going to go home and die. Given his reaction and stated goals of care, Mr. B's oncologist delayed palliative care referral despite pain and other symptom burden. In time, Mr. B reluctantly agreed to a referral to the oncology/palliative care social worker.

The social worker identified that Mr. B was experiencing depression, anxiety, and grief related to his loss of independence. His unwillingness to discuss pain was tied to his perception that pain was something to endure coupled with mistrust of the clinical team. His wife reported being overwhelmed by his increasing care needs and concerned about his decline. After reframing and providing education, the couple became more open to additional support and interventions. A serious illness conversation was conducted, during which Mr. B expressed that he was amenable to palliative care services. The palliative care team provided symptom management and support to both Mr. B and wife as cancer treatment proceeded. As he declined and his functional limitations increased, he continued to discuss care goals and agreed to transition to a community partner providing home palliative care services. After a brief time on home palliative care during which he received symptom management and support for his emotional and spiritual distress, Mr. B transitioned to in-home hospice services.

Guiding Best Practices for the Future

Early palliative care referrals can mitigate symptoms and enhance support as well as foster relationship building that can facilitate earlier and more comprehensive discussions about goals of care as illness progresses. Palliative care teams can also assist in grief and legacy work and other forms of meaning-making as patients and families navigate end-of-life issues. Using a lens of cultural humility, palliative care teams can explore barriers to care for underserved populations.

Pearls

- Every patient with advanced cancer would benefit from access to palliative care services. When specialty palliative care is not available, clinicians can still implement primary palliative care skills and approaches.
- Social workers should maintain an active role in pain and symptom management, using clinical assessments and interventions to address distress, trauma, and suffering along with barriers related to social determinants of health.
- Clinicians need to practice cultural humility to learn the nuances of cultural, religious, and spiritual beliefs as they impact patients' perceptions of illness, care, and death.

Pitfalls

- If palliative care teams do not make a concerted effort to build rapport with their oncology providers, it will result in less trust and collaboration as well as fewer referrals.
- Avoiding prognostic awareness discussions affects care decisions and crucial opportunities for meaning-making at end of life.
- Late referrals to palliative care result in decreased hospice use.

Additional Resources

Center to Advance Palliative Care: www.capc.org
National Hospice and Palliative Care Organization: www.nhpco.org
Serious Illness Conversation Guide: https://www.ariadnelabs.org/serious-illness-care/

References

Altilio, T., Otis-Green, S., & Cagle, J. (2011). The social work role in pain and symptom management. In T. Altilio & S. Otis-Green (Eds.), *Oxford textbook of palliative social work* (pp. 271–286). Oxford University Press.

Abernethy, E. R., Campbell, G. P., & Pentz, R. D. (2019). Why many oncologists fail to share accurate prognoses: They care deeply for their patients. *Cancer*, *126*(6), 1163–1165. https://doi.org/10.1002/cncr.32635

Bickel, K. E., McNiff, K., Buss, M. K., Kamal, A., Lupu, D., Abernethy, A. P., Broder, M. S., Shapiro, C. L., Acheson, A. K., Malin, J., Evans, T., & Krzyzanowska, M. K. (2016.) Defining high-quality palliative care in oncology practice: An American Society of Clinical Oncology/ American Academy of Hospice and Palliative Medicine guidance statement. *Journal of Oncology Practice, 12*(9), e828–e838. https://doi.org/10.1200/JOP.2016.010686

Boles, J. C., & Jones, M. T. (2021). Legacy perceptions and interventions for adults and children receiving palliative care: A systematic review. *Palliative Medicine, 35*(3), 529–551. https://doi.org/10.1177/0269216321989565

Cathcart-Rake, E., O'Connor, J., Ridgeway, J. L., Breitkopf, C. R., Kaur, J. S., Mitchell, J., Leventakos, K., & Jatoi, A. (2020). Patients' perspectives and advice on how to discuss sexual orientation, gender identity, and sexual health in oncology clinics. *American Journal of Hospice and Palliative Medicine, 37*(12), 1053–1061. https://doi.org/10.1177/1049909120910084

Center to Advance Palliative Care. (n.d.). *About* palliative *care*. Retrieved December 4, 2021, from https://www.capc.org/about/palliative-care/

Dillon, E. C., Meehan, A., Nasrallah, C., Lai, S., Colocci, N., & Luft, H. (2021). Evolving goals of care discussions as described in interviews with individuals with advanced cancer and oncology and palliative care teams. *American Journal of Hospice and Palliative Medicine, 38*(7), 785–793. https://doi.org/10.1177/1049909120969202

Ferrell, B. R., Temel, J. S., Temin, S., & Smith, T. J. (2017). Integration of palliative care into standard oncology care: ASCO clinical practice guideline update summary. *Journal of Oncology Practice, 13*(2), 119–121. https://doi.org/10.1200/jop.2016.017897

Griggs, J. J. (2020). Disparities in palliative care in patients with cancer. *Journal of Clinical Oncology, 38*(9), 974–979. https://doi.org/10.1200/jco.19.02108

Givler, A., Bhatt, H., & Maani-Fogelman, P. A. (2022, Jan.). The importance of cultural competence in pain and palliative care. *StatPearls*. Updated May 8, 2022. https://www.ncbi.nlm.nih.gov/books/NBK493154/

Halpern, J. J. (Ed.). (2020, February). *Core curriculum for palliative and hospice social work*. Social Work in Hospice and Palliative Care Network. https://swhpn.memberclicks.net/assets/Core%20Curriculum%20Preview%20Ed01%20030520.pdf

Hui, D., & E. Bruera. (2020). Models of palliative care delivery for patients with cancer. *Journal of Clinical Oncology, 38*(9), 852–865. https://doi.org/10.1200/jco.18.02123

Krawczyk, M., Wood, J., & Clark, D. (2018) Total pain: Origins, current practice, and future directions. *Omsorg: Norwegian Journal of Palliative Care, 2018*(2). http://eprints.gla.ac.uk/167847/

Lawrie, K., Charow, R., Giuliani, M., & Papadakos, J. (2020). Homelessness, cancer, and health literacy: A scoping review. *Journal of Health Care for the Poor and Underserved, 31*(1), 81–104. https://doi.org/10.1353/hpu.2020.0010

LoPresti, M. A., Dement, F., & Gold, H. T. (2016). End-of-life care for people with cancer from ethnic minority groups. *American Journal of Hospice and Palliative Medicine, 33*(3), 291–305. https://doi.org/10.1177/1049909114565658

Morrison, R. S., Meier, D. E., & Arnold, R. M. (2021). What's wrong with advance care planning? *Journal of the American Medical Association, 326*(16), 1575. https://doi.org/10.1001/jama.2021.16430

National Coalition for Hospice and Palliative Care. (2018). Clinical *practice guidelines for quality palliative care* (4th ed.). Retrieved from https://www.nationalcoalitionhpc.org/wp-content/uploads/2020/07/NCHPC-NCPGuidelines_4thED_web_FINAL.pdf

National Hospice and Palliative Care Organization. (2020, July 13). *History of hospice*. Retrieved from https://www.nhpco.org/hospice-care-overview/history-of-hospice/

Patel, M. N., Nicolla, J. M., Friedman, F. A. P., Ritz, M. R., & Kamal, A. H. (2020). Hospice use among patients with cancer: Trends, barriers, and future directions. *JCO Oncology Practice, 16*(12), 803–809. https://doi.org/10.1200/op.20.00309

Rego, F., Gonçalves, F., Moutinho, S., Castro, L., & Nunes, R. (2020). The influence of spirituality on decision-making in palliative care outpatients: A cross-sectional study. *BMC Palliative Care*, *19*(1). https://doi.org/10.1186/s12904-020-0525-3

Smith, C. B., Phillips, T., & Smith, T. J. (2018, October 29). Using the new ASCO clinical practice guideline for palliative care concurrent with oncology care using the team approach. *American Society of Clinical Oncology Educational Book*, *37*, 714–723. https://doi.org/10.1200/edbk_175474

Watts, K. J., Meiser, B., Zilliacus, E., Kaur, R., Taouk, M., Girgis, A., Butow, P., Kissane, D. W., Hale, S., Perry, A., Aranda, S. K., & Goldstein, D. (2018). Perspectives of oncology nurses and oncologists regarding barriers to working with patients from a minority background: Systemic issues and working with interpreters. *European Journal of Cancer Care*, *27*(2), e12758. https://doi.org/10.1111/ecc.12758

Weng, K., Shearer, J., & Grangaard Johnson, L. (2022). Developing successful palliative care teams in rural communities: A facilitated process. *Journal of Palliative Medicine*, *25*(5), 734–741. https://doi.org/10.1089/jpm.2021.0287

Wu, C. C., Hsu, T. W., Chang, C. M., Lee, C. H., Huang, C. Y., Lee, C. C. (2016, June). Palliative chemotherapy affects aggressiveness of end-of-life care. *Oncologist*, *21*(6), 771–777. https://doi.org/10.1634/theoncologist.2015-0445.

15

Grief, Loss, and Bereavement in Oncology and Palliative Care

Kimarie Knowles, Abigail Nathanson, Danetta Hendricks Sloan, and Grace Christ

Key Concepts

- Bereavement care is an integral part of oncology and palliative care.
- Theoretical grounding is important when working with bereft individuals.
- A comprehensive assessment is vital in understanding the unique grief experience of the client and to guide appropriate clinical intervention.
- Assessment should include one's history, biopsychosocial factors, cultural context, and social location.
- Clinicians must be aware that their own privilege and biases have an impact on assessment and treatment.
- While most bereft individuals adjust and cope well without the need for professional help, a subset of grievers may develop psychological distress that warrants professional intervention.
- Current recommendations for bereavement treatment include tiered levels that can be incorporated into oncology and palliative care settings.

Keywords: assessment, bereavement, grief, intervention, loss, prolonged grief disorder, theory

Oncology and palliative care social workers support patients, caregivers, and communities experiencing loss, grief, and bereavement throughout the illness trajectory. This work spans from time of diagnosis through end of life and into bereavement. As such, social workers witness patients' and caregivers' experiences of illness, help enhance coping techniques, and provide support for those with whom they work.

While the experiences of loss are universal, comprehending the nuanced ways that providers integrate those experiences in treatment plans may be

Kimarie Knowles, Abigail Nathanson, Danetta Hendricks Sloan, and Grace Christ, *Grief, Loss, and Bereavement in Oncology and Palliative Care* In: *Oncology and Palliative Social Work*. Edited by: Susan Hedlund, Bryan Miller, Grace Christ, and Carolyn Messner, Oxford University Press. © Oxford University Press 2024. DOI: 10.1093/oso/9780197607299.003.0015 useful in formulating assessment and interventions. Whereas *bereavement* is defined as the state of having experienced a loss from death, *grief* is defined as the response (emotional, affective, somatic, spiritual, existential, and so on) associated with loss (PDQ Supportive and Palliative Care Editorial Board [PDQ], 2020). *Mourning* is the outward expression of grief, driven largely by sociopolitical identities and socialization (for example, age, gender, culture, and socioeconomic status), that occurs during a period of bereavement. Social workers can understand losses temporally—in other words, whether they occur before a death (predeath grief) or in anticipation of losses later (anticipatory grief). Losses may also be understood to be physical or symbolic, concrete or ambiguous, and socially acknowledged or disenfranchised. All these categorizations speak to the ways in which each person's experience both within their society and with their loss will affect how they process and integrate bereavement, grief, and mourning. In this chapter, we focus primarily on grief associated with a loss due to death from cancer. We begin with a brief overview of anticipatory grief and theoretical models of bereavement to help conceptualize our understanding of grief. This is followed by an in-depth discussion on the importance of a thorough bereavement assessment. Finally, we present a tiered intervention approach.

Anticipatory Grief

Grief begins at the moment of awareness that something significant has changed—this moment could be experiencing a symptom, receiving a worrying test result or a crisis, or hearing of an actual death. We may think of grief along a timeline trajectory: preloss, anticipatory, or bereavement. Preloss grief refers to the losses people experience before death, such as the loss of roles or functions, health, relationships, and so on. People experience anticipatory grief in the present, in anticipation of losses to follow with worsening health or death, including future experiences and relationships that will likely not be realized (Caserta et al., 2019). In bereavement, grief occurs after a death, and includes both the entirety of the losses that occurred during illness and the sense of loss for the life not lived by or with the person who died. Any of these losses may be concrete (death, a role, a function), symbolic (connection, history), or ambiguous (as with dementia, a psychological absence while still living).

When working with anticipatory grief, clinicians must carefully balance adaptive avoidance and the compartmentalization that aids in daily functioning, with the very real benefit of advance preparation. Many interventions appropriate for bereavement, such as naming, normalizing, facilitating social support, and allowing opportunities for sharing and venting, also apply during anticipatory grief. Sometimes, patients and families need more practical guidance with financial and legal matters, funeral planning, or anticipating the ways in which a loss will impact their lives (Caserta et al., 2019). Social workers should be mindful that not every patient or family member needs to actively anticipate future losses; in fact, depending on both culture and personal temperament, this may be contraindicated. A good place to begin assessing where a patient or family member is and what they may need, is to ask them how they feel they are coping, how much they want to know about what illness and grief may look like, and what their thoughts are about the future. Often, letting families know that bereavement can be a shock, even if it is not a surprise, can help normalize the flood of emotions that may come after death.

Theoretical Models

While there are many valuable theoretical models of grief and bereavement, we focus here on three approaches with high utility for oncology and palliative care social workers, the dual process model (DPM) (Stroebe & Schut, 2010), attachment theory, and meaning reconstruction theories (Neimeyer et al., 2009). These approaches are largely developmental and existential in nature, while the other commonly held theories of grief may be in a stage/phase/task models and provide different perspectives.

The DPM posits that healthy and adaptive grief is an oscillation process between loss-oriented and restoration-oriented activities (Stroebe & Schut, 2010). Loss orientation refers to the process of focusing on and expressing the loss experience itself. Activities during this process might include telling the story of the death, talking about one's experience in grief, looking at photos of the person who died, visiting the grave or special spaces that remind the individual of the person, or any other action that focuses on the death and absence of the person. Restoration orientation refers to the ways in which an individual copes with changes brought about by the loss or begins to restore their life. Restoration-orientated activities might include taking on new roles and responsibilities (a new job, learning home skills—laundry, cooking, finances), engaging in activities that provide distance from the intense grief feelings (distraction, learning something new), and taking on new identities and relationships. One of the most important aspects of the DPM is that the griever oscillates back and forth between these two orientations (Stroebe & Schut, 2010). This model is particularly useful to help the bereaved normalize the waves of grief they experience rather than feel they are regressing every time they return to process the loss. Unlike many other models that focus on a White, male, Western view of decathexis (withdrawal of emotional and mental energy from the deceased) to deal with loss, the DPM also holds a wide frame for people who grieve both instrumentally and intuitively, to maintain continuing bonds and allowing people to mourn in whatever ways are culturally and temperamentally appropriate for them.

Grief is an outcome of love or connection. Thus, by understanding the ways in which we love and connect, we can better understand the ways in which we grieve. As such, attachment theory is important to understanding grief. Every person has an attachment system formed in childhood that continues into adulthood. Attachment figures influence our sense of being protected, supported, loved, and cared for (when things go well), and contribute to how we think about others, how we see ourselves in relation to others, and how we understand relationships in general (Zech & Arnold, 2011). When our attachment figures are present and consistent enough throughout childhood, we have a sense of being cared for by others, being safe in our bodies, and being able to trust that our needs will be met. When someone we are attached to dies, our feelings of security and safety may be disrupted along with our concept of who we are and how we engage with the world. From this perspective, grieving might involve a renegotiation of the attachment to the deceased person as well as the formation of attachments that help create feelings of safety, security, and protection.

The final theoretical model of bereavement we highlight here is a meaning-making or constructivist model. This perspective holds that people create meaning in their lives, which assists each individual in understanding oneself and navigating the world. When a person experiences a loss due to death, the griever enters a complex process of adapting to their changed reality. In this model, we can understand grieving as the process by which individuals reconstruct the meaning of who they are, what the world is like, and how they operate in the world in light of this loss (Neimeyer et al., 2009). This may involve finding a new sense of meaning and purpose, redefining what relationships look like, leaning into familiar roles and rituals to assimilate the loss, or expanding worldviews to accommodate the loss.

The DPM provides a way to view adaptive grieving as an oscillation process between grief and restoration. We can understand that the ways people engage in that oscillation is driven by both attachment paradigms and meaning-making efforts. Clinicians must engage with curiosity and empathy when working with a bereft individual, family, or community in order to understand the ways in which attachment bonds were formed and meaning was constructed around the life and death of the person who died.

Assessment

Assessing bereft individuals is an important aspect of treatment. Each patient and each caregiver system is unique. Each grieving individuals' experience, even within the same family, social, or cultural system, will also be unique. As such, ongoing assessment should consider one's history, biopsychosocial factors, and cultural context, all of which combine to inform an individual's and family's experience of grief and guide appropriate clinical intervention.

Physical/Somatic

Common physical and somatic symptoms of acute grief may include changes in sleep, appetite, fatigue, cognition, muscle tension or aches, abdominal/digestive distress, palpitations, headaches, and tearfulness (Killikelly et al., 2018; PDQ, 2020; Table 15.1). Some symptoms may be culturally based, and clinicians from a culture that is different from the bereft individual/family should be mindful of cultural context in their assessments of symptoms as functional or pathological.

Table 15.1 Common/Typical Grief Symptoms

Emotions	Cognitions	Behaviors	Physical Symptoms
Sadness Anger/irritability	Changes in executive function (disorganization, "grief brain")	Avoidance of or seeking out reminders of the loss/deceased	Changes in energy level (fatigue, hyperactivity)
Despair Anxiety	Preoccupation with thinking about the deceased	Crying	Changes in sleep patterns
Yearning/longing for deceased	Intrusive images of the illness and death		Changes in appetite
Guilt			
Regret	Cognitive changes		Abdominal/digestive distress
Relief		Withdrawal from social interactions or not wanting to be alone.	
Numbness	Attempts to understand illness and death		Muscle tension/aches
Shock			Headaches
Disbelief	Re-experiencing the deceased (visions, voices, dreams)		Palpitations
Gratitude		Short temper	Sexual changes
Connection	Ruminations/racing thoughts		

Sources: Jerome, 2017; Killikelly et al., 2018; Lichtenthal et al., 2020; PDQ, 2020; University of Nottingham, 2010.

Box 15.1

M.J. self-referred for bereavement services after the loss of her mother to breast cancer. When the clinician inquired about M.J.'s physical/somatic symptoms and her own health care needs, M.J. shared that in addition to changes in her sleep and eating patterns, she also had not had her yearly mammogram or followed up with a genetic counselor. Her mother was BRCA positive, placing her at increased risk for getting cancer herself, and she expressed fear around facing her own risk as well as the risk her children may face.

Fully assessing how the caregiving and grief experience has affected one's health is important (Box 15.1). While significant changes to sleep, appetite, and energy are more common than not, bereft individuals should be encouraged to follow up with their doctors regarding their own health needs, which may have been postponed due to the focus on the deceased person's care to make sure there is not a concurrent medical condition or concern about physical health. In addition to assessing the caregiver's health, it is also important to understand the deceased person's illness experience and any family history and narrative of cancer.

Psychological/Relational

In addition to common physical and somatic symptoms of grief are typical emotional reactions, including emotional numbness, shock, disbelief, yearning for the deceased, anxiety, anger, sadness, despair, guilt, disorganization, preoccupation with thinking about the deceased, intrusive images of the death, and reexperiencing the deceased (visions, voices, dreams) (Killikelly et al., 2018; PDQ, 2020). These symptoms can feel distressing and overwhelming but change in their level of intensity and frequency for most individuals over time. While there is no set time frame for grief, many people experience a decrease in the intensity of their symptoms after the first 6 to 12 months; this decrease usually continues over the first few years (PDQ, 2020). It is important to note that symptoms and time frames vary between and within cultures.

While most bereft individuals do feel better over time, a subset of grievers (15%–30%) (PDQ, 2020) may develop psychological distress, including major depressive disorder (MDD), post-traumatic stress disorder (PTSD), and prolonged grief disorder (PGD) (Lichtenthal et al., 2020). Research has confirmed that these disorders are distinct diagnoses with unique treatment recommendations (PDQ, 2020).

PGD, a newly recognized mental health disorder, was included in the World Health Organization's (WHO) 11th edition of the *International Classification of Diseases* (ICD-11) (WHO, 2018) and the 5th edition (Text Revision) of the American Psychological Association's (APA) *Diagnostic and Statistical Manual* (DSM-5-TR) (APA, 2022). PGD is characterized by a longing for or preoccupation with the deceased that is accompanied by intense emotional pain (sadness, guilt, anger, denial, blame, difficulty accepting the death, feeling one has lost a part of oneself, an inability to experience positive mood, emotional numbness, and difficulty in engaging with social or other activities). The death must have occurred at least 6 months prior (ICD-11) or 12 months prior (DSM-5-TR), and the symptoms must lead to substantial impairment that exceeds the norms for the individual's social, cultural, or religious context (APA, 2022; WHO, 2018).

Some concerns exist regarding this new diagnosis of PGD, including questions about the applicability of the PGD criteria outside the Global North (Stelzer et al., 2018). The current understanding and approach to grief and bereavement treatment is founded on Western models of psychological health, which historically have been based on the experiences of White, European men (Granek & Peleg-Sagy, 2017). Studies have demonstrated variability among diverse cultures in terms of the types of symptoms and frequency with which the criteria for PGD are met (Granek & Peleg-Sagy, 2017; Stelzer et al., 2020). Oncology and palliative social workers should use caution when thinking about diagnosing a bereft individual. Additional research with diverse populations as well as cultural adaptations may improve the utility of this diagnosis.

Box 15.2

The inpatient social worker was paged immediately following the death of a patient in the hospital. The referring staff member reported "abnormal" behavior, with family members crying and screaming loudly over the body and refusing to leave the room. Upon entering the room, the social worker recognized the communal wailing as part of this family's culturally congruent expression of grief. A plan was made for the hospital to provide adequate space and time for the family to mourn prior to moving the patient to the morgue. The social worker stayed with the family at their request and allowed time for each family member to express their grief through words honoring the deceased as well as ritual communal wailing.

Because such deep cultural differences can exist in bereavement and mourning, social workers should conduct a nuanced psychological and relational assessment. Assessing bereft individuals will provide the clinician with a wealth of understanding about the individual's grief experience and help direct the level of intervention (Box 15.2). Certain psychological and relationship factors have been identified that can be protective or can increase risk for mental health challenges in bereavement. Areas important to explore include the bereft person's relationship with the deceased as well as their current mental state and any history of mental health challenges and trauma (Strada, 2019). Relational areas that can increase one's risk of PGD include a conflictual or dependent relationship with the deceased, conflict with family members, avoidant or ruminative coping styles, insecure attachment, and isolating oneself from others. Current and past mental health diagnoses, previous traumatic experiences, current or past suicidal ideation or attempt, and current feelings of regret, guilt, and avoidance can also increase one's risk (Roberts et al., 2017; Strada, 2019). Protective factors include having a strong social support network, secure attachment style, and older age (above 60) (PDQ, 2020).

Social/Societal

A social and societal assessment of a bereft individual starts with understanding whether and how one's basic needs for survival are being met. It also includes the ways in which the circumstances of the death along with current and historical societal systems of oppression intersect with one's grief. In what areas does the bereft person have or perceive a lack of resources? Is there financial, food, housing, and health insurance security or did the death impact some or all these areas? How have systems of oppression, including discrimination, racism, sexism, homophobia, inequality, poverty, and immigration status, affected the patient's life and death, and how is the grieving individual making meaning within this context?

Certain factors related to the social situation and circumstances of the illness and death are associated with greater psychological distress in bereavement. Social factors that contribute to greater distress include financial hardship, severity of stressful life events, and lack of perceived available social support (PDQ, 2020). Circumstances of the illness and death include poor patient quality of life at the end of life; illness and death that are perceived as painful, traumatic, or unexpected; and difficulty with advanced care planning (Roberts et al., 2017).

Studies have shown that in oncology and palliative care settings at end of life, Black Americans have poorer outcomes, are offered less pain management, have fewer end-of-life and advanced-care planning discussions, have a lower quality of life, and die earlier than White patients (Jones et al., 2021). Racism and discriminatory practices affect housing, jobs, and financial security, which in turn can lead to delays in diagnosis and poorer treatment outcomes (Rosenblatt & Wallace, 2005). In addition, some bereft individuals carry with them cultural and historical traumas perpetuated by systemic racism and structural barriers that have led to understandable mistrust of the medical system. Medical racism and neglect (racism and discriminatory practices related to the health care system) will have an impact on a loved one's grief experience (Bordere, 2016). One qualitative study of Black American adults found that 40% of participants believed their loved one's death was related to medical racism. Medical racism may include denial of services, inadequate informed consent discussions, being offered minimal or substandard care, or care from underqualified providers (Rosenblatt & Wallace, 2005) (Box 15.3).

Understanding how each grieving individual makes meaning of the life and death of the person who died, including the contributing factors that affected the death, is vital to a clinician's assessment. While not every individual who is part of a community that has been historically marginalized will attribute the death to the impacts of social injustice, it is imperative that clinicians, especially White clinicians, actively reflect and invite discourse and discussion in these areas.

Box 15.3

Social worker reached out to the patient's partner (L.S.) to offer bereavement support. During the initial phone call, L.S. stated that her partner suffered traumatic and uncontrollable pain at the end of life. She expressed anger and frustration with the medical system, stating that in the last 3 weeks of the patient's life, she asked the medical team to increase the pain medication or change it to something that might work better. She felt that her advocacy was ignored because her partner was Black and had been active in Narcotics Anonymous for the past 20 years. The subsequent feelings of powerlessness, injustice, and trauma in bearing witness to so much needless suffering left L.S. deeply distressed and symptomatic in her bereavement. She described the traumatic images and nightmares that she now experiences related to witnessing her partner's pain and suffering.

Spirituality

Religion and spirituality play a vital role in many grievers' lives and will affect the ways in which they understand and cope with bereavement. Possessing a comprehensive understanding of what *spirituality* includes is helpful to the clinician and the client with whom they are working. Dimensions of spirituality include connectedness, meaning, purpose, beliefs, values, peace, community, and faith (Ribeiro Miller et al., 2019). Just as each individual's grief is unique, so too are their spiritual beliefs (Box 15.4). Affiliation with any specific organized religion should not prevent the clinician from engaging in a thorough spiritual assessment. For some, the rituals and traditions by which certain spiritual practices abide after a death (sitting shiva, attending a wake, belief in an afterlife) along with community support and deeper existential connection provides a sense of comfort after a loss. For others, a death can create a crisis in faith that leads to a sense of meaninglessness and distress during a difficult time.

Box 15.4

In the fourth session of a bereavement group for the loss of a sibling, a quiet member tentatively asked if anyone else had experienced signs that their sibling was present. She went on to share that although she was raised Christian, she had always been drawn to the idea of reincarnation. Over the last week, she went for a hike and came to a stream where a beaver was building a dam. She described sitting and watching the beaver as it built and interacted with her (looking at her, coming close without fear, being playful). She felt a deep sense of connection to her brother in that moment and believed the beaver was actually her brother who always loved nature. She took comfort in the experience but worried others would judge her.

Cultural

Grief is a universal experience; however, the ways in which it is expressed are culturally bound and influenced by one's beliefs, attitudes, values, behaviors, and practices (Box 15.5). To fully assess a bereft individual's experience with grief, clinicians must attend to the social locations (ethnicity, race, religion/spirituality, sexuality, nationality, age, gender identity, family structure, ability, education, socioeconomic status, and more) (Bordere, 2016; Granek & Peleg-Sagy, 2017) in which the bereft person exists while also acknowledging their own social location and its impact on the clinical relationship. Clinicians should endeavor to continually evaluate their own biases and privileges as well as seek out clinical supervision in order to practice cultural awarenessand humility.

Box 15.5

In a closed bereavement group for the loss of a parent, a daughter (J.B.) shared a photo of her mother who died of cancer. She explained that her mother was White, and her father was Black. J.B. shared that until her mother's death, she was able to straddle and feel comfortable in two worlds. "My mother was my membership card to the White world. Even when spending time in familial spaces with progressive and racially conscious White people, my mother created an umbrella of safety and acceptance around me. When she died, my membership card was revoked, and I became a guest in these spaces." Within the group experience, it was important to allow for exploration and acceptance around the impact that the death had on J.B.'s racial identity and how this change was connected to her unique experience of loss and grief.

Interventions

The *Clinical Practice Guidelines for Quality Palliative Care* (National Consensus Project for Quality Palliative Care [NCPQPC], 2018) recommends that bereavement support be available to caregivers for a minimum of 13 months after a patient's death. The guidelines further recommended that bereavement services be available directly or through referral and should include access to support (grief counseling, spiritual support, peer support), educational resources, and commemorative services. The palliative care team should seek to identify individuals at risk of PGD and provide "interventions in accordance with developmental, cultural, and spiritual needs" (NCPQPC, 2018).

Over the past 3 years, the world has been changed by the COVID-19 pandemic with over 6.5 million deaths worldwide (over 1 million in the United States) as of this writing. Due to the nature of the pandemic and the increased risk of infection to those treated by palliative care and oncology teams, necessary safety measures will have impacted the end of life for patients and caregivers as well as the grieving experience. Many grievers were unable to engage in cultural and ritual activities meant to provide support and guidance when mourning. In addition, there were disparities among historically marginalized communities in COVID-19 cases, deaths, access to care, and vaccinations (Johns Hopkins University, 2022). Increased psychological challenges such as increased levels of anxiety, depression, and traumatic stress are already evident (Mental Health America, 2022). With these unprecedented levels of loss worldwide, it is imperative that oncology and palliative care social workers enhance their skills in this area, provide clinically appropriate interventions, and advocate for governmental leadership to support bereft individuals.

In a comprehensive synthesis of the literature related to bereavement services commissioned by the United Kingdom Department of Health, three levels of intervention were identified: "(i) acknowledgement and information-based services; (ii) one to one support and/or peer support; and (iii) more intensive therapeutic and structured bereavement interventions for more complex grief reactions" (University of Nottingham, 2010). These categories fit well with Lichtenthal et al.'s (2020) recommendations to use the CARE (*Communicate* compassionately, *Assess* risk for acute bereavement challenges, *Refer* when appropriate, and *Educate* about resources) framework.

Combining these two frameworks, the first level of bereavement support would include acknowledgment, education, and commemorative services. This would include compassionately offering condolences, listening to the caregiver's experience, holding commemorative services, and providing psychoeducation, validation, and normalization around grief and bereavement. Education around typical grief reactions, self-care strategies, and the value of social support can help facilitate adjustment for the majority of grievers who are not at higher risk for mental health complications. The clinician must be mindful of the language they use and take care to normalize and validate the grief experience without labeling grievers' reactions as out of the ordinary or pathological. Anyone on the health care team with sufficient grief literacy can provide interventions at this first level.

The second level of intervention includes supportive counseling and participation in bereavement groups. We distinguish *supportive counseling* from *mental health therapy* (in Level 3; Table 15.2) in that supportive counseling focuses on venting, validation, and focusing on ego strengths rather than more intensive therapeutic work that involves processing long-standing personality development and trauma. Palliative or oncology social workers with some postgraduate specialty training in their field and sufficient grief literacy are best suited to provide this supportive level of intervention. Research on the effectiveness of bereavement interventions is variable (Currier et al., 2008) but some studies have shown that individuals who self-refer or are clinically referred to individual bereavement counseling or bereavement support groups have better treatment outcomes compared to participants who were recruited

Table 15.2 Bereavement Intervention: Three Levels of Care

	Level #1: General	Level #2: Moderate	Level #3: Intensive
Description	Information and guidance for most of the population and for most losses	Supportive counseling and bereavement groups for losses with moderate distress	Skilled intervention by trained specialists for major distress
Who Provides	Any grief-literate health care team member	Palliative and oncology-trained social workers (or similar)	Mental health providers with advanced, specialty training in bereavement disorders
Indications	Awareness of experiencing a loss Tolerating oscillation Able to engage social supports Uninterested in more intensive support Anticipatory or bereavement	Bereaved person feels they want or need more support Existing social supports are compromised for this need Rigidity in oscillation Significant concurrent psychosocial stressors	Bereaved persons express either concern about how they are coping or a need for more individual, specialized therapy Any immediate safety risk to self, others, ability to care for self Level 1 & 2 interventions are inadequate Meet criteria for PGD, PTSD, or other significant mental health diagnoses
Interventions	Compassionate acknowledgment and condolences Rituals and commemorative services Psychoeducation, validation, normalization	Assess risk and ability to cope Supportive services (individual counseling, support group, bereavement group) Increase social connections and support	Specialized bereavement interventions (e.g., complicated grief therapy) or other evidence-based interventions with empirical support for PGD (CBT, Eye Movement Desensitization and Reprocessing Therapy, Acceptance and Commitment Therapy, etc.)
Barriers	Grief literacy of providers Institutional: funding, role delineation, infrastructure Cultural variations	Accessible, culturally congruent services and providers Organizational barriers (financial constraints, fears of liability in assuming responsibility in outreach or assessing risk)	Accessible care (financially, logistically) Trained specialty providers Lack of awareness of existence, need Stigma, overnormalization Generalist therapists not aware of need for specialists in this area

using less personal outreach methods (for example, using death records to find and contact participants) (Jerome, 2017). Individual and group counseling can provide additional support that may promote the natural and adaptive grieving process. Bereavement groups have been noted to help grieving individuals in numerous ways, including reducing social isolation, increasing a sense of community, allowing for emotional expression, exchanging information and advice, instilling hope, and sharing in the universal experience of grief (Yalom & Leszcz, 2005). Additional factors that contribute to more positive (albeit small to moderate) treatment effects for bereavement support groups include homogeneity of group membership (in terms of type of loss) (Yalom & Leszcz, 2005), participating in more than six group sessions (Kustanti et al., 2021), and delivery by health care professionals trained in grief (Kustanti et al., 2021).

Clinicians should reserve the third and final level of intervention for individuals who have been assessed to be at higher risk of acute and prolonged bereavement challenges and require specialized mental health treatment for disorders such as depression, PTSD, and PGD. Only highly trained grief and trauma specialists should provide these interventions. Despite inconsistent findings and debate within the bereavement field around the effectiveness of interventions overall, research indicates that treatments targeting high-risk individuals have a more significant impact (Currier et al., 2008). Psychosocial interventions focusing on PGD are adaptations of cognitive behavioral therapy (CBT) that incorporate strategies from exposure therapy, cognitive restructuring, interpretive therapy, and interpersonal therapy (PDQ, 2020).

Guiding Best Practices for the Future

Bereavement care is part of oncology and palliative care. Continuity of services for caregivers, families, and communities is vital to assisting in the adaptive grief experience as well as identifying at-risk individuals and connecting them with higher-level care. Currently, financial and legal (fears around assuming liability for bereft caregivers) barriers can prohibit palliative care and oncology agencies from creating the needed infrastructure to offer a fully integrated three-level treatment approach. Addressing and reducing these barriers in addition to ensuring that accessible and culturally congruent services are provided are important first steps in providing comprehensive care. Oncology and palliative care social workers are uniquely positioned to advocate for these changes in infrastructure and to provide bereavement support to bereft individuals, families, and communities.

Pearls

- Grief is a natural response to loss. A range of biopsychosocial spiritual symptoms that may be culturally influenced are common and usually decrease in intensity over the first few years after a death.
- Conducting a thorough assessment to understand the unique experience and needs of each individual, family, or community is crucial.
- Racism, discriminatory practices, and systems of oppression negatively contribute to patient outcomes at end of life and therefore, affect the experience of grief.

Pitfalls

- The historical understanding of grief and bereavement is founded on Western models of psychological health, which historically have been based on the experiences of White, European men and focus on individualism over a collective identity. Additional research with diverse populations is needed to develop cultural understanding of grief and bereavement.
- When working with bereft individuals, families, and communities, clinicians should be mindful of the language they use as there is a wide range of typical grief responses based on social, cultural, and religious norms.
- Financial and legal barriers in palliative care and oncology settings and a lack of grief literacy in the community contribute to the scarcity of culturally congruent comprehensive bereavement services.

Additional Resources

Healing from grief [Audio podcast]. Huberman Labs. https://hubermanlab.com/the-science-and-process-of-healing-from-grief/

Alexander, Elizabeth. (2016). *The light of the world*. Grand Central.

Bonanno, George. (2009). *The other side of sadness*. Basic.

Harris, D. L., & Bordere, T. C. (2016). *Handbook of social justice in loss and grief: Exploring diversity, equity, and inclusion*. Routledge.

Gerbino, S., & Raymer, M. (2022). Holding on and letting go: The red thread of adult bereavement. In T. Altilio, S. Otis-Green, & J. G. Cagle (Eds.), *The Oxford textbook of palliative social work* (2nd ed.). Oxford University Press.

Neimeyer, R. A. (Ed.). (2015). *Techniques of grief therapy: Assessment and intervention*. Taylor & Francis.

References

American Psychiatric Association. (2022). *Diagnostic and statistical manual of mental disorders* (5th ed., Text Revision). American Psychiatric Association.

Bordere, T. C. (2016). Social justice conceptualizations in grief and loss. In D. Harris & T. Bordere (Eds.), *Handbook of social justice in loss and grief* (pp. 29–40). Routledge.

Caserta, M., Utz, R., Lund, D., Supiano, K., & Donaldson, G. (2019). Cancer caregivers' preparedness for loss and bereavement outcomes: Do preloss caregiver attributes matter? *Omega, 80*(2), 224–244. https://doi.org/10.1177/0030222817729610

Currier, J. M., Neimeyer, R. A., & Berman, J. S. (2008). The effectiveness of psychotherapeutic interventions for bereaved persons: A comprehensive quantitative review. *Psychological Bulletin, 134*(5), 648–661. https://doi.org/10.1037/0033-2909.134.5.648

Granek, L., & Peleg-Sagy, T. (2017). The use of pathological grief outcomes in bereavement studies on African Americans. *Transcultural Psychiatry, 54*(3), 384–399. https://doi.org/10.1177/1363461517708121

Jerome, H. (2017). *Outcomes of cancer bereavement therapeutic support groups* (Doctoral dissertation). University College London. https://discovery.ucl.ac.uk/id/eprint/1574714/

Jones, K. F., Laury, E., Sanders, J. J., Starr, L. T., Rosa, W. E., Booker, S. Q., Wachterman, M., Jones, C. A., Hickman, S., Merlin, J. S., & Meghani, S. H. (2021). Top ten tips palliative care clinicians should know about delivering antiracist care to Black Americans. *Journal of Palliative Medicine, 22*(3), 479–487. https://doi.org/10.1089/jpm.2021.0502

Johns Hopkins University. (n.d.). *Coronavirus resource center*. Retrieved September 26, 2022, from https://coronavirus.jhu.edu/

Killikelly, C., Bauer, S., & Maercker, A. (2018). The assessment of grief in refugees and post-conflict survivors: A narrative review of etic and emic research. *Frontiers in Psychology, 9*, 1957. https://doi.org/10.3389/fpsyg.2018.01957

Kustanti, C. Y., Fang, H. F., Linda Kang, X., Chiou, J. F., Wu, S. C., Yunitri, N., Chu, H., & Chou, K. R. (2021). The effectiveness of bereavement support for adult family caregivers in palliative care: A meta-analysis of randomized controlled trials. *Journal of Nursing Scholarship, 53*(2), 208–217. https://doi.org/10.1111/jnu.12630

Lichtenthal, W. G., Roberts, K. E., & Prigerson, H. G. (2020). Bereavement care in the wake of COVID-19: Offering condolences and referrals. *Annals of Internal Medicine, 173*(10), 833–835. https://doi.org/10.7326/M20-2526

Mental Health America. (2022). *Mental health and COVID-19*. Retrieved September 26, 2022, from https://mhanational.org/mental-health-and-covid-19-two-years-after-pandemic#:~:text=COVID%2D19%20has%20had%20a,and%20other%20mental%20health%20concerns

National Consensus Project for Quality Palliative Care. (2018). *Clinical practice guidelines for quality palliative care* (4th ed.). National Coalition for Hospice and Palliative Care. https://www.nationalcoalitionhpc.org/wp-content/uploads/2020/07/NCHPC-NCPGuidelines_4thED_web_FINAL.pdf

Neimeyer, R. A., Burke, L. A., Mackay, M. M., & van Dyke Stringer, J. G. (2009). Grief therapy and the reconstruction of meaning: From principles to practice. *Journal of Contemporary Psychotherapy, 40*, 73–83.

PDQ Supportive and Palliative Care Editorial Board. (2020). *Grief, bereavement, and coping with loss (PDQ®): Health professional version*. PDQ Cancer Information Summaries. National Cancer Institute. Retrieved December 16, 2021, from https://www.cancer.gov/about-cancer/advanced-cancer/caregivers/planning/bereavement-hp-pdq

Ribeiro Miller, D., Stewart, M., & Sumser, B. (2019). Spiritual, religious, and existential dimensions of care in palliative care: A guide for health social workers. In B. Sumser, M.

Leimena, & T. Altilio (Eds.), *Palliative care: A guide for health social workers* (pp. 122–147). Oxford University Press.

Roberts, K., Holland, J., Prigerson, H. G., Sweeney, C., Corner, G., Breitbart, W., & Lichtenthal, W. G. (2017). Development of the Bereavement Risk Inventory and Screening Questionnaire (BRISQ): Item generation and expert panel feedback. *Palliative & Supportive Care, 15*(1), 57–66. https://doi.org/10.1017/S1478951516000626

Rosenblatt, P., & Wallace, B. (2005). Racism as a cause of death. In P. Rosenblatt & B. Wallace (Eds), *African American grief* (pp. 7–18). Routledge/Taylor & Francis.

Stelzer, E. M., Zhou, N., Maercker, A., O'Connor, M. F., & Killikelly, C. (2020). Prolonged grief disorder and the cultural crisis. *Frontiers in Psychology, 10*, 2982. https://doi.org/10.3389/fpsyg.2019.02982

Stroebe, M., & Schut, H. (2010). The dual process model of coping with bereavement: A decade on. *Omega, 61*(4), 273–289. https://doi.org/10.2190/OM.61.4.b.

Strada, E. A. (2019). Psychosocial issues and bereavement. *Primary Care, 46*(3), 373–386. https://doi.org/10.1016/j.pop.2019.05.004

University of Nottingham. (2010). Bereavement care services: A synthesis of the literature. https://webarchive.nationalarchives.gov.uk/ukgwa/20130502195344/https://www.gov.uk/government/publications/bereavement-care-services-a-synthesis-of-the-literature

Yalom, I. D., & Leszcz, M. (2005). *The theory and practice of group psychotherapy*. Basic.

World Health Organization. (2018). *International classification of diseases for mortality and morbidity statistics* (11th rev.). https://icd.who.int/browse11/l-m/en#/http://id.who.int/icd/entity/1183832314

Zech, E., & Arnold, C. (2011). Attachment and coping with bereavement: Implications for therapeutic interventions with the insecurely attached. In R. A. Neimeyer, D. L. Harris, H. R. Winokuer, & G. F. Thornton (Eds.), *Grief and bereavement in contemporary society: Bridging research and practice* (pp. 23–35). Routledge/Taylor & Francis.

SECTION III

POPULATION HIGHLIGHTS: UNDERREPRESENTED, UNDERSERVED, AND VULNERABLE POPULATIONS

Guadalupe Palos

Access to palliative care is a basic human right. The core ethics, values, and standards of the social work profession provide a road map for serving multicultural and at-risk populations during their palliative care journey. Yet, social workers are painfully aware of groups of people who receive inadequate or no palliative care. This inequity is highly prevalent among specific groups, which are underrepresented, underserved, and vulnerable. Limited published evidence suggests that lack of access to adequate palliative care exists among children, adolescents, the elderly, disabled, sexual and gender minorities, and those with diverse ethnicity, race, or tribal characteristics.

The authors of each chapter in this section cover specific groups in critical need of age- or culturally appropriate social work interventions. To achieve this goal, each chapter presents key concepts, case studies, resources, and "take home messages" in the form of pearls and pitfalls. Chapter 16 provides a broad overview of the unique challenges encountered and models of practice used when working with older adults. Chapter 17 addresses the numerous hardships that affect middle-aged adults, often referred to as the "sandwich generation," throughout their palliative care experience. Chapter 18 introduces the reader to the unfulfilled needs of three vulnerable groups: children, adolescents, and young adults. Chapter 19 focuses on LGBTQI communities, for whom there is scarce published evidence of the challenges and opportunities that occur during the stage of one's life when palliative care is most needed. Chapter 20 provides an informative overview of the multicultural and diverse populations who are changing the demographic landscape of America, and the implications for oncology and palliative social work practice. The authors in this section offer their chapters in hopes the reader will better understand the challenges and joys social workers face in providing the basic human right of high-quality palliative care to underrepresented, underserved, and vulnerable populations.

16

The Older Person With Cancer

Danielle Saff, Sarah Kelly, and Lisa Petgrave-Nelson

Key Concepts

- Age is a significant risk factor for a cancer diagnosis, and older adults are the fastest growing segment of the United States population.
- Older adults face myriad challenges ranging from comorbid health issues to negative societal attitudes that have a negative effect on the medical care received and treatment options presented to them.
- Understanding how minority populations are frequently disadvantaged due to a history of systemic, institutional, and environmental racism can help social workers understand an individual's feelings and reactions toward cancer, palliative care, and mortality.
- Social workers play a key role in advocating and empowering cancer patients in understanding and exploring decisions regarding quality of life while promoting social justice and the dignity and worth of humans.

Keywords: ageism, Black Americans, disparities, geriatrics, older adults, palliative care, racism

Older adults are the fastest growing segment of the population in the United States and the leading segment of the population diagnosed with cancer. Age is a significant risk factor for a cancer diagnosis. Approximately 60% of cancers and 70% of deaths occur in this population (Estape, 2018). As the older adult population increases, cancer incidence will increase with the largest percentage occurring among adults aged 85 years or older (DeSantis et al., 2019).

Older adults may also be managing comorbid health issues, age-related cognitive challenges, and psychological and social issues related to aging. Negative societal attitudes, such as racism and ageism, affect many older adults, which has repercussions that extend into the medical care received and treatment options presented to them, including palliative care. Older adult patients also find themselves in an increasingly complex medical system,

Danielle Saff, Sarah Kelly, and Lisa Petgrave-Nelson, *The Older Person With Cancer In: Oncology and Palliative Social Work.* Edited by: Susan Hedlund, Bryan Miller, Grace Christ, and Carolyn Messner, Oxford University Press.
 DOI: 10.1093/oso/9780197607299.003.0016

where they are expected to take an active role in managing their care and may face challenges in doing so.

Lastly, Black, Indigenous, people of color (BIPOC) and other minority populations are frequently disadvantaged due to a history of systemic, institutional, and environmental racism. A cancer diagnosis only exacerbates the injustices these individuals encounter.

A multidisciplinary approach addressing the multifaceted experience of older adult patients is essential as this segment of the population grows. Health care professionals must stay abreast of the challenges older cancer patients face and attempt to navigate.

Psychosocial Needs of Older Adults

Eighty percent of older adults aged 65 and older have at least one chronic condition; 68% have two or more (Healthy Aging Team, 2021). It is important to understand how these comorbid medical conditions affect the cancer diagnosis and treatment options presented, as well as their ability to complete activities of daily living (ADLs) and instrumental activities of daily living (IADLs). Older adults' comorbid medical conditions and level of functioning should be fully explored and assessed prior to treatment choices being presented and recommended. As physical changes occur, the older adult patient may be coping with feelings of loss—specifically, the loss of their health and independence. The treatment team members must be knowledgeable of the multitude of challenges that cancer patients and their caregivers navigate in this new normal or changed reality.

In addition, older adults may also present with cognitive changes. Social workers must consider two specific groups. First, older adults who present with normal cognition at diagnosis, and second, older adults with preexisting cognitive impairments. While there is increasing evidence about the cognitive impacts of cancer treatment, few studies address older adults. Treatment team members need to counsel patients in order to help them understand the potential for cognitive-related effects of cancer treatments, their effect on independence, and the importance of advanced directives (Magnuson et al., 2019).

Older adults diagnosed with cancer face specific financial challenges as they are more likely to have a fixed income or limited financial sources and are at risk for financial toxicity. The challenges of financial toxicity to cancer patients have been well documented in relation to quality of life and cancer outcomes. In a study analyzing Medicare Part D coverage, researchers found that older adults still have high out-of-pocket costs, which negatively affects their ability to continue treatment (Davis & Fugett, 2018).

Older Adults' Societal Perceptions

Despite the prevalence of cancer in older adults, they are frequently undertreated and often excluded from clinical trials when compared to younger cancer patients. Ageism and other negative societal attitudes affect the options that medical professionals present to them. Age is not a contraindication for receiving treatment, yet breast cancer studies show that older adults don't receive recommendations for chemotherapy despite their clinical situations being similar to those of a 55-year-old. Ageism affects the ways in which health care professionals communicate with older adults. "Elderspeak," which is characterized by speaking louder and/or more slowly, can have a negative impact on older adult patients' views of their treatment team (Schroyen et al., 2014).

Interventions

Currently, limited interventions exist that specifically address older adults. The geriatric assessment (GA) evaluates ADLs and IALDs while also assessing such important domains as cognition, social support, depression, and nutrition (Mohile et al., 2018). Social workers can intervene in patients' needs for transportation, financial assistance, home health, caregiver support, and emotional support.

The Cancer and Aging Research Group developed what is known as the chemotherapy toxicity calculator, a tool used to guide conversations with patients and help medical providers understand chemotherapy toxicity risk. The chemo toxicity calculator assesses age, height, and weight as well as ADLs, hemoglobin levels, and chemotherapy agents. Ultimately, it allows for shared decision-making among the patient and members of the treatment team as they weigh the benefits and risks.

Patient-Centered Care Model

Patient-centered care is a collaborative partnership between patients and their health care providers in making shared decisions about personalized treatment plans. The Institute of Medicine (IOM) recommends addressing six dimensions in patient-centered care: understanding the patient's values, ensuring care coordination and integration, psychoeducation, physical comfort, and emotional support (Tzelepis et al., 2015).

Social workers should place importance on providing patients with information about communication skills, quality-of-life wishes, and end-of-life planning. For example, few older adults have completed important advanced directives such as outlining and formalizing a durable power of attorney, living will, and medical directives (Bern-Klug & Byram, 2017). The patient-centered care model puts the responsibility on patients to voice their concerns, but when patients do speak up, the treatment must listen.

Social workers strive to enhance human well-being, promote social justice, and support the dignity and worth of all humans. Oncology social workers can help by providing psychoeducation on the comprehensive geriatric assessment and chemotherapy toxicity tool while also encouraging older adults to discuss and share their needs and quality-of-life wishes with the treatment team. However, the patient-centered care model also requires social workers to advocate for the medical team to explore patient's wishes and treatment options and ultimately to lead with empathy and compassion. Treatment team members and social workers must provide interventions that encompass the assessment of practical, emotional, social, and financial challenges. Patients should receive information about all options when navigating a chronic illness that includes palliative care (Box 16.1).

Box 16.1

Being a woman of color and having worked in various oncology settings, I have personally experienced and have been included in conversations with interdisciplinary teams to discuss and find solutions related to barriers among Black cancer patients. Facilitating palliative care and hospice referrals during the pandemic was also quite involved, while being personally affected by COVID-19 and experiencing similar losses and fear by societal upheavals.

The experiences of Black patients during the pandemic resonated deeply, sometimes painfully, with me, but I also found within them empathy, insight, and joy. Helping these patients during a challenging time proved to be an important process of self-discovery, allowing me to home in on broader questions related to oncology, barriers, culture, health disparities, and health equity.

Older Adults and Palliative Care

Over the past 20 years, the integration of palliative care in oncology has required an expanded understanding of the intersections among palliative care, oncology, and geriatric care. The IOM, American Society of Clinical Oncology (ASCO), and International Society of Geriatric Oncology (SIOG) provide guidelines and recommendations for palliative care and older adults (Extermann et al., 2005; Ferrell et al., 2017; IOM, 2013). While these guidelines provide a path toward further integration of palliative care and geriatric oncology, there are still gaps to be bridged.

Access to Palliative Care Services

Access to palliative care services can be challenging for all age groups. Research in the challenges that exist for older adults is limited; however, the studies that have been done show that the palliative and supportive needs of older adults are often unmet due to significant barriers to care. A recent review of the literature noted such barriers as race, gender, and marital status; socioeconomic status; geographic location; health insurance/financial factors; negative perceptions of palliative care; confusion regarding the difference between palliative and hospice care; the misconception that discussing palliative care will diminish hope; and issues in prognostication and timing of palliative care referrals (Parajuli et al., 2020).

Despite this, research clearly indicates the benefits to older adults of an early referral to palliative care services. IOM and ASCO include this in their guidelines; however, implementation of early intervention remains limited and older adult cancer patients often are referred to palliative care later in their cancer trajectory than younger patients (Brighi et al., 2014). Early referral can assist in symptom management and improving a patient's psychosocial, spiritual, and financial outlook. Patient–provider collaboration can result in earlier referral to palliative care, as well as continued success in decision-making and intervention through the illness trajectory.

Assessment in Palliative Care

A comprehensive approach to assessment that addresses the multidimensional needs of older adult cancer patients can also assist in collaborative decision-making. We have discussed two important assessment tools: the GA and the chemo toxicity calculator. Additionally, social workers use several other screening tools across settings to inform more in-depth assessments. As care moves forward, a social worker can revisit various screenings and assessments with the patient and then review, reassess, or make changes (if needed), all of which are vital.

Social workers must address supportive care needs, including psychosocial needs, as an integral part of assessment and care, both at time of diagnosis and throughout the trajectory of care. The IOM recommends the importance of assessing and treating the psychosocial issues that accompany a cancer diagnosis (Adler et al., 2008). Screening and assessment may vary depending on settings; however, using tools like the distress thermometer can guide a more comprehensive psychosocial assessment and intervention. Screening and assessment combined with informal assessment and observation is also key.

Disparities in Palliative Care

Disparities in access to palliative care and referral are seen in many underserved populations; evidence suggests that disparities also exist in quality of care (Elk et al., 2018). Studies consistently document lower rates of hospice use for minority older adults than for Whites across diagnoses, geographic areas, and settings of care, including nursing homes (National Hospice and Palliative Care Organization, 2020). A disproportionate gap in knowledge about palliative care among minority older adults has been well documented. Despite evidence showing the benefits of hospice and palliative care, Black and Hispanic patients often underuse these services. Institutional and cultural factors that account for this include medical mistrust, lack of knowledge surrounding palliative care, the idea that acknowledging illness hastens death, and the desire to seek aggressive care. Minority patients often have a mistrust in the medical system that leads to racial differences in end-of-life care (Rhodes et al., 2013).

Blacks and Palliative Care

Black people in the United States experience significant disparities with chronic conditions, access to care, preventive screenings, and mental health. In addition, Blacks have the highest incidence and mortality rates of any ethnic group for several types of cancer (National Cancer Institute, n.d.). The cause of these disparities is complex and rooted in a long history of segregation, unequal access to medical care, poverty, and medical mistrust.

The pandemic cast a spotlight on the inequities of the health care system and exacerbated the challenges marginalized communities face. According to the American Public Media Research Lab, COVID-19 claimed nearly 171,000 American lives through mid-August 2020, with the heaviest losses among Black and Indigenous Americans (Gawthrop, 2022). With higher death rates and increased suffering, where does palliative care fit in for patients of color?

Black communities whose members have suffered through generations of segregation and discrimination often cite the Tuskegee syphilis experiments for their ongoing distrust and fear. Blacks often refer to the "study"—along with AIDS, the "crack epidemic," and COVID-19—as proof of a U.S.-government–backed genocidal plot. Otado et al. reported in 2015 that "it is well-documented that minority populations do not trust researchers and the research establishment and have expressed fear of being used as guinea pigs" (p. 460).

Historical Roots of Mistrust

Incidents of historical references that have involved racism, paternalism, deception, exploitation, and injustice include the following cases.

- Tuskegee Syphilis Experiment: Conducted from 1932 to 1972. The U.S. Public Health Service ran this study to observe the natural history of untreated syphilis, without notifying the participants about their disease or offering them treatment that was available (Park, 2017).
- Henrietta Lacks (HeLa Cells): Cancer cells were harvested and used for scientific experiments at John Hopkins without her consent. These HeLa cells were in high demand by other researchers and were put into mass production. According to Vernon (2020), "They were mailed to scientists around the globe, and the cell line would be used to make many important breakthroughs in biomedical research." Ironically, HeLa cells were used to develop the first vaccine for polio and used for the treatment of White patients while Black patients were excluded from treatment options.

The dark history of medical experimentation on Black bodies has had a lasting, negative impact on Black people and often contributes to lethal health outcomes within this community. Another contributing factor is the deeply religious and strong spiritual taboos African Americans have surrounding death and dying. Studies have shown that Black people are more likely to express discomfort discussing death, more willing to go to heroic measures to extend their lives, and have spiritual beliefs that can conflict with the goals of palliative care (Rhodes et al., 2013). Older Black patients often view referrals to palliative and hospice care with suspicion due to past injustices and ongoing disparities (Box 16.2).

Box 16.2

J.B. was a 68-year-old Black farmer from Alabama diagnosed with renal failure who visited the clinic to explore renal transplant. Patient disclosed to the oncology social worker his distrust and fear seeking and obtaining care from the predominantly all-White staff at the medical institution. Patient grew up in the segregated south and at 15 years old, had his left arm amputated without anesthesia by a White doctor. The last words J.B. heard prior to the amputation were, "Cut that nigger's arm off."

While cancer is challenging for everyone, it is often most challenging for disadvantaged or minority patients who are seeking treatment or for those who have had traumatic experiences and suffered injustices from providers and health care organizations. The physician and social work workforce continues to struggle with inadequate representation of racial and ethnic minorities.

Social work is a field that is "majority white" (68.8%) and female (83%) (Salsberg et al., 2017). This racial and gender imbalance requires improvement. Oncology centers need staff members who both reflect the diversity to be found in clinics and share the same cultural norms and diverse backgrounds as their patients. Social workers are uniquely positioned to educate, advocate, and implement policies addressing health disparities where applicable. Supporting and educating minority patients on the benefits of palliative care is essential as is bringing awareness and openness into each therapeutic relationship.

Reducing disparities and ensuring equity is incumbent on the awareness of providers to acknowledge and control our own implicit biases. Cultural humility asserts that none of us are exempt from biases but that we must be willing to "do the work" to overcome how those biases affect our relationships with patients. Social workers (indeed, all medical practitioners) must undertake this important self-journey, being always open to learning more about ourselves and the patients we serve (Box 16.3).

Box 16.3

C.G. was a 65-year-old Black female diagnosed with metastatic breast cancer. Patient met with the treatment team to discuss hospice care. Patient became visibly upset and informed the oncology social worker, "God has the final say. You can't tell me God can't heal me." Patient requested to receive ongoing treatment and declined hospice care. In Black cancer patients, spiritual beliefs often influence treatment—for example, patients often share beliefs in divine intervention and miracles.

As providers, we must be willing to learn about and be respectful of our patients' cultural influences and the way those experiences contribute to the way patients respond, cope, and adhere to their treatment plans. As the demographics in our oncology centers continue to grow and become more diverse, shifting to a patient-centered model, we must seek opportunities to embrace diversity while valuing the strength in our differences.

Oncology social workers play a unique and dynamic role in addressing the needs of the older adult cancer patient. Through a multifaceted social work lens, oncology social workers can use their knowledge of the psychosocial factors of illness to assess individual patients' needs, provide psychoeducation, help patients navigate systems and barriers to care, improve communication across disciplines, and provide care coordination. Additionally, oncology social workers both advocate for their clients and work collaboratively to include and empower patients and caregivers as part of the care team. Strengths-based approaches that are patient centered and acknowledge the older adult patient as the expert of their own situation are integral in ensuring the older adult patient is an active participant in both assessment and intervention. More diversity in the social work profession will support these strengths-based and patient-centered approaches, as well as the necessary awareness and exploration of social workers' implicit bias in understanding their clients' experiences particularly with regard to racism, discrimination and inequity.

Guiding Best Practices for the Future

Older adult cancer patients require an interdisciplinary approach that is truly patient centered, supportive, and addresses their individual needs. Interdisciplinary, team-based care should be standard with social workers in an integral role. While this is an aim for a standard of care, the barriers discussed in this chapter mean it's not always possible to take this comprehensive interdisciplinary approach. One recommendation is to ensure that providers across disciplines receive training in both geriatric oncology and palliative care. Training would ensure that the older adult cancer patient is receiving informed care and care coordination is completed as early as possible. The interdisciplinary approach could also have implications in research and expand knowledge of the older adult cancer patient's needs and possible inclusion in clinical trials.

Pearls

- Understanding and assessing the older adult's level of functioning is important when discussing treatment options, which should always include palliative care.
- As palliative care continues to expand its integration into oncology there are opportunities for the intersection of palliative care and geriatric oncology.
- Practicing cultural humility can decrease barriers by building trust around end-of-life conversations.

Pitfalls

- Minority cancer patients have many experiences of medical distrust and suspicion.
- Oncology social workers and providers may not be knowledgeable of cultural humility or aware of their own implicit biases.
- Older adult cancer patients may not have access or be referred for palliative care services, and when they are referred, it may be late in their disease trajectory.

References

Adler, N. E., Page, A. E. K., & Institute of Medicine Committee on Psychosocial Services to Cancer Patients/Families in a Community Setting (Eds.). (2008). *Cancer care for the whole patient: Meeting psychosocial health needs. National Academies Press* (pp. 23–49). National Academies Press.

Bern-Klug, M., & Byram, E. A. (2017). Older adults more likely to discuss advance care plans with an attorney than with a physician. *Gerontology and Geriatric Medicine*, 3, 1–5. https://doi.org/10.1177/2333721417741978

Brighi, N., Balducci, L., & Biasco, G. (2014). Cancer in the elderly: Is it time for palliative care in geriatric oncology? *Journal of Geriatric Oncology*, *5*(2), 197–203.
Davis, M. E., & Fugett, S. (2018). Financial toxicity. *Clinical Journal of Oncology Nursing*, *22*(6), 43–48. https://doi.org/10.1188/18.CJON.S2.43-48
DeSantis, C. E., Miller, K. D., Dale, W., Mohile, S. G., Cohen, H. J., Leach, C. R., Sauer, A. G., Jemal, A., & Siegel, R. L. (2019). Cancer statistics for adults aged 85 years and older, 2019. *CA: A Cancer Journal for Clinicians*, *69*(6), 452–467. https://acsjournals.onlinelibrary.wiley.com/doi/full/10.3322/caac.21577
Elk, R., Felder, T. M., Cayir, E., & Samuel, C. A. (2018, August). Social inequalities in palliative care for cancer patients in the United States: A structured review. *Seminars in Oncology Nursing*, *43*(3), 305–315.
Estape, T. (2018). Cancer in the elderly: Challenges and barriers. *Asia-Pacific Journal of Oncology Nursing*, *5*(1), 40–42. https://doi.org/10.4103/apjon.apjon_52_17
Extermann, M., Aapro, M., Bernabei, R., Cohen, H. J., Droz, J.-P., Lichtman, S., Mor, V., Monfardini, S., Repetto, L., Sørbe, L., & Topinkova, E. (2005). Use of comprehensive geriatric assessment in older cancer patients: Recommendations from the task force on CGA of the International Society of Geriatric Oncology (SIOG). *Critical Reviews in Oncology/Hematology*, *55*(3), 241–252. https://doi.org/10.1016/j.critrevonc.2005.06.003
Ferrell, B. R., Temel, J. S., Temin, S., Alesi, E. R., Balboni, T. A., Basch, E. M., Firn, J. I., Paice, J. A., Peppercorn, J. M., Phillips, T., Stovall, E. L., Zimmerman, C., & Smith, T. J. (2017). Integration of palliative care into standard oncology care: American Society of Clinical Oncology clinical practice guideline update. *Journal of Clinical Oncology*, *35*(1), 96–112. https://doi.org/10.1200/JCO.2016.70.1474
Gawthrop, E. (2022, June 16). *Color of coronavirus: COVID-19 deaths analyzed by race and ethnicity*. Retrieved from APM Research Lab website: https://www.apmresearchlab.org/covid/deaths-by-race
Healthy Aging Team. (2021, April 23). *The top 10 most chronic conditions in older adults*. National Council on Aging. https://www.ncoa.org/article/the-top-10-most-common-chronic-conditions-in-older-adults
Institute of Medicine (U.S.) Committee on Improving the Quality of Cancer Care: Addressing the Challenges of an Aging Population, Board on Health Care Services. (2013). Patient-centered communication and shared decision making. In L. Levit, E. Balogh, S. Nass, & P. A. Ganz (Eds.), *Delivering High-Quality Cancer Care: Charting a New Course for a System in Crisis* (Section 3). Retrieved from the National Library of Medicine website: https://www.ncbi.nlm.nih.gov/books/NBK202146/
Magnuson, A., Sattar, S., Nightingale, G., Saracino, R., Skonecki, E., & Trevino, K. (2019). A practical guide to geriatric syndromes in older adults with cancer: A focus on falls, cognition, polypharmacy, and depression. *American Society of Clinical Oncology Education Book*, *39*, e96–e109. https://doi.org/10.1200/EDBK_237641
Mohile, S. G., Dale, W., Somerfield, M. R., Schonberg, M. A., Boyd, C. M., Burhenn, P. S., Canin, B., Cohen, H. J., Holmes, H. M., Hopkins, J. O., Janelsins, M. C., Khorana, A. A., Klepin, H. D., Lichtman, S. T., Mustian, K. M., Tew, W. P., & Hurria, A. (2018). Practical assessment and management of vulnerabilities in older patients receiving chemotherapy: ASCO guideline for geriatric oncology. *Journal of Clinical Oncology*, *36*(22), 2326–2347. https://ascopubs.org/doi/10.1200/JCO.2018.78.8687
National Cancer Institute. (n.d.). *Cancer disparities*. Retrieved July 3, 2022, from https://www.cancer.gov/about-cancer/understanding/disparities
National Hospice and Palliative Care Organization. (2020, August 17). *Hospice facts & figures*. Retrieved from https://www.nhpco.org/hospice-facts-figures
Otado, J., Kwagyan, J., Edwards, D., Ukaegbu, A., Rockcliffe, F., & Osafo, N. (2015). Culturally competent strategies for recruitment and retention of African American populations into

clinical trials. *Clinical and Translational Science*, *8*(5), 460–466. https://doi.org/10.1111/cts.12285

Parajuli, J., Tark, A., Jao, Y. L., & Hupcey, J. (2020). Barriers to palliative and hospice care utilization in older adults with cancer: A systematic review. *Journal of Geriatric Oncology*, *11*(1), 8–16. https://doi.org/10.1016/j.jgo.2019.09.017

Park, J. (2017). Historical origins of the Tuskegee experiment: The dilemma of public health in the United States. *Korean Journal of Medical History*, *26*(3), 545–578. https://doi.org/10.13081/kjmh.2017.26.545

Rhodes, R. L., Batchelor, K., Lee, S., & Halm, E. (2013). Barriers to end-of-life care for African Americans from the providers' perspective. *American Journal of Hospice and Palliative Medicine*, *32*(2), 137–143. https://doi.org/10.1177/1049909113507127

Salsberg, E., Quigley, L., Mehfoud, N., Acquaviva, K., Wyche, K., & Sliwa, S. (2017). *Profile of the social work workforce*. George Washington University Health Workforce Institute. https://www.cswe.org/Centers-Initiatives/Initiatives/National-Workforce-Initiative/SW-Workforce-Book-FINAL-11-08-2017.aspx

Schroyen, S., Adam, S., Jerusalem, G., & Missotten, P. (2014). Ageism and its clinical impact in oncogeriatry: State of knowledge and therapeutic leads. *Clinical Interventions in Aging*, *10*, 117–125. https://doi.org/10.2147/CIA.S70942

Tzelepis, F., Sanson-Fisher, R. W., Zucca, A. C., & Fradgley, E. A. (2015). Measuring the quality of patient-centered care: Why patient-reported measures are critical to reliable assessment. *Patient Preference and Adherence*, *9*, 831–835. https://doi.org/10.2147/PPA.S81975

Vernon, L. F. (2020). Tuskegee syphilis study not America's only medical scandal: Chester M. Southam, MD, Henrietta Lacks, and the Sloan-Kettering research scandal. *Online Journal of Health Ethics*, *16*(2). https://doi.org/10.18785/ojhe.1602.03

17
Cancer in Middle Age

Meredith Cammarata, Samantha Fortune, and Carissa Hodgson

Key Concepts

- Middle adulthood brings a plethora of different life perspectives, experiences, and responsibilities, which has an impact on risk factors, early prevention, treatment decisions, and coping techniques.
- Common challenges middle-aged patients encounter include psychosocial and systemic factors, financial burdens, caregiving stress, and health care disparities.
- A thorough biopsychosocial assessment is an essential first step for social workers in identifying the specific needs of this population of people to appropriately tailor specific therapeutic interventions.

Keywords: body image, caregiving, children, cognitive behavioral therapy (CBT), employment, end of life, family, fertility, finances, grief work, health care disparities, intimacy, middle adulthood, middle age, partners, sandwich generation, sexuality, spirituality, teens

The priorities and responsibilities of the middle-aged cancer patient are unique and can be vastly different from those of young adult or older adult cancer patients. While those in middle age have surpassed most of the inaugurating encounters that characterize young adulthood, they often feel far removed from the factors that distinguish old age. Furthermore, middle-aged adults commonly feel like they are in the prime of their lives, which can make a cancer diagnosis difficult to navigate. Defining middle adulthood is subjective, with age ranges varying within the literature, among agencies, and between individuals who all have unique perceptions of their age group. This chapter defines middle adulthood using the age range designated by the Centers for Disease Control and Prevention (2021).

Meredith Cammarata, Samantha Fortune, and Carissa Hodgson, *Cancer in Middle Age* In: *Oncology and Palliative Social Work*. Edited by: Susan Hedlund, Bryan Miller, Grace Christ, and Carolyn Messner, Oxford University Press. © Oxford University Press 2024. DOI: 10.1093/oso/9780197607299.003.0017

What We Have Learned So Far: Psychosocial and Systemic Factors

While middle adulthood comprises a diversity of experiences, roles, and identities, essential psychosocial and systemic factors contribute to a cancer experience during this developmental stage. These factors should be addressed during psychosocial assessments with cancer patients in middle age, as well as incorporated into client-centered interventions to support overall well-being.

Sexuality, Body Image, and Intimacy

A cancer diagnosis can have a significant effect on sexuality and intimacy, which are central aspects of quality of life. Treatments such as surgery, chemotherapy, radiation, and hormonal therapies can change the way a body looks, functions, and feels. Cancer and treatment can cause significant damage to both emotional and physical systems that are needed for one to have a sexual response. Such damage can interfere with sexual functioning and have a negative impact on sexual orientation and relationships (Reisman & Gianotten, 2017). Middle-aged adults with cancer may have significant concerns about how cancer and its treatment will impact their sexual interest, sexual response, relationship to their body, current intimate relationships, and ability to find a future partner. Completing a thorough psychosocial assessment is important for oncology social workers who wish to explore issues of sexuality, intimacy, and body image with patients. Social workers can address concerns through counseling or education. Additionally, oncology social workers play a role in advocating for the patient's sexual health needs with the medical team, who may refer the patient to a sexual health program.

Fertility

While fertility is not typically thought of as a concern for cancer patients in middle age, it should be recognized that many people are postponing having children well into their forties. Cancer treatment can seriously impair fertility, which can come as a significant loss for a middle-aged person who had still hoped to have children (Reisman & Gianotten, 2017). Oncology social workers should ask if patients are still considering biological parenthood and explore options that may preserve fertility during cancer treatment. Issues of grief and loss may be explored if fertility cannot be preserved.

Partners and Caregivers

Roughly 64% of middle-aged Americans are married (U.S. Census Bureau, 2021). When a middle-aged person is diagnosed with cancer, the responsibility for caregiving often falls to the spouse or partner. While many marriage vows speak of caring for each other in sickness, most spouses do not expect this responsibility to start as early as middle adulthood.

Caregivers often work full-time, balancing caring for their partner with their job responsibilities. Middle-aged adults are typically too young to qualify for retirement, yet they may need to take time away from work to care for their partner. During an already challenging time, the added financial strain can add significant stress to a couple's relationship (Junkins et al., 2020). Both partners and primary caregivers experience their own psychological distress and negative health outcomes (Northouse et al, 2012; Shin et al., 2019).

Oncology social workers should be aware of the significant stressors for this group of caregivers and how they may affect the patient's well-being. They can support primary caregivers by sharing information, providing psychoeducation, referring them to support services, and facilitating counseling sessions (within agency guidelines). Institutional policies may limit how partners can be included in services; oncology social workers should address issues of caregiving to the extent their organization allows.

Parenting

Around 80% of middle-aged Americans have children under age 18 living with them (U.S. Census Bureau, 2020). The diagnosis of a parent with cancer has a profound effect on every member of the family and can create significant stress for parents who often focus on how the diagnosis will affect their children. Given the potential risk of psychosocial distress associated with a parent's diagnosis, it is critical to recognize the preventive role of supportive interventions for the parent with cancer. Research has shown that it is important for parents and caregivers to appropriately communicate and support children during this overwhelming time. Effective parent–child communication is thought to help families adjust more easily during stressful events such as parental cancer (Gazendam-Donofrio et al., 2009).

Oncology social workers should listen to the concerns of parents and assist them in having conversations with their children. They may role-play difficult conversations, provide books and resources (see Box 17.1), and connect them with other families facing cancer to reduce a sense of isolation and connect them with peer support.

Box 17.1 Suggested Websites for Patients With Children and Teenagers

CancerCare: https://www.cancercare.org/tagged/children
Cancer Support Community: https://www.cancersupportcommunity.org/virtual-home/what-do-i-tell-kids
Children's Treehouse Foundation: https://childrenstreehousefdn.org
Camp Kesem: https://www.kesem.org
Well Beings Studio: https://www.wellbeings.studio/

Sandwich Generation

A common life experience for middle-aged adults is caring for aging parents while also having dependent children. Adults in this so-called sandwich generation often feel squeezed between the caregiving obligations coming from both their parents and children, an experience that may be emotionally, mentally, and financially exhausting.

Many systemic factors contribute to the experience of familial caregiving, including gender, ethnicity, culture, economics, geography, availability, resource accessibility, and trust in welfare institutions. Women commonly experience the "double burden" of being sandwiched, as they tend to maintain unpaid household duties and relational obligations beyond paid employment. Notably, sandwiched women experience more chronic health conditions, including depression (Alburez-Gutierrez et al., 2021).

While assessing the middle-aged cancer patient, oncology social workers should explore their caregiving responsibilities for their parents in addition to dependent children. This information may prove valuable when identifying support systems, creating a treatment plan, and providing emotional support to the patient.

Employment and Finances

Roughly 81% of middle-aged Americans are employed (U.S. Bureau of Labor Statistics, n.d.). While some patients can maintain their work schedule throughout their cancer treatment, many others will need to take a leave of absence from their job or request accommodation. The need for time off can result from the time and travel demands of the patient's treatment schedule as well as side effects such as fatigue, pain, and cognitive impairment that can negatively affect work efficiency. The Americans with Disabilities Act (ADA) as well as the Family Medical Leave Act (FMLA) are two essential laws that can protect and support patients who wish to maintain their job. Patients may need to apply for Social Security Disability Insurance (SSDI) or complete other forms that will get them enrolled in other financial assistance programs while they are unable to work.

Family members often must take leave from or stop work altogether to be a caregiver to the cancer patient, which may financially burden the family. Many people fear losing health insurance if either the cancer patient or spouse/partner is unable to work. At this age, many adults have partners, children, or elderly family members they financially support. A cancer diagnosis during this stage of life can have serious financial effects. Cancer treatment costs are increasing at alarming rates. Many people are uninsured or underinsured, preventing them from "receiving optimal cancer prevention, early detection, and treatment" (American Cancer Society [ACS], 2022a). A lack of or limits to health care insurance can result in additional costs to patients for medications, medical appointments, treatment, and scans. Furthermore, patients may have added expenses of transportation, gas, lodging, and childcare while they are in treatment. While there are some resources for temporary financial aid, many patients find themselves ineligible due to incomes higher than federal poverty guidelines.

Oncology social workers can offer valuable support to patients by helping them navigate and understand their insurance plans, ADA, FMLA, SSDI, and other relevant financial resources. They should advocate for patients with their employers, health insurance, and other financial assistance programs. They may assist patients in establishing boundaries and expressing needs in the workplace when appropriate. Patients may also need emotional and mental health support as they respond to transitions or losses in employment and financial distress.

Spirituality

Middle adulthood is often perceived as a time of reflection—a period to take inventory of one's life and adjust to find more meaning. This audit can be a productive, positive experience. For others, it may precipitate a dreaded midlife crisis that can result in regressive behaviors rooted in a desire to relive or regain youth.

A cancer diagnosis at any age typically inspires introspection, and in middle age, one may find the effects multiplied. Patients may benefit from support in their existential evaluation, which is often tied closely to religion and spirituality. While some providers are hesitant to breach these topics with patients, they are core components of many people's lives that shape the way in which they perceive a cancer diagnosis, make medical decisions, access resources, and use coping skills. Key medical and mental health professional organizations support the integration of religion and spirituality into patient care (Kelly et al., 2020).

A thorough patient psychosocial assessment includes an exploration of the patient's religion and spirituality. While standard instruments exist, Doka encourages flexibility in gathering information about a patient's spiritual dimension, namely allowing the patient to use narrative in sharing about their unique values and practices (2017). Once discovered, aspects of religion and spirituality should be included in the patient's treatment plan and care.

Health Care Disparities

Research has shown that early detection and treatment can reduce cancer mortality (Lee et al., 2020). Middle age—especially between the ages of 40 and 49—is typically the time when recommended cancer screenings start (ACS, 2022b). Despite evidence of early cancer screening and its improvement for survival, low-income and minority communities experience delayed diagnosis and treatment. Once diagnosed with cancer, people of color face additional obstacles including provider bias, institutional racism, and medical treatments formulated from clinical trials that have severely underrepresented their race and ethnicity (Fortune, 2021).

Socioeconomic factors such as a lack of education, lower income, or the community in which a patient resides can contribute to a patient's distrust of medical providers and institutions, which can have a significantly negative effect on the patient's quality of care. Some patients may have a difficult time understanding medical terms and simultaneously have a medical team that consistently overlooks or even dismisses their psychosocial needs. Especially among people of color, patients have expressed feeling a lack of respect and consideration from their health care team due to their low-income status (Duke & Stanik, 2016). Understandably, these patients will be hesitant to seek guidance from their team, which can in turn reduce their ability to make informed decisions regarding treatment and quality of life.

Oncology social workers must support patients in navigating socioeconomic factors and their resultant psychosocial obstacles through emotional support, education, and advocacy work. Oncology workers can educate patients about their rights and encourage patients to educate themselves about their cancer through workshops and easy-to-read, accessible literature. Oncology social workers should provide space for patients to ask questions and specifically check in with them along the way to ensure their needs are being met. There are many ways oncology social workers can advocate on behalf of patients—an important one is helping a patient communicate with their treatment team in a way that makes the patient feel heard and validated. Encouraging patients to seek second opinions when appropriate may help patients feel more comfortable with a potential treatment plan and more in control of their situation.

Oncology social workers must educate themselves about a patient's culture and its potential effect on patient communication, treatment beliefs, and support systems. They must continuously reflect on how their internal biases affect their own communication and response to patients and encourage the larger team and institution to do the same.

Specific Interventions for the Middle-Aged Cancer Patient

Cognitive Behavioral Therapy

Cognitive behavioral therapy (CBT) is a useful method that can enable patients with long-term illnesses such as cancer to better cope with psychosocial stressors (Sage, 2008). Patients may express negative thoughts and cognitive distortions about their cancer or treatment, including polarized thinking ("My life will never get better now that I have cancer"), discounting the positive ("Even though they caught the cancer early, it is going to come back"), or personalization ("If I got tested earlier or ate healthier, this would not have happened to me") (Chi, 2016). CBT interventions can help patients challenge these thought distortions and help them deal more effectively with their cancer stressors. For example, a female patient may express negative thoughts of feeling unlovable and unattractive due to hair loss from chemotherapy. An oncology social worker can use CBT to help the patient reframe how she sees herself by outlining her positive traits and helping her feel more in control of her looks. This could be done by encouraging her to learn new make-up tricks or wearing colorful headscarves that are meaningful to her. Particularly for middle-aged adults, CBT interventions can be implemented when a patient is struggling with feelings of worthlessness due to being unable to provide for their families either financially or through caregiving responsibilities. In this situation, an oncology social worker can work with a patient to reconstruct how they see themselves in their past roles and highlight other important familial contributions. Implementing such interventions can help patients build their confidence and feel more empowered and in control while they are navigating perceived losses during treatment.

End-of-Life Interventions

Death is an uncomfortable topic for most people, especially those in middle age who believe it is not yet their time. This population of cancer patients may be forced into practical and existential conversations about death much earlier than their peers (Junkins et al., 2020). When examining end-of-life issues with a patient, oncology and palliative social workers should be mindful of the middle-aged person and their life stage. Inquiring about aspects of the patient's identity such as career, family relationships, community roles, and caregiving responsibilities for children and older parents will be important.

Patients may wish to address concerns relating to end of life and death regardless of their prognosis. They may desire support in discussing their thoughts and feelings relating to death or need assistance with advance care planning. They may benefit from facilitated discussions with family to discuss their wishes. Special attention may be required for parents who have dependent children, especially if they are the sole parent. Referrals to spiritual care and legal services may be especially valuable.

Meaning-centered psychotherapy is an empirically based treatment that can be an effective intervention for improving quality of life, enhancing spiritual well-being, and reducing psychological distress in patients with advanced cancer (Breitbart et al., 2018). Similarly, dignity therapy is an empirically validated intervention for patients who wish to explore end-of-life issues and leaving a legacy. Dignity therapy has proven to decrease anxiety, depression, and the sense of burden family members may feel while their loved one is dying (Cuevas et al., 2021).

Grief Work

Grief is a normal response to all loss not just a reaction to death. As people enter middle age, they have already encountered losses associated with aging, identity, and relationships. A cancer diagnosis may introduce additional losses—pieces of anatomy, physical functioning, energy, motivation, cognitive capacity, employment, financial security, intimacy, fertility, ability to parent or care for family, faith, and sense of safety.

Grief work begins with a thorough assessment that explores the diverse losses the patient may be experiencing. For some people, the simple act of identifying and labeling losses allows them to acknowledge their grief; this may be the only intervention required. Others may benefit from grief interventions that alleviate distress and help them increase their understanding of the loss. Research has well documented post-traumatic growth (PTG) in cancer survivors (Cormio et al., 2017). Interventions that assist patients in finding meaning through their loss may contribute to their experience of PTG. Individual counseling, spiritual services, or participation in a support group may be valuable interventions in achieving these goals.

Rituals are a particularly effective intervention in loss. A ritual is a symbolic act done with intention and can be tailored to any unique situation. Used in grief, a person may engage in a meaningful gesture to recognize their loss and ceremoniously let it go. A ritual can incorporate a person's preference for art, writing, music, movement, or any type of creative process. It can be done in solitude or with a group of loved ones. Some examples of rituals used by middle-aged cancer patients may include writing a letter to cancer and burning it in a fire, having a party for a piece of the body that will be removed, or creating art/music/dance based on the loss.

Box 17.1 Learning Exercise

Identify the relevant factors in the following case scenario and outline effective interventions to support the patient.

Donna is a 52-year-old Black woman with stage III breast cancer. Donna is the primary wage earner in her family but has had to stop working due to her treatment. However, due to her salary, Donna is not eligible for several financial assistance programs, which is putting financial strain on her and her family. Donna further feels like a burden to her husband, who has become her caregiver. She feels guilty that she is not as present in her children's lives as she was before the cancer diagnosis. Additionally, Donna is struggling with her identity as she no longer looks like herself due to hair loss and a mastectomy. She is experiencing several losses in her life as a result of cancer, including her social life and independence. Donna has concerns about treatment and prognosis and feels as though she doesn't have a good understanding of her care plan. However, her doctor often rushes during appointments, which prevents her from asking questions. Donna became more anxious when she sought out information online. Due to all these stressors from her cancer and treatment, Donna has become depressed and discouraged. When Donna expressed these feelings to her treatment team, they dismissed her feelings saying, "You are strong."

Middle-aged adulthood brings unique challenges and life experiences that can make a cancer diagnosis difficult to navigate. Psychosocial and systemic factors, finances, caregiving responsibilities, and access to resources including cancer screenings can affect how this population of individuals cope during treatment in comparison to young adults or older cancer patients. Oncology social workers can take an active role in effectively supporting this specific age group of patients by implementing tailored interventions. This includes a thorough biopsychosocial assessment that is mindful of the unique psychosocial challenges, roles, and responsibilities of this population of patients. Additionally, social workers must be aware of the specific health disparities, including access to preventive medicine, people in this age group face. Awareness of these significant assessment factors will help guide oncology social workers as they make referrals to resources and provide counseling (Box 17.1).

Guiding Best Practices for the Future

Middle-aged patients experience unique challenges, including financial challenges, psychosocial factors, and physical side effects. While cancer in middle-adulthood shares many common themes, oncology and palliative social workers must continue to provide culturally relevant, person-centered care to each patient. It is essential to assess each patient's unique beliefs, traditions, customs, strengths, resources, and needs and incorporate these into the care plan. Furthermore, oncology and palliative social workers have a responsibility to advocate on the patient's behalf that all members of the medical team seek to understand and respect the uniqueness of each patient.

Health care disparities, provider bias, and systemic racism are significant problems that all oncology social workers should work to eliminate. They must use their power to advocate for individual clients, as well as push for policy changes within their institution, community, and government. Oncology social workers can also work to increase representation of minorities in research and clinical trials.

Pearls

- Middle adulthood comprises of a diversity of experiences, roles, and identities, and psychosocial and systemic factors contribute to a cancer experience during this developmental stage.
- A thorough biopsychosocial assessment is a key component of and should be the first step when providing clinical interventions to middle-aged cancer patients.
- Identifying cancer health disparities among this age group can help reduce cancer risk and increase early detection and treatment.

Pitfalls

- Middle-aged adults face unique challenges throughout the cancer journey due to being part of the sandwich generation and having to care not only for themselves financially and emotionally but also for their children and their parents.
- While this is the age when most people should start receiving screens for cancer, many middle-aged adults are prevented from doing so due to several social and economic factors, including health care disparities.
- Oncology social workers should take an active role in assisting patients in advocating for themselves as well as supporting patients as they cope with conflicts. However, social workers will have to do so while also encountering provider bias, limited resources, and systemic racism.

Additional Resources

- American Cancer Society: https://www.cancer.org
- Cancer*Care*: https://www.cancercare.org
- Cancer and Careers: https://www.cancerandcareers.org
- Cancer Legal Resource Center: https://thedrlc.org/cancer/
- Cancer Support Community: https://www.cancersupportcommunity.org
- Caring Bridge: https://www.caringbridge.org/
- Imerman Angels: https://www.imermanangels.org/
- Livestrong: https://www.livestrong.org/
- Triage Cancer Center: https://www.triagecancer.org

References

Alburez-Gutierrez, D., Mason, C., & Zagheni, E. (2021). The "sandwich generation" revisited: Global demographic drives of care time demands. *Population and Development Review*, 1–27. https://doi.org/10.1111/padr.12436

American Cancer Society. (2022a). *2022 Cancer facts and figures*. Retrieved from https://www.cancer.org/content/dam/cancer-org/research/cancer-facts-and-statistics/annual-cancer-facts-and-figures/2022/2022-cancer-facts-and-figures.pdf

American Cancer Society. (2022b). *Cancer screening guidelines by age*. Retrieved from https://www.cancer.org/healthy/find-cancer-early/screening-recommendations-by-age.html

Breitbart, W., Pessin, H., Rosenfeld, B., Applebaum, A. J., Lichtenthal, W. G., Li, Y., Saracino, R. M., Marziliano, A. M., Masterson, M., Tobias, K., & Fenn, N. (2018). Individual meaning-centered psychotherapy for the treatment of psychological and existential distress: A randomized controlled trial in patients with advanced cancer. *Cancer*. *124*(15), 3231–3239. https://doi.org/10.1002/cncr.31539

Chi, M. (2016, July 27). Using cognitive-behavioral therapy principles in daily patient interactions. *Oncology Nurse Advisor*. https://www.oncologynurseadvisor.com/home/departments/navigation/using-cognitive-behavioral-therapy-principles-in-daily-patient-interactions/#:~:text=For%20people%20with%20cancer%2C%20cognitive

Centers for Disease Control and Prevention. (2021, September 1). *Cancer prevention during midlife*. https://www.cdc.gov/cancer/dcpc/prevention/midlife.htm

Cormio, C., Muzzatti, B., Romito, F., Mattioli, V., & Annunziata, M. A. (2017). Posttraumatic growth and cancer: A study 5 years after treatment end. *Supportive Care in Cancer: Official Journal of the Multinational Association of Supportive Care in Cancer*, *25*(4), 1087–1096. https://doi.org/10.1007/s00520-016-3496-4

Cuevas, P. E., Davidson, P., Mejilla, J., & Rodney, T. (2021). Dignity therapy for end-of-life care patients: A literature review. *Journal of Patient Experience*, *8*. https://doi.org/10.1177/2374373521996951

Doka, K. J. (2017). Spiritual care: An essential aspect of cancer care. In L. Berk (Ed.), *Dying and death in oncology* (pp. 67–76). Springer. https://doi.org/10.1007/978-3-319-41861-2_6

Duke, C. C., & Stanik, C. (2016, August 11). Overcoming lower-income patients' concerns about trust and respect from providers: *Health Affairs* forefront. *Health Affairs*. https://www.healthaffairs.org/do/10.1377/forefront.20160811.056138/full/

Fortune, S. (2021, September 28). Barriers in BIPOC populations diagnosed with breast cancer. *Oncology Nursing News*. https://www.oncnursingnews.com/view/barriers-in-bipoc-populations-diagnosed-with-breast-cancer

Gazendam-Donofrio, S., Hoekstra, H., van der Graaf, W., van de Wiel, H., Visser, A., Huizinga, G., & Hoekstra-Weebers, J. (2009). Parent–child communication patterns during the first year after a parent's cancer diagnosis: The effect on parents' functioning. *Cancer. 115*(18), 4227–4237. https://doi.org/10.1002/cncr.24502

Junkins, C. C., Kent, E., Litzelman, K., Bevans, M., Cannady, R. S., & Rosenberg, A. R. (2020). Cancer across the ages: A narrative review of caregiver burden for patients of all ages. *Journal of Psychosocial Oncology, 38*(6), 782–798. https://doi.org/10.1080/07347332.2020.1796887

Kelly, E. P., Parades, A. Z., Tsilimigras, D. I., Hyer, J. M., & Pawlik, T. M. (2020). The role of religion and spirituality in cancer care: An umbrella review of the literature. *Surgical Oncology*, 101389–101389. https://doi.org/10.1016/j.suronc.2020.05.004

Lee, D. C., Liang, H., Chen, N., Shi, L., & Liu, Y. (2020). Cancer screening among racial/ethnic groups in health centers. *International Journal of Equity in Health, 19*(1), 43. https://doi.org/10.1186/s12939-020-1153-5

Northouse, L., Williams, A. L., Given, B., & McCorkle, R. (2012). Psychosocial care for family caregivers of patients with cancer. *Journal of Clinical Oncology, 30*(11), 1227–1234.

Reisman, Y., & Gianotten, W. L. (2017). *Cancer, intimacy, and sexuality: A practical approach* (1st ed.). Springer.

Sage, N. (2008). *CBT for chronic illness and palliative care: A workbook and toolkit*. Wiley-Interscience.

Shin, J. Y., Steger, M. F., Shin, D. W., Kimn, S. Y., Yang, H. K., Cho, J., Jeong, A., Park, K., Kweon, S. S., & Park, H. P. (2019). Patient–family communication mediates the relation between family hardiness and caregiver positivity: Exploring the moderating role of caregiver depression and anxiety. *Journal of Psychosocial Oncology, 37*(5), 557–572. https://doi.org/10.1080/07347332.2019.1566808

U.S. Bureau of Labor Statistics. (n.d.). *Employment projections. Table 3.3. Civilian labor force participation rate by age, sex, race, and ethnicity 2000, 2010, 2020, and projected 2030 (in percent)*. Retrieved February 13, 2022, from https://www.bls.gov/emp/tables/civilian-labor-force-participation-rate.htm

U.S. Census Bureau. (2021). *America's families and living arrangements: 2021. Table A1. Marital status of people 15 years and over, by age, sex, and personal earnings: 2021*. Retrieved from https://www.census.gov/data/tables/2021/demo/families/cps-2021.html

U.S. Census Bureau. (2020). *America's families and living arrangements: 2020. Table A3. Parents with coresident children under 18, by living arrangement, sex, and selected characteristics: 2020*. Retrieved from https://www.census.gov/data/tables/2020/demo/families/cps-2020.html

18

Children, Adolescents, and Young Adults With Cancer

Nancy Cincotta, Sarah Paul, and Arika Patneaude

Key Concepts

- Children and adolescents and young adults (AYAs) each embody cognitive, spiritual, cultural, familial, and physical attributes consistent with their age and development—their journey with cancer is affected by these domains.
- Language, communication, and educational efforts with these populations need to be tailored to their developmental level.
- Children's knowledge and desire for involvement in decision-making around their treatment may be underappreciated, which can negatively affect their ability to cope with their illness.
- Cancer can thwart children and AYAs' movement toward autonomy and growth, which needs to be cultivated and centered on the individual's needs and wishes.
- Children and AYAs with cancer need to be heard in the context of their lives and their interests, e.g., connecting with peer groups, establishing age-appropriate growth experiences (school, recreation, work, and relationships), and creative endeavors (expressive arts and social media), as they are crucial in helping them live and grow through these developmentally significant stages.
- Cancer in the young is a "family affair" unique to each family and culture and involves parents, siblings, partners, friends, grandparents, extended family, and others in their support network.

Keywords: adolescents, children, development, pediatrics, young adults

Nancy Cincotta, Sarah Paul, and Arika Patneaude, *Children, Adolescents, and Young Adults With Cancer* In: *Oncology and Palliative Social Work*. Edited by: Susan Hedlund, Bryan Miller, Grace Christ, and Carolyn Messner, Oxford University Press.
 DOI: 10.1093/oso/9780197607299.003.0018

Box 18.1

The baby feels pain and the changes in routine but does not have a way to react beyond crying or withdrawing. The 4-year-old begins to understand that their life is different when they enter school and learns that not everyone has a "tubey" (port). The 6-year-old fears that someone is coming to steal all the blood in her body when a nurse says someone will be in to "take" her blood. The 9-year-old sibling whose parents cannot attend their dance recital because their sister is hospitalized with chickenpox forever sees that moment as an indicator that they are the less-loved child. The 12-year-old who is dying shares a bed with their 13-year-old sibling—the two had vowed never to sleep in separate rooms. The 15-year-old is rejected from a camp program because their neutrophil counts are too low. The 18-year-old dreams of a rural college experience, only to learn that she cannot attend school away from a major medical center because of her diagnosis. The 20-year-old is accepted for a summer internship and must withdraw from it and return to his parents' home so he can begin an experimental treatment protocol. The 25-year-old gets married in the hospital while awaiting a bone marrow transplant so she can evade the hospital rules, which only allow family members to stay over. The 28-year-old woman arranges for egg retrieval, stopping treatment during the process, only to see her ovarian cancer spread as her dreams of surviving to be a mother diminish. All understand the cancer experience at their developmental stage and the stress and isolation it can impose.

A cancer diagnosis at any age can be devastating, but when it occurs earlier in life, it can carry a greater burden (Box 18.1). Cancer and its treatment risk altering the life course of children, adolescents, and young adults; dismantling dreams; and preventing individuals from reaching their fullest potential. For those who are still maturing emotionally, physically, and cognitively, a cancer diagnosis becomes a family disease, with an impact on each family member. In this chapter, we refer to adolescents and young adults ages 15–29 as AYAs.

Although great strides have been made in pediatric and AYA oncology care, these vulnerable populations continue to face vastly different challenges from those of other age groups. In this chapter, we note the implications of a cancer diagnosis and its treatment on the developmental trajectories of young people; the holistic impact on the entire family, including siblings; and disruptions in the life cycle and developmental progression, causing physical, emotional, and social challenges.

Due to the unique confluence of these life disruptions, oncology and palliative care social workers with their knowledge of development and family

Table 18.1 Development, Disruption, and Coping During the Cancer Journey for Children, Adolescents, and Young Adults

Age at Diagnosis	Primary Developmental Tasks	Possible Disruption Due to Cancer Diagnosis and Treatment	Coping/Adaptation	Issues to Consider	Quotations from Practice
Infancy	Secure attachments Bonding with caregiver(s) Exploring the environment (sensory exploration) Discovering physical self Trust, learning that the world is "safe" Comfort-seeking, self-soothing behavior Feeding Expressive self: crying, smiling, laughter	Bonding and normal routine interrupted Separation issues: insecure attachments Delays in development, regressive behavior Increased irritability, emotional withdrawal Introduction to physical pain Absence of touch, sensory exploration interrupted Physical restraint—restriction of movement Physical symptoms impeding feeding (nausea) Disrupted consistency: unstable environment, presence of strangers, or caregiver stress/volatility	Calm, supportive environment with attention to basic needs Recognition, reduction, and alleviation of pain Mitigation against discomfort, unnecessary strangers, loud sounds Unrestricted family visiting Ongoing physical contact	Pain is often less readily recognized in infants—proactive management of pain, uncomfortable situations, and positioning Caregiver support: anxiety and guilt in caregiver Enable caregiver's comfort	*I ushered my baby into life, and I feel privileged to usher my child from life.*

Toddler/ Preschool	Exploration and mastery of the environment Trust Testing boundaries Expressive self: language, laughter, tears Parallel play Cognitive advances Physical exploration Self-discovery Magical thinking	Delays in development Physical achievements impacted by treatment: feeding, walking, toileting, or sleeping Limitation of opportunities to explore the environment Curiosity decreases Situational anxiety Lack of caregiver confidence Physical, emotional, social, and cognitive challenges Fears and imagination prevail	Supportive environment Opportunities for mastery of feasible tasks Support for caregiver Affording appropriate play and growth opportunities Maintain strong physical contact Illness identity/naming Engagement around illness activities, routines Illness (cancer) programming/fun initiatives Age-appropriate education Play activities and intervention to complement development	Recognition and management of pain and discomfort Parent and sibling education and support Address fear of being left alone in the hospital—establish a plan	*Doesn't everyone get chemo?* *Do I need to brush my teeth in heaven?*

(*continued*)

Table 18.1 Continued

Age at Diagnosis	Primary Developmental Tasks	Possible Disruption Due to Cancer Diagnosis and Treatment	Coping/Adaptation	Issues to Consider	Quotations from Practice
School Age Decision-making: Provision of Assent to treatment	Cognitive growth Community development/ School identity Development of new routines	"Play dates" deferred, limitation in social and emotional development Illness and treatment-related fear, anxiety, and pain Reduction in confidence School absences More contact with adults then peers Fewer boundaries around sleep schedules and routines	Age-appropriate interventions such as game playing, skill-building, and cancer education Mutually agreed on school/ education plan Maintain and create joyful activities (baking, crafting) Increased decision-making as allowable in light of physical autonomy Illness peer-based activities (camps, wishes, or other adventures) Illness peer cohorting Psychoeducation Illness-related discussions, education, and assent in medical decision-making	Managing fears of the unknown Age-appropriate education Wish programs Pain management Maximizing family time Family memory making	*Will they take all my blood when they take blood?* *Do you have to take tests in heaven?*

Preteens Decision-making: Provision of Assent to treatment	Dramatic cognitive growth Understanding of oneself in relationship to others Self-esteem, body image, and puberty/sexual self	Disruptions in social interactions, friendship insecurity Challenges to identity and basic tenets of adolescence Peer-group limitations, identification with cancer More limited exploration of interests, less autonomy Less involvement with team/club activities Challenges to physical growth and sexual awareness Struggle between rebellion versus guilt following all medical instructions	Provide education, choice, and control in medical treatment activities Create an education plan and maintain academic tracking Create and maintain developmentally affirming skill- and competence-building activities, team opportunities Connect to peer networks within cancer community Sustain friendships, encourage visiting and activities Develop opportunities for life-affirming growth and achievement beyond cancer Honest dialogues Shared decision-making Explore emotions and allow for independent thinking and choice-making	Children engaging parents Continuing to find joy Creating memories Legacy building—leaving behind something to be remembered by	*I would not change the fact that I had cancer, I like who I am.* *Take care of my parents for me after I die, I worry about them.*

(*continued*)

Table 18.1 Continued

Age at Diagnosis	Primary Developmental Tasks	Possible Disruption Due to Cancer Diagnosis and Treatment	Coping/Adaptation	Issues to Consider	Quotations from Practice
Adolescents Decision-making <18 Assent ≥18 Consent	Identity development, sense of self Peers, friendships Self-esteem/body image Personal sense of identity Physical sense of self/ sexuality Increased cognitive abilities and demands Peer relationships Vocational goals	Complicated sense of self, higher risk for anxiety/ depression Isolation and fear of missing out Lessening of trust in one's own body Feelings of immortality minimized Disruptions in social development, education, friendship, peer communication, romantic opportunities, sports, and recreational programs More limited autonomy More time with parents and family; less time with peers and friends Delay in normative activities (e.g., college visits, college attendance)	Help in navigating multiple identities (patient, survivor, etc.) Address challenges in disclosure and implications for friendships, romantic relationships Romantic relationships (when to disclose?) Establish and maintain transparency at diagnosis through treatment Communication with the patient first Sustain relationships of support Encourage strong partnerships with medical team Explore attainable educational and career goals	Screening and support to address emotional symptoms Honest communication regarding prognosis and addressing fears/concerns Delineate focus on curative versus palliative care Structured advance care planning tools Help facilitate conversations about choices in general and ongoing end-of-life conversations Facilitate conversations about fertility preservation "Poor timing" of end-of-life conversations and "poor timing" for the end of life to be at the beginning of life.	*Mail this postcard to my father after I die—I wanted to tell him I would be okay.*

Twenties	Achieving autonomy Establishing identity Career building Romantic/intimate relationships Community building Family building Decision-making; life choices Integration of autonomy/independence and parental support/family involvement Conformity with peer development Support and alliance transitions with parents, caregivers, friends and partners	Regression Altered sense of self Interruptions in life tasks and milestones Less autonomy (AYAs may move back home with family) Loss of identity/sense of self (activities may have to change) Loss of financial stability (changes in employment) Disruption and delays in education/career Disruption or shifts in relationships (peer and romantic) Loss of community, increased isolation Risk of infertility, disruption to family building	Risk of anxiety, depression, PTSD Normalize life-cycle disruptions and being in a different place than peers Establish relationships with illness-connected peers Developing avenues to increase autonomy and independence Encouraging involvement in illness community-based activities to minimize isolation and increase socialization (peer groups, cancer support groups, outdoor adventure programming) Navigating role changes (parents, siblings, friends, or partners) Coping with loss of fertility and other potential losses Adapting to the loss of developmental milestones reached by peers that they may/will not achieve Loss of potential Accepting changes in dreams and fulfillment of reframed goals	Reframing hope as appropriate to the situation Transparent and honest communication about concerns Conversations earlier in the illness trajectory (introduction of palliative care; planning for the future) Allow for and connect with emotions: avoidance/denial, acceptance, anger, hope, expectation, loneliness, and community Exploration of age-related values (How do they want to spend their remaining time?)	*Cancer is like a school—it has taught me many things.* *I want the life I dreamed of.* *I want to have this child to keep my legacy alive.*

systems are well suited to contribute to the care of children, adolescents, and young adults with cancer, whether treatment is curative or ends in palliative or hospice care (Table 18.1).

Facts and Figures

Although rare, cancer is the leading cause of death by disease among children and adolescents past infancy in the United States. In 2022, it was estimated that 10,470 children (birth to 14 years) and 5,480 adolescents (15–19 years) would be diagnosed with cancer and 1,050 and 550, respectively, would die from the disease (Siegel et al., 2022). Although research efforts with this vulnerable population have increased in the last decade, many childhood and AYA-specific cancer needs remain unmet (Miller et al., 2020).

Support Networks

We define *family* here as any individual, dyad, or group involved in the care, love, nurturance, and support of a child, adolescent, or young adult. The authors recognize that this is different from the legal definition of *guardian* or *decision-maker*; *family* does not necessarily equal decision-maker. In addition, it is possible that the minor's legal guardian may not be a member of the nuclear family and that decision-makers designated by older AYAs may not be family members.

A cancer diagnosis in children and AYAs can have a significant effect on the family system, emotionally and financially. Bona et al. (2014) reported on the economic impact of progressive, recurrent, or nonresponsive cancer in the children of 71 families followed at three children's hospitals. Families of lower socioeconomic status were affected disproportionately, especially when the patient was a child with a special health care need.

Families of children and AYAs with cancer now face additional fear related to COVID-19. A study of 45 parents of children with cancer that examined the psychological impact of the COVID-19 pandemic on them, their stress levels and anxiety, and how they perceived the quality of their children's lives, found that 75% exhibited significant anxiety symptoms that existed well beyond the "typical" three-month time period post-diagnosis (Guido et al., 2021). While we acknowledge the impact of COVID-19, the authors are focusing on the overall impact of cancer.

Decision-Making

Decision-making regarding the course of treatment for children, adolescents, and young adults can look different depending on family values, experiences, and cultural norms. For some families, decision-making is a collective process; in others, the legal guardian(s) (most often the parents) make decisions. Depending on the family, culture, or other circumstances, the decision-maker may be someone other than the patient or parent: a family elder, spiritual leader, spouse, partner, best friend, and in some circumstances, a court-ordered proxy.

Decision-making can serve as a paradigm for the course of cancer treatment from childhood through young adulthood. In the days immediately following diagnosis, parents must decide to give their consent for treatment, taking a leap of faith as they seek to learn everything about the condition in an effort to save their child's life. Communication with children is affected by a child's age and their ability to understand both language and meaning around illness. The youngest children often have the youngest, most inexperienced parents. Those whose first child is diagnosed with cancer may just be learning how to be parents, much less "cancer parents."

Box 18.2

A 9-year-old was approaching the end of his life. His mother chose to ask him his thoughts about his "Do Not Resuscitate" status. He told her that if everyone who wanted to say goodbye to him had not had a chance to visit, he would agree to be resuscitated but if they had, he would not need to be resuscitated.

The patient's age can and often does affect the treatment course. A teen with more autonomy is often expected to be involved in decision-making, whereas younger children are less often included in major decisions (note, however, that in some treatment centers, the age of assent begins as young as 7 years). Decisions of the youngest patients can at times be unexpected, revealing, and speak to self-determination (Box 18.2). Young adults who have come of age (18 years) may be expected to make decisions independently, depending on the philosophy of their treatment team/center.

Siblings

Brothers' and sisters' lives are forever altered by a sibling's cancer diagnosis, but limited attention may be focused on their concerns. Jealousy over the attention given to the sibling; guilt about those feelings or of being unaffected by cancer; worry and fear; and the enormity of changes in the homeostasis of family life can impose a silent burden on siblings. They may be temporarily displaced from home and familiar support, excluded from hospital visits, and have less access to professional resources and medical information than other family members. Siblings live parallel experiences and face lifelong consequences (Cincotta, 2015). Pediatric cancer can have a greater impact on siblings' family relationships than those of the child undergoing treatment (Erker et al., 2018).

Families must consider treatment decisions for not only the patient but also the patient's siblings. What does support look like for siblings? Who cares for them during long hospitalizations when primary caregivers may be at the patient's bedside? A pediatric cancer diagnosis has a significant impact on siblings (Oberoi et al., 2020). Their developmental stage combined with a lack of complete information may lead to misperceptions. *I do not understand why my parents stopped treatment and killed my brother* (the parents decided to stop treatment because it was not working).

Special Programs

Children, adolescents, and young adults learn and grow in groups, at school, in sports programs, bands/choirs, clubs, through religious affiliations and rites of passage, and in concert with their siblings. These natural outlets provide social and emotional stability and growth by creating environments in which friendships and identities form, support is present, and feelings are validated. Young people facing cancer have the same emotional and social needs as those without cancer, and treatment teams should implement programs to address those needs.

Special programs and recreational activities (camps, family retreats, outdoor adventures) for children and AYA populations serve to provide experiences consistent with their developmental age otherwise limited by chemotherapy schedules, immune suppression, and attendant risk of infection. Interfacing with others who might not view safety as a priority or understand feelings associated with the cancer experience can become an emotional burden for the person with cancer. Recreational programming and developmentally sensitive activities enrich lives, minimize isolation, and open the door to building personal networks of peers with cancer.

Medical Care for the AYA With Cancer

Adolescents and young adults with cancer represent a cohort at a time of life transition, emerging into adulthood. The Children's Oncology Group (COG) currently provides treatment protocols through age 26 (https://childrenoncologygroup.org). Whether these young adults have been recently diagnosed, aged out of pediatric care but have recurrent disease, or are born with an illness that predisposes them to cancer, the AYA cancer experience comes with its own emotional sequelae.

For those diagnosed in their late teens and early twenties, a pediatric oncology service can feel like an inappropriate place for care, yet an adult setting with significantly older patients may also be isolating and emotionally overwhelming. Programs for AYAs are essential in managing the physical and emotional sequelae of cancer, as they can help mitigate the anxiety, sadness, and loneliness that emerges from the redirection of attendant life tasks (Table 18.2).

Table 18.2 Questions According to Age

Developmental Age/ Age at Diagnosis	Who has the question?	Questions
Infants	Parents/Caregivers	*What did I do to cause this? Did the glass of wine I had before I knew I was pregnant cause this?*
Toddlers	Parents/Caregivers	*I thought the bruising was because he's learning how to walk and keeps falling down. Why didn't I get this checked sooner?!*
Preschoolers	Parents/Caregivers	*Is it because I smoke? Is it because a power line runs over our house?*
School-Age	Parents/Caregivers/ Patient/ Sibling	*Am I going to die? Will my parents be able to afford this? Will I be a burden? What about the sleepover that is scheduled next week? Do they love my sick sibling more than me? They spend all their time with her.*
Adolescents	Patient	*Will I be able to go to prom? I'm applying to college; will I have to delay it? Will I be able to play basketball? I have college recruiters looking at me.*
Young Adult	Patient	*I'm supposed to get married next year. What about my career? Can I keep up with my peers?*

Selected Developmental Issues

Identity/Sense of Self

Cancer affects identity development regardless of the age at diagnosis. Children, adolescents, and young adults face different "identity crises" as they begin treatment. Because a child's sense of self develops through positive relationships, shared memories, and experiences of belonging, children diagnosed with cancer may struggle with their identity. Being removed from daily life and everyday peer interactions can hinder socialization. Sense of self continues to be established in adolescence through experimentation with identity, trying new things, and developing new skills and hobbies. A cancer diagnosis often disrupts the "normal" teenage experience, resulting in adolescents who are wise beyond their years but may exhibit social and developmental delays. Young adults struggle to maintain a sense of self when diagnosed with cancer. Their cancer journey sets them apart from their peers and makes it difficult for them to feel understood. In each age group, isolation and separation from peers and activities integral to social development may have an adverse effect on the formation of identity and autonomy.

Children, adolescents, and young adults with cancer often feel misunderstood by peers at a time when social experiences play an integral role in identity development. A recurring theme for children and AYAs with cancer is dealing with profound isolation, changes in peer relationships, or compromised friendships (Fainsilber Katz et al., 2011).

Body Image

Body image and self-esteem go hand in hand. For children and AYAs with cancer, body image concerns vary depending on the diagnosis, nature of its treatment, and long-term side effects. Regardless of age, it is essential for pediatric and oncology social workers to understand how a negative body image can increase emotional distress. Younger children may be more concerned about looking "different" from their peers. For adolescents, body image heavily impacts identity formation and sense of self. For young adults, sexual orientation, gender identity, and self-esteem directly correlate to positive or negative body image.

Fertility Preservation

Conversations about infertility and fertility preservation play an essential role for children, adolescents, and young adults diagnosed with cancer. While studies have shown that effective communication regarding fertility preservation options improves patients' quality of life (Assi et al., 2018), patients report that these conversations do not always take place in a timely manner. Providing information early to patients regardless of their gender, age, or relationship status is an integral step to improving psychosocial outcomes. For young children, parents must take the initiative to connect with the medical team for referral to a reproductive specialist if needed. While younger children may lack understanding regarding fertility preservation, it makes sense developmentally to begin discussion of the topic around the time of puberty. Infertility affects young male and female cancer patients, many of whom fear that their choice to have biological children will be out of their control. Resource management and navigation are critical in the early stages of diagnosis, while there may still be an opportunity to initiate the fertility preservation process.

Survivorship

Long-term effects and quality-of-life issues for children and AYAs can have prolonged implications (emotionally and physically). Growing up with a cancer identity is complicated; psychosocial programming can help with adherence to medical care, supportive peer networking, and resilience. Some specific diagnoses (e.g., brain tumors), age, gender, and long-term effects can all influence the quality of life of children and AYAs and increase the risk of social isolation (Pahl et al., 2021). Psychoeducation, age-appropriate interventions, career and academic counseling, activities promoting socialization and skill development, and family planning serve as adjuncts to treatment and are invaluable to the ongoing well-being of patients.

End-of-Life Conversations

Many people consider death a taboo topic, especially for children, adolescents, and young adults. Providers often avoid conversations about death due to the emotional distress they perceive they might cause patients, families, and even themselves. Stigma and avoidance can lead to children being left out of advance care planning and discussions regarding prognosis and end of life. Narratives from bereaved parents indicate that ongoing open, honest, and "stepwise disclosure of prognostic information," an avenue for hope and realism, anticipatory guidance for end-of-life planning, and support from the medical team are essential themes in conversations around death and dying (Robert et al., 2022). Regardless of the prognosis, many adolescents and young adults have shared that they think about the prospect of death and want to discuss it. AYAs report that they may feel sad, worried, or angry in the short term when engaging in advance care planning. However, research indicates discussing and being involved in end-of-life planning leads to decreased levels of emotional distress and improved quality of life (Rosenberg et al., 2016). In a pilot study of a structured advance care planning program for adolescents with cancer, Lyon et al. (2013) found that although 24% of those surveyed said that early conversations about a possible poor prognosis made them sad, 71% said that the conversations were also valuable and 91% said they were helpful. Such critical conversations may not be easy for clinicians, yet it remains important to anticipate and support the unique needs of children, adolescents, and young adults.

Parents, partners, and siblings need to communicate about the journeys of children and AYAs at the end of life. Notably, the choice to die at home creates permanent, specific memories in the space within which family members feel safe. Children may die in their parents' bed, a shared bedroom, or the living room. Considerations need to be made for how surviving siblings will feel after experiencing death where they continue to live. Feelings conceived in these moments will become embedded in the memories of family members.

Adults leave legacies through their shared experiences, accomplishments, and all they have accumulated. Helping a family experience joyful activities, the products of which may be seen as a part of the young person's "legacy," is an important aspect of oncology and palliative social workers' role throughout treatment and at the end of life. With the youngest of children, social workers can offer to help the family create memories. With older children, it is more of a collaborative process, while teens can be encouraged to explore their creativity. Working with young adults is a parallel endeavor. In each case, the object is to enable each individual to identify what they might want to physically/emotionally explore, create, achieve, or leave behind.

The "essence" of a child can be found embodied in sensory experiences related to memories made as they grow up. Activities that focus on a child's or AYA's physical presence can serve as ways to maintain a tangible connection to the deceased. Examples of these include recording a heartbeat (sometimes to the "beat" of a favorite song), capturing the sounds of breath in a song or in the playing of a wind instrument, plaster casts of the individual's hand, foot/hand/thumb prints, voice recordings, and visual memories (photographs and videos). Saving unwashed garments (to retain the individual's smell) or creating a quilt of the child's clothing each create memories unique to the essence of the person. Such memories link the past to the future (Cincotta, 2022).

Children, just as adults, benefit from being given permission to let go. The youngest children want to be held and not to be alone at the end of life. Older children, teens, and young adults value the ongoing support, physical presence, and contact of those who love them.

While a family's focus is understandably on the young person who is dying, bereaved siblings endure more "silent" losses, including the loss of roles that had provided security and identity formation, emotional distance from parents during the illness and after the death, changes in family systems, and involuntary changes in birth role (becoming the oldest), which can affect future communication, development, and achievement. For example, a young man leaving for college described to his peers in a bereavement group that he got a tattoo of his deceased sister's name so that it would bring her into the conversation in his new environment. For the young woman whose life partner (soulmate) dies in their twenties or the parents who lose their oldest child, the challenge to their identity and the promise of what might have been becomes woven into the future.

Reflections on Working With Children and AYAs

Among the general population, it can be difficult to acknowledge that children, adolescents, and young adults not only are diagnosed with cancer but also die from cancer. Some of the most rewarding yet emotionally laden therapeutic work can happen between a social worker and a family navigating a cancer diagnosis and treatment. Social workers' value is in the skills they bring to the table: empathy, cultural humility, developmental knowledge, specific therapeutic skills, support for treatment/medication adherence, and the ability to facilitate honest conversations from diagnosis to those unfortunate times when interventions cease to work and end-of-life conversations begin.

When a young person dies, it affects everyone in that individual's community and symbolizes the loss of a shared future. The homeostasis of the family is altered. Family patterns and life expectations change. Connections between others who have experienced a similar loss are among the most helpful bonds social workers can enable.

Guiding Best Practices for the Future

Genetic Implications

Genetic testing may have individual and global implications in the care of children, adolescents, and young adults with cancer. It may hold crucial insights leading to precision medicine solutions for the newly diagnosed child and also provide answers for future treatment, unlocking solutions that have thwarted researchers for decades.

Testing for genetic cancer markers raises developmentally informed questions: At what age do you test? When do you give a child/AYA results? And who makes those choices? As this field progresses rapidly, one might speculate that soon everyone will know their genetic profile from birth. Such knowledge will influence decision-making and the challenges today's children face as tomorrow's adults (Box 18.3).

Consider the challenges for those with cancer predisposition syndromes, born into an unusual trajectory, who live knowing that cancer may be part of their future and aware that they may need oncology care throughout their lives. They begin their lives in pediatric care but eventually leave the physicians, researchers, and care teams that they have known their whole lives, a tremendous loss at a complicated, transitional time in their illness experience. Social workers can be of great assistance in helping young adults with decision-making around salient life issues.

Box 18.3 Kyle's Story

Kyle, a healthy 20-year-old with no known preexisting conditions, began to experience abnormal digestive symptoms that affected his ability to eat and caused rapid weight loss. After many laboratory investigations and biopsies, he was diagnosed with severe gastritis. Two months later, he began to have trouble walking and breathing. While hospitalized, the medical team determined that he had an aggressive gastric cancer that had already metastasized to his bones and lungs. Kyle's health quickly declined, and he died during a procedure to improve his breathing. Shortly after his death, genetic testing revealed that Kyle's gastric cancer had developed due to a mutation in the CDH1 gene. The discovery of this mutation led to testing his remaining two siblings, one of whom tested positive. At 13, his younger brother, Tim, began undergoing annual monitoring, knowing the high-risk factors that accompany this gene mutation. Four years later, during a routine endoscopy, he was diagnosed with signet ring cell carcinoma. Fortunately, he was able to undergo surgery before the cancer spread and continues to be monitored regularly.

Cultural Humility and Responsiveness

Social workers are obligated through training rooted in social justice and through the National Association of Social Workers Code of Ethics (2021), which governs the social work profession in responding to patients and families in a competent manner. Culture is vast and broad yet as unique as each patient and family that we encounter. Debate is ongoing as to whether one can truly become culturally "competent." Thus we choose to use the term "*cultural responsiveness*" to describe the intersection of cultural humility and competence in which social workers must engage with children, AYAs, and their loved ones to provide the best assessment and care possible. Patneaude (2021) defines cultural humility and responsiveness as the ability to see and authentically accept another who is different from oneself—for example, race and ethnicity, gender identity, national origin, religion, sexual orientation—essentially, how one navigates the world. Cultural humility allows one to remain open to these differences despite socially implicit and explicit outside influences encouraging otherwise (Patneaude, 2021).

When working with children and AYAs with cancer, it is important to not only explore with the family what culture, inclusive of spirituality (separate from religion), means to them as a family but also with the patient themselves. When focusing on spirituality, one can ask a child about the things that are most important to them, who or what they turn to when they are afraid, what brings them joy. For younger children, it might be their caregiver, their special stuffed animal or blanket. For teens and young adults, it may mean contemplating what spirituality means to them, whether it be connecting with friends and/or listening to music. For young adults, it could be talking with a spouse, trusted friend, social worker, and/or chaplain about what having cancer means to them within the larger context of spirituality and/or religion. For patients of all ages creating a space to have these conversations is of utmost importance in providing holistic cultural care.

Pearls

- Cancer in childhood, adolescence, and young adulthood is a family affair, affecting everyone in the individual's immediate family and community. Family-centered care recognizes that those early in life are reliant on their nuclear family/caregivers and partners.

- Direct (developmentally appropriate, culturally sensitive) communication is essential whether the person with cancer is a child, adolescent, or young adult.
- Siblings are very much participants in the cancer journey, with distinct needs to be recognized and supported.
- The information an individual receives about the diagnosis and the stage of illness they are facing needs to become more sophisticated as they age. Children and AYAs with cancer require information to make decisions consistent with what they understand, want, and need.
- Children, teens, and young adults need opportunities for support to advance their social and emotional growth and education and to enhance their coping throughout the cancer journey.

Pitfalls

- Societal aversion to conversations with children and AYAs about difficult medical situations and end-of-life issues is an ongoing concern.
- Cultural humility requires a constant awareness to understand the impact of culture on children, AYAs, and their families' illness experience. Patients and families and the way "culture" shows up for them are all unique. It is impossible to be fully culturally responsive without understanding the context in which the patient/family synthesize their experience at any given moment.
- Compliance with medical care and follow-up decreases as childhood cancer patients get further removed in time from treatment. Not all children or AYAs want to remain connected to the cancer experience, limiting comprehensive follow-up data and creating difficulty in establishing short- and long-term programming/standards.
- Referrals to palliative care or hospice in all the younger age groups are often late.
- Collaboration among systems that serve children and AYAs (on treatment and off treatment along the continuum of care) is limited.
- Patient-centered qualitative studies that address the unique needs of children and AYAs during and after treatment are limited.

Additional Resources

Alex's Lemonade Stand Foundation for Childhood Cancer. *SuperSibs!*: https://www.alexslemonade.org/childhood-cancer/for-families/supersibs
American Childhood Cancer Organization: http://www.acco.org
Cancer*Care*. *Cancer*Care *for Kids*®: https://www.cancercare.org/forkids
Cancer*Care*. *Coping with cancer as a young adult*: https://www.cancercare.org/publications/164-coping_with_cancer_as_a_young_adult
Center to Advance Palliative Care. *On-demand webinars: Embracing cultural humility in palliative care*: https://www.capc.org/events/recorded-webinars/embracing-cultural-humility-in-palliative-care
Children's Oncology Camping Association, International: https://www.cocai.org
Courageous Parents Network: https://courageousparentsnetwork.org
Dear Jack Foundation: https://www.dearjackfoundation.org.
Provides quality-of-life programs to AYA cancer patients and survivors and their families.
National Institutes of Health. (2015, September). *Children with cancer: A guide for parents*. NIH Publication No. 15-2378: https://www.cancer.gov/publications/patient-education/guide-for-parents
The Samfund: https://www.thesamfund.org
Supports young adults through financial assistance, free online support, and education.
Stupidcancer: https://stupidcancer.org. (empowering AYAs affected by cancer)
Teen Cancer America: https://teencanceramerica.org

Grief Resources

Experience Camps: https://www.experiencecamps.org
For grieving children who have experienced the death of a parent, sibling, or primary caregiver.
Bo's Place: https://www.bosplace.org
Compassionate Friends: https://www.compassionatefriends.org
Dougy Center: The National Grief Center for Children & Families: https://www.dougy.org
Judi's House/JAG Institute: https://www.judishouse.org
National Alliance for Children's Grief: https://www.childrengrieve.org
Sesame Street in Communities: Helping Children Grieve: https://www.sesamestreetincommunities.org/topics/grief/

References

Assi, J., Santos, J., Bonetti, T., Serafini, P. C., Motta, E., & Chehin, M. B. (2018). Psychosocial benefits of fertility preservation for young cancer patients. *Journal of Assisted Reproduction and Genetics*, *35*(4), 601–606. https://doi.org/10.1007/s10815-018-1131-7
Bona, K., Dussel, V., Orellana, L., Kang, T., Geyer, R., Feudtner, C., & Wolfe, J. (2014). Economic impact of advanced pediatric cancer on families. *Journal of Pain and Symptom Management*, *47*(3), 594–603. https://doi.org/10.1016/j.jpainsymman.2013.04.003
Cincotta, N. F. (2015). Helping siblings of pediatric cancer patients. In G. Christ, C. Messner, & L. Behar (Eds.), *Handbook of oncology social work: Psychosocial care for people with cancer* (pp. 473–483). Oxford University Press.

Cincotta, N. F. (2022). Bereavement in the beginning phase of life: Grief in children and their families. In T. Altilio, S. Otis-Green, & J. Cagle (Eds.), *Oxford textbook of palliative social work* (2nd ed., pp. 714–725). Oxford University Press. https://doi.org/10.1093/med/9780197537855.001.0001

Erker, C., Yan, K., Zhang, L., Bingen, K., Flynn, K. E., & Panepinto, J. (2018). Impact of pediatric cancer on family relationships. *Cancer Medicine*, *7*(5), 1680–1688. https://doi.org/10.1002/cam4.1393

Fainsilber Katz, L., Leary, A., Breiger, D., & Friedman, D. (2011). Pediatric cancer and the quality of children's dyadic peer interactions. *Journal of Pediatric Psychology*, *36*(2), 237–247. https://doi.org/10.1093/jpepsy/jsq050

Guido, A., Marconi, E., Peruzzi, L., Dinapoli, N., Tamburrini, G., Attinà, G., Balducci, M., Valentini, V., Ruggiero, A., & Chieffo, D. P. R. (2021). Psychological impact of COVID-19 on parents of pediatric cancer patients [Brief research report]. *Frontiers in Psychology*, *12*. https://doi.org/10.3389/fpsyg.2021.730341

Lyon, M. E., Jacobs, S., Briggs, L., Cheng, Y. I., & Wang, J. (2013). Family-centered advance care planning for teens with cancer. *JAMA Pediatrics*, *167*(5), 460–467. https://doi.org/10.1001/jamapediatrics.2013.943

Miller, K. D., Fidler-Benaoudia, M., Keegan, T. H., Hipp, H. S., Jemal, A., & Siegel, R. L. (2020). Cancer statistics for adolescents and young adults, 2020. *CA: A Cancer Journal for Clinicians*, *70*(6), 443–459. https://doi.org/10.3322/caac.21637

National Association of Social Workers (NASW). (2021). *Code of ethics of the National Association of Social Workers*. NASW Press.

Oberoi, A. R., Cardona, N. D., Davis, K. A., Pariseau, E. M., Berk, D., Muriel, A. C., & Long, K. A. (2020). Parent decision-making about support for siblings of children with cancer: Sociodemographic influences. *Clinical Practice in Pediatric Psychology*, *8*(2), 115–125. https://doi.org/10.1037/cpp0000324

Pahl, D. A., Wieder, M. S., & Steinberg, D. M. (2021). Social isolation and connection in adolescents with cancer and survivors of childhood cancer: A systematic review. *Journal of Adolescence*, *87*(1), 15–27. https://doi.org/10.1016/j.adolescence.2020.12.010

Patneaude, A. (2021, May 18). *Cultural humility in palliative care: A journey from the professional to the personal*. Center to Advance Palliative Care. https://www.capc.org/events/recorded-webinars/embracing-cultural-humility-in-palliative-care

Robert, R., Razvi, S., Triche, L. L., Bruera, E., & Moody, K. M. (2022). Bereaved parent perspectives on end-of-life conversations in pediatric oncology. *Children (Basel, Switzerland)*, *9*(2), 274. https://doi.org/10.3390/children9020274

Rosenberg, A. R., Wolfe, J., Wiener, L., Lyon, M., & Feudtner, C. (2016). Ethics, emotions, and the skills of talking about progressing disease with terminally ill adolescents: A review. *JAMA Pediatrics*, *170*(12), 1216–1223. https://doi.org/10.1001/jamapediatrics.2016.2142

Siegel, R. L., Miller, K. D., Fuchs, H. E., & Jemal, A. (2022). Cancer statistics, 2022. *CA: A Cancer Journal for Clinicians*, *72*(1), 7–33. https://doi.org/10.3322/caac.21708

19

Palliative Care for Lesbian, Gay, Bisexual, Transgender, Queer, and Intersex (LGBTQI) Persons Coping With Cancer

Mandi L. Pratt-Chapman, Gary Stein, Cathy Berkman, and Andre Pruitt

Key Concepts

- Lesbian, gay, bisexual, transgender, queer, and intersex (LGBTQI) people have historically experienced criminalization, discrimination, and denial of health care.
- Some LGBTQI people have a higher risk for certain cancers.
- LGBTQI people with cancer deserve respectful, dignified care near the end of life.

Keywords: LGBTQI, nondiscrimination, palliative care, psychosocial support, spiritual support

By 2030, approximately 7 million people over age 50 will identify as lesbian, gay, bisexual, transgender, or queer (LGBTQ). Another 1.7% of the population have intersex (I) conditions. Those who came of age in the 1950s and early 1960s faced criminalization through so-called sodomy laws, employment discrimination, and involuntary psychiatric care. Many people were forced to remain closeted. Those who grew up in the late 1960s and into the 1970s participated in the gay and other civil rights movements. These experiences have directly affected how LGBTQI individuals perceive health care providers and what they anticipate when in need of health care services.

Mandi L. Pratt-Chapman, Gary Stein, Cathy Berkman, and Andre Pruitt, *Palliative Care for Lesbian, Gay, Bisexual, Transgender, Queer, and Intersex (LGBTQI) Persons Coping With Cancer* In: *Oncology and Palliative Social Work*. Edited by: Susan Hedlund, Bryan Miller, Grace Christ, and Carolyn Messner, Oxford University Press.
DOI: 10.1093/oso/9780197607299.003.0019

This chapter provides an overview of palliative care needs and recommendations to advance health equity for LGBTQI cancer patients and their families. Fundamental to the purpose here is recognition of the agency of LGBTQI individuals in making health care choices, acknowledgment of the diversity of LGBTQI individuals, and assertion of the social worker's ethical requirement to optimize health and minimize harm over the course of individual lives. The chapter summarizes what is known about LGBTQI cancer palliative care needs and approaches that vary based on diverse lived experiences.

Palliative care includes the continuum of specialty care, from diagnosis to end of life, that focuses on pain and symptom management and improving quality of life. Hospice is delivered in a patient's final months, weeks, or days. Thus, the chapter considers communication and support for medical decisions aligned with patients' and families' goals of care, as well as physical, psychosocial, and spiritual support for patients and their families.

LGBTQI Discrimination and Cancer Disparities

The LGBTQI community deserves health care and social services that are respectful and free from stigma; yet discrimination persists. Evidence shows that LGBTQI patients and their partners experience elevated levels of disrespectful and discriminatory hospice and palliative care (Stein et al., 2020). Concerns about long-term care are particularly troubling, with reports of mistreatment, harassment, and denial of care. Transgender individuals may also face discrimination in health care and health insurance (James et al., 2016). As a result, many LGBTQI individuals, especially older adults and transgender people, may be hesitant to disclose their sexual orientation or gender identity (SOGI) and may delay or avoid health care, fearing they will be poorly received or mistreated.

LGBTQI persons experience elevated risk for some cancers due to a range of social determinants of health (SDOH). Specifically, lesbian and bisexual women have higher tobacco and alcohol use than their heterosexual counterparts, and men who have sex with men (MSM) are more likely to engage in "chemsex" (sexual practices that involve drug use to heighten stimulation). These behavioral risks often reflect maladaptive responses to chronic stress due to societal stigma, stress that is magnified when persons are multiply minoritized and stigmatized (Pratt-Chapman & Potter, 2019). Maladaptive health behaviors, including alcohol and tobacco use, put lesbian and bisexual women at greater risk for breast, cervical, vaginal, and vulvar cancers (American Cancer Society, 2021). Anal-receptive sex partners are at highest risk for anal cancer, making HPV vaccination an LGBTQI health priority. Gender dysphoria and fear of discrimination also can lead transgender and genderqueer people to avoid cancer screenings discordant with their identity. Recommendations to reduce these inequalities include providing a safe, inclusive environment; affirming communication; ensuring comprehensive palliative care; and focusing on patient-centered end-of-life planning.

Affirming Care Environments for LGBTQI Patients and Families

Leaders of health care programs should assess their nondiscrimination and employment policies, intake practices, and community outreach and marketing (Acquaviva, 2017). Creating an affirming care environment includes obtaining input from LGBTQI staff and community members. Ensuring that LGBTQI-affirming policies are in place supports LGBTQI staff in being open with their colleagues and service community and provides a safe space for patients and families to openly discuss health, personal, and family matters with the health care team. This is especially important for many older adults who may fear the bullying and other stigmatizing behaviors they experienced in the past. Unless they observe that it is safe and comfortable to be their true selves, elder LGBTQI patients may "return to the closet" in residential and long-term care settings to avoid revisiting the discrimination they faced when they were younger.

Nondiscrimination Policies

Institutional policies should clearly protect employees and patients/clients from discrimination based on SOGI. Federal, state, and local civil rights laws promote fairness and equity for LGBTQI people in employment and access to and provision of services. Twenty-two states and the District of Columbia protect against discrimination based on SOGI (Movement Advancement Project, 2022). In 2020, the U.S. Supreme Court expanded the definition of "gender" in employment cases brought under Title VII of the Civil Rights Act of 1964 to include SOGI. The federal Department of Health and Human Services forbids discrimination in its programs (U.S. Department of Health and Human Services, 2021). Institutional policies should reflect these legal requirements. Nondiscrimination policies should be explicit and visible in the organization's educational and marketing materials—including on its website.

Employment Policies

Organizations should display respect for their LGBTQI employees. LGBTQI palliative care providers have reported elevated levels of discrimination based on SOGI (O'Mahony et al., 2020). Institutions should have a clear nondiscrimination policy that applies to all aspects of employment including hiring, compensation, benefits, and organizational culture. All staff should receive cultural competency training on SOGI to promote respectful employee relations and patient care.

Intake Practices

As the first points of contact for LGBTQI people diagnosed with cancer, intake staff must be welcoming to both patients and their families. Staff should receive training in how to create a safe and respectful environment for LGBTQI patients. Intake forms should be inclusive to communicate an awareness of community needs. Inclusive forms can remind staff to consider the full-service needs of their LGBTQI patients. Forms should ask about SOGI, chosen names and pronouns, and patient-identified next of kin and caregivers.

Community Outreach and Marketing

Organizations frequently engage with clients through their website, flyers, and brochures. They may reach out to the public through health fairs and educational fora using volunteer or paid subject matter experts with lived LGBTQI experience. Leaders of these organizations should use such platforms to demonstrate a visible commitment to equality, inclusion, and nondiscrimination. Photographs or other images of clients and services should reflect LGBTQI individuals, couples, and families across a range of ages, races, ethnicities, and gender identities. Organizations may consider advertising in LGBTQI publications and media and having a presence at community events.

Affirming Communication

A key component of high-quality palliative care is patient-centered, affirming communication. For LGBTQI cancer patients, this means understanding basic terminology (see Table 19.1) and providing space for SOGI disclosure. Remember, terms evolve over time. For example, differences in sex development (DSD) were historically pathologized as disorders of sex development (DSD), and many people with these conditions prefer the term "*intersex*" over "*DSD*." Terms also vary among subpopulations. Black people with Afrocentric roots typically use the term "*same gender loving*" over "*gay*" or "*lesbian*," the latter of which White people tend to prefer. Finally, terminology varies across regions and generations. Younger people may be more comfortable with the term "*queer*" than older populations. Younger people may also have a wider variety of terms to describe sexual attraction, including terms like *demisexual*, *pansexual*, and *sapiosexual*. An overarching recommendation is to listen to the words patients use and mirror those words—including what the patient

Table 19.1 Basic Terminology

Asexual: term describing lack of sexual attraction or low interest in sexual activity
Bisexual: person who has a sexual attraction to people regardless of sex or gender
Bottom surgery: gender-affirming genital surgical intervention
Cisgender: person whose gender identity aligns with sex assigned at birth
Gay: person who primarily identifies romantic and sexual feelings toward same-sex persons
Gender: socially constructed term to describe characteristics perceived as "male" or "female"
Gender identity: distinct from sex, the gender a person feels through their lived experience
Gender dysphoria: significant distress from discordance between sex and gender identity
Genderqueer: challenging gender norms
Heterosexism: beliefs and/or systems that assume opposite-sex sexuality is the norm
Homophobia: a range of negative reactions to same-gender attraction or behavior
Intersex: preferred term for people whose sex falls between male- and female-typical forms
Lesbian: woman who identifies primary romantic and sexual feelings toward women
Queer: umbrella term referencing nonmainstream SOGI
Sex: sex karyotype and phenotype at birth
Sexual orientation: complex construct comprising sexual identity, attraction, and behavior
Top surgery: gender-affirming surgical intervention on breasts/chest
Transgender: persons whose gender is discordant with sex assigned at birth
Transitioning: process of adopting and/or affirming gender identity; does not always include hormonal and/or surgical interventions
Transphobia: range of negative reactions toward gender nonconforming people

wishes to be called, their pronouns, and how they refer to body parts. Best practices suggest that practitioners should simply ask patients how they would like to be addressed and listen carefully as they share their concerns.

Engaging in affirming communication also means suspending heterosexual and cisgender (het/cis) assumptions. This does not mean that providers should instead assume people are gay, bisexual, or transgender but rather that providers should self-reflect and consider what kind of communication will lead to a positive patient encounter and care that is best for the patient. Allowing patients opportunities to disclose their lived experiences, including SOGI, along with other aspects of identity that may inform patient values, preferences, and needs in palliative care is fundamental. Essential to suspending assumptions is critically examining language—such as gendered terms like *women's centers*. Even when offering space for disclosure, some patients may remain covert due to a lifetime of discrimination and fear. In addition, asking about and acknowledging patients' sources of support and understanding who their preferred caregivers and medical decision-makers is critical to patient-centered care.

A primary goal of palliative care is supporting a person's dignity at end of life. Practitioners should seek to help LGBTQI patients die with dignity by documenting key decisions—including health care proxies, advance directives, custodial relationships, and other decisions important to the patient—before the end of life is imminent. LGBTQI elders are more likely to rely on caregivers who are not biologically related to them (Maingi et al., 2021). In states without legal protections for same-sex partners or with laws allowing for discrimination in health care practices toward LGBTQI people, providers should refer patients to colleagues who know which documents are necessary to protect their care preferences and formalize who the patient wants involved in decision-making to ensure their last wishes are respected and honored. Documentation of disclosure or nondisclosure to other health care and social service professionals throughout care transitions is also important—remember, patients may not want to risk being "out" to all providers.

Comprehensive Palliative Care Services

Comprehensive palliative care means attention to the physical, psychosocial, and spiritual needs of LGBTQI patients and families.

Physical Care

LGBTQI elders often have significant concerns about long-term care—including fears of isolation, lost autonomy, mistreatment, and physical health care denial (Kortes-Miller et al., 2018). Transgender persons in long-term care are vulnerable to harassment, to being called by their dead name and incorrect pronouns, and to the compromising or discontinuation of hormonal treatments. For example, in 2007, a gay caregiver reported that his partner's feeding tube had been "accidentally" removed and his catheter manipulated aggressively. This callous treatment resulted in multiple emergency department visits for the patient (National Senior Citizens Law Center [NSCLC], 2010).

Physical health needs include attention to self-care and sexual health. A recent systematic review of cancer survivorship research focused on LGBTQI populations found that women who had sex with women (WSW) had better mental health following breast cancer treatment than MSM did following prostate cancer treatment (Pratt-Chapman et al., 2021). This may be due to different cultural connotations of body image between WSW and MSM compared to heterosexual peers. In a systematic review, sexual minority women reported less body image disturbance than heterosexual women while sexual minority men reported more body image disturbance than heterosexual men (Dahlenburg et al., 2020). Additionally, MSM mentioned sexual challenges after prostate cancer that were exacerbated by the lack of available pharmacotherapies available to treat erectile dysfunction for anal-penetrative sex (Pratt-Chapman et al., 2021).

Psychosocial Care

LGBTQI people experience unique stressors, including discrimination, violence, self-stigma, concealment, family rejection, negative social attitudes, and physical and psychological victimization, all of which are associated with higher rates of mental health disorders and substance use compared with het/cis people (Barrett & Wholihan, 2016; Mustanski et al., 2016). The adverse effects of these experiences result in higher rates of stress-sensitive mental health issues, including anxiety, depression, suicidality, post-traumatic stress disorder, isolation, distress, low self-esteem, and low life satisfaction, as well as higher risk for alcohol and illicit drug use (Chidiac & Connolly, 2016).

Transgender individuals are even more likely than sexual minority persons to have been a victim of sexual violence or a hate crime at some point in their life (Witten, 2015), and transgender older adults have reported poorer mental health than cisgender adults and higher risk of depressive symptomatology compared with sexual minority persons (Fredriksen-Goldsen et al., 2014).

Negative past experiences of LGBTQI people can reduce their ability to deal with the stress a serious illness brings to their lives. Such experiences also may lead to nondisclosure of their SOGI to health care professionals, resulting in suboptimal care throughout the course of their illness. Furthermore, negative past experiences can trigger post-traumatic stress disorder at the end of life. Some transgender individuals have reported they would consider suicide if faced with deteriorating health. Coping with the stress of a life-limiting illness and end of life is even more challenging for LGBTQI people when health care providers and health care systems are insensitive or discriminatory, thereby compounding the lifelong stressors they have experienced (Arthur, 2015).

Some LGBTQI people may hope for reconciliation with estranged family at end of life, but such reunions may generate conflict with the family of origin and exacerbate the patient's feelings of grief and loss (World Health Organization, 2015). The biological family may initiate the reconciliation but not be willing to acknowledge or accept a same-sex partner or the patient's family of choice, which may be distressing for patients at an already vulnerable time. Addressing the increased risk of psychosocial distress and mental health problems, including suicide risk, is important (Maingi et al., 2018). Health care providers should refer patients having difficulty coping with serious illness to an LGBTQI-affirming mental health professional, support group, chaplain, or other source of support.

Despite the fact that experiencing multiple life stressors around their SOGI can lead to a greater risk of mental health disorders among LGBTQI people with serious illness, many have also developed resilience and robustness (Javier, 2021). LGBTQI patients will be better served by health care providers who are aware of positive coping mechanisms, including resiliency, community support groups, and affirming spiritual affiliations. Assessments of LGBTQI patients should include exploring the strengths and resources they have developed as well as their preferences around and needs for coping with serious illness. Including the spouse/partner or other caregivers results in better treatment and mental health for patients (Kamen et al., 2020).

The lifetime of stressors experienced by some LGBTQI people can put them at higher risk for negative bereavement outcomes, necessitating additional support. This need may be greater among older LGBTQI people whose SOGI was criminalized or pathologized. Survivors of an unrecognized or unaccepted same-sex relationship may experience disenfranchised grief—hidden or invalidated grief. Disenfranchised grief can result in diminished support for a bereaved partner, including the inability to find culturally competent bereavement services (Inventor et al., 2022).

The death of a partner may also result in an LGBTQI person's loss of identity, especially if the bereaved partner's identity was defined through their relationship with the deceased. The survivor may feel that their LGBTQI identity is now hidden because they are no longer in a relationship with another LGBTQI person. Health care professionals can minimize this by encouraging discussions with the patient about loved ones that will need bereavement support. Offering bereavement services to members of a patient's chosen family and making referrals to welcoming and affirming services is essential. Referrals to a bereavement group should be appropriate to the specific LGBTQI identity of the survivor. Participating in a mostly het/cis bereavement group may be uncomfortable for an LGBTQI person; similarly, someone who is lesbian or transgender might also be uncomfortable in a gay male group. Providers should identify a group in which the bereaved individual is most likely to feel understood, safe, and supported (Acquaviva, 2017).

Spiritual Considerations

When assessing spiritual needs, providers should be mindful of the unfortunate history of spiritual abuse that religious organizations have enacted on LGBTQI people. While it is critical to meet patients' (and caregivers') spiritual needs, it is equally paramount to take cues from the patient regarding their faith and spirituality.

Spirituality incorporates values, beliefs, and practices and has an irreducible dynamic with a holistic quality that can be either religious or nonreligious (Canda et al., 2019). Spirituality includes religious, atheist, and other forms of meaning-seeking expression, ranging from organized religion (Christianity, Judaism, Islam, Hinduism, Afro-Caribbean, Afro-Brazilian, shamanism) to nonreligious spirituality (agnosticism, atheism, existentialism, humanism) to traditional Indigenous ways (African, Native American/First Nations, South American, shamanism) and Eastern philosophies (Buddhism, Confucian). Some spiritual practices include a belief in multiple deities or polytheism (WICCA, Yoruba religion, Santeria, and vodun). Environmental factors, sociocultural identities, and lived experiences also influence spirituality.

Social workers define spirituality as the process of making meaning of one's existence, which includes profound relationships with ourselves and others, morality, well-being, and transcendence (Canda et al., 2019). Patients face potential disruption in their spiritual practices due to being excluded or attacked for identifying as LGBTQI (Barringer, 2020). Denial of access to spirituality may internalize shame and affect a person's ability to manage the psychological impacts of facing cancer and end of life. Despite potential disruptions, patients' yearning to find meaning in their lives, to experience profound relationships with the self and others, and to find spiritual connection typically persists. However, because of past negative experiences surrounding SOGI, LGBTQI patients may keep silent this quest for wholeness.

Providing high-quality palliative care includes supporting the diversity of spiritual practices patients may embrace as they deal with the reality of cancer and potential end of life. Providers should follow a patient's lead and allow them space in which to explore spirituality. Meaningful palliative care honors the wholeness of the individual; connects patients and families to affirming organizations and providers; and guards against the influence of those who may further stigmatize or shame the patient (Lau et al., 2021). Providers should ensure that they ask questions in the best interest of the patient's well-being, not out of personal curiosity. Finally, if a provider makes a mistake, they should apologize and ask for feedback to do better in the next patient encounter.

End-of-Life Planning

Seriously ill LGBTQI individuals who have disclosed their SOGI to their biological family may experience a distancing from them and choose to rely on alternative sources of caregiving and support (Acquaviva, 2017). Families of choice may include close friends, as well as LGBTQI community organizations and affirmative religious groups. Elderly LGBTQI persons are more likely than het/cis seniors to be single and childless, to live alone, to be estranged from biological family, and to be socially isolated. Patients may worry that care providers will not recognize their family of choice. Transgender people may have additional concerns that their biological family will identify them as their birth gender and not bury or memorialize them under their proper gender. Conflict over care decisions between families of choice and biological relatives can be challenging for health care professionals to navigate. The complex dynamics of these relationships can be stressful for the LGBTQI patient at a time when they are quite vulnerable. Health care providers can help the LGBTQI patient receive care and support based on their preferences.

This also underscores the importance of advance care planning for LGBTQI persons to ensure that health care providers and members of the patient's social support network know the patient's preferences for care and who they want to communicate these preferences for them if they become unable to do so. It is important for LGBTQI patients to name a surrogate in a timely manner to avoid having decisions made by default individuals (likely biological family members) as specified in statutes or regulations. Advance directives are critically important in ensuring that providers strictly follow LGBTQI patients' preferences for care and not ignore their partners and spouses (Maingi et al., 2021). It may also be necessary for the provider to help the patient complete a visitation directive, which specifies whom the patient wants to receive as a visitor during hospital stays, to prevent estranged family members from intruding on the patient and attempting to direct their care when the patient is unable to advocate for themselves.

LGBTQI people are also more likely than cis/het people to rely on formal care services if they are estranged from biological family. LGBTQI individuals who do not have a traditional support system are more likely to be placed in a long-term care facility. Because most of these facilities are heterocentric and gender normative, LGBTQI residents, particularly those who came of age before the gay rights movement and enactment of legal protections, may feel the need to hide their SOGI. They may also be concerned about allowing formal care providers into their home due to fear of neglect, harm, judgment, or outing to their family of origin (NSCLC, 2010).

Providers should be observant and assess potentially complex family dynamics while keeping the patient's preferences central. However, providers should not assume an LGBTQI patient has difficult relations with family or is estranged. Many have supportive and loving relationships with biological family.

This chapter has provided an overview of palliative care considerations for LGBTQI patients and families when dealing with a critical illness, such as cancer. LGBTQI people have faced a history of criminalization, institutionalization, discrimination, and alienation—and yet each person experiences different reactions to these harms. Older generations may experience more fear and remain closeted in a health care setting (Table 19.2). Younger generations may be more open to expressing their SOGI without shame or fear of harm. Key to providing affirming, patient-centered care is ensuring safe, welcoming environments; communicating with respect and active listening; and attending to the physical, psychosocial, and spiritual needs of patients. Finally, respecting patient caregiver choices and documenting medical and end-of-life decisions can ensure dignity in life and death for LGBTQI patients.

Table 19.2 Resources for LGBTQI Elders

Resource	Link
Lambda Legal Tools for Life, Burial, and Financial Planning	http://www.lambdalegal.org/publications/take-the-power
LGBT Community Centers	http://lgbtcenters.org
National Resources Center on LGBT Aging to Find LGBT-Affirming National and Local Resources	http://lgbtagingcenter.org/resources
SAGE: Services and Advocacy for GLBT Elders	http://sageusa.org

Guiding Best Practices for the Future

- Champion culture change to advance LGBTQI health equity.
- Collect SOGI and intersectionality data in clinical care and health services research.
- Advocate for ongoing LGBTQI cultural and clinical competency training.
- Promote a safe environment with a zero-tolerance policy for discriminatory language or behaviors.
- Train staff to increase competence and comfort with LGBTQI patients.

Pearls

- Provide open and welcoming space for patient disclosure of SOGI.
- Acknowledge patients' social support network.
- Respond to personal care concerns of transgender persons, such as providing hormone therapy through end of life.
- Challenge antigay and transphobic behaviors.
- Ensure advance directives, burial rights, and other legal decisions are documented.
- Be open to nontraditional family arrangements, but do not assume estrangement from biological family.

Pitfalls

- Do not assume all patients are heterosexual and cisgender.
- Do not assume patients will tell you about their SOGI.

- Do not dismiss experiences of stigma or discrimination.
- Do not perpetuate stereotypes of LGBTQI people.

References

Acquaviva, K. (2017). *LGBTQ-inclusive hospice and palliative care: A practical guide to transforming professional practice*. Harrington Park.

American Cancer Society. (2021). *Lifestyle-related breast cancer risk factors*. Retrieved from https://www.cancer.org/cancer/breast-cancer/risk-and-prevention/lifestyle-related-breast-cancer-risk-factors.html

Arthur, D. P. (2015). Social work practice with LGBT elders at end of life: Developing practice evaluation and clinical skills through a cultural perspective. *Journal of Social Work in End-of-Life and Palliative Care*, *11*(2), 178–201. https://doi.org/10.1080/15524256.2015.1074141

Barrett, N., & Wholihan, D. (2016). Providing palliative care to LGBTQ patients. *Nursing Clinics of North America*, *51*(3), 501–511. https://doi.org/10.1016/j.cnur.2016.05.001

Barringer, M. N. (2020). Lesbian, gay, and bisexual individuals' perceptions of American religious traditions. *Journal of Homosexuality*, *67*(9), 1173–1196. https://doi.org/10.1080/00918369.2019.1582221

Canda, E. R., Furman, L. D., & Canda, H.-J. (2019). *Spiritual diversity in social work practice: The heart of helping*. Oxford University Press.

Chidiac, C., & Connolly, M. (2016). Considering the impact of stigma on lesbian, gay and bisexual people receiving palliative and end-of-life care. *International Journal of Palliative Nursing*, *22*(7), 334–340. https://doi.org/10.12968/ijpn.2016.22.7.334

Dahlenburg, S. C., Gleaves, D. H., Hutchinson, A. D., & Coro, D. G. (2020). Body image disturbance and sexual orientation: An updated systematic review and meta-analysis. *Body Image*, *35*, 126–141. https://doi.org/10.1016/j.bodyim.2020.08.009

Fredriksen-Goldsen, K. I., Cook-Daniels, L., Kim, H. J., Erosheva, E. A., Emlet, C. A., Hoy-Ellis, C. P., Goldsen, J., & Muraco, A. (2014). Physical and mental health of transgender older adults: An at-risk and underserved population. *Gerontologist*, *54*(3), 488–500. https://doi.org/10.1093/geront/gnt021

Inventor, B. R., Paun, O., & McIntosh, E. (2022). Mental health of LGBTQ older adults. *Journal of Psychosocial Nursing and Mental Health Services*, *60*(4), 7–10. https://doi.org/10.3928/02793695-20220303-01.

James, S. E., Herman, J. L., Rankin, S., Keisling, M., Mottet, L., & Anafi, M. (2016). *The report of the 2015 U.S. Transgender Survey*. National Center for Transgender Equality.

Javier, N. M. (2021, September 9). Palliative care needs, concerns, and affirmative strategies for the LGBTQ population. *Palliative Care and Social Practice*, *15*. https://doi.org/10.1177/26323524211039234

Kamen, C., Pratt-Chapman, M. L., & Quinn, G. (2020). "Sex can be a great medicine": Sexual health in oncology care for sexual and gender minority patients. *Current Sexual Health Reports*, *12*(4), 320–328. https://doi.org/10.1007/s11930-020-00285-1

Kortes-Miller, K., Boulé, J., Wilson, K., & Stinchcombe, A. (2018). Dying in long-term care: Perspectives from sexual and gender minority older adults about their fears and hopes for end of life. *Journal of Social Work in End-of-Life and Palliative Care*, *14*(2–3), 209–224. https://doi.org/10.1080/15524256.2018.1487364

Lau, J., Khoo, A. M., Ho, A. H., & Tan, K. (2021). Psychological resilience among palliative patients with advanced cancer: A systematic review of definitions and associated factors. *Psycho-Oncology*, *30*(7), 1029–1040. https://doi.org/10.1002/pon.5666

Maingi, S., Bagabag, A. E., & O'Mahony, S. (2018). Current best practices for sexual and gender minorities in hospice and palliative care settings. *Journal of Pain and Symptom Management, 55*(5), 1420–1427. https://doi.org/10.1016/j.jpainsymman.2017.12.479

Maingi, S., Radix, A., Candrian, C., Stein, G. L., Berkman, C., & O'Mahony, S. (2021). Improving the hospice and palliative care experiences of LGBTQ patients and their caregivers. *Primary Care, 48*(2), 339–349. https://doi.org/10.1016/j.pop.2021.02.012

Movement Advancement Project. (2022). *Nondiscrimination laws.* https://www.lgbtmap.org/equality-maps/non_discrimination_laws

Mustanski, B., Andrews, R., & Puckett, J. A. (2016). The effects of cumulative victimization on mental health among lesbian, gay, bisexual, and transgender adolescents and young adults. *American Journal of Public Health, 106*(3), 527–533. https://doi.org/10.2105/ajph.2015.302976

National Senior Citizens Law Center. (2010). *LGBT older adults in long-term care facilities: Stories from the field.* https://www.lgbtagingcenter.org/resources/pdfs/NSCLC_LGBT_report.pdf

O'Mahony, S., Maingi, S., Scott, B. H., & Raghuwanshi, J. S. (2020). Perspectives on creating an inclusive clinical environment for sexual and gender minority patients and providers. *Journal of Pain and Symptom Management, 59*(3), e9–e11. https://doi.org/10.1016/j.jpainsymman.2019.11.025

Pratt-Chapman, M. L., Alpert, A. B., & Castillo, D. A. (2021). Health outcomes of sexual and gender minorities after cancer: A systematic review. *Systematic Reviews, 10*(1), 183. https://doi.org/10.1186/s13643-021-01707-4

Pratt-Chapman, M. L., & Potter, J. (2019). Cancer care considerations for sexual and gender minority patients. *Oncology Issues, 34*(6), 26–36. https://doi.org/10.1080/10463356.2019.1667673

Stein, G. L., Berkman, C., O'Mahony, S., Godfrey, D., Javier, N. M., & Maingi, S. (2020). Experiences of lesbian, gay, bisexual, and transgender patients and families in hospice and palliative care: Perspectives of the palliative care team. *Journal of Palliative Medicine, 23*(6), 817–824. https://doi.org/10.1089/jpm.2019.0542

U.S. Department of Health and Human Services. (2021). *HHS announces prohibition on sex discrimination includes discrimination on the basis of sexual orientation and gender identity.* https://www.hhs.gov/about/news/2021/05/10/hhs-announces-prohibition-sex-discrimination-includes-discrimination-basis-sexual-orientation-gender-identity.html

Witten, T. M. (2015). Elder transgender lesbians: Exploring the intersection of age, lesbian sexual identity, and transgender identity. *Journal of Lesbian Studies, 19*(1), 73–89. https://doi.org/10.1080/10894160.2015.959876

World Health Organization. (2015). *Transgender people and HIV: Policy brief.* http://apps.who.int/iris/bitstream/handle/10665/179517/WHO_HIV_2015.17_eng.pdf;jsessionid=49DD94DE23337B5AB8BC7A1484959396?sequence=1

20
America's Growing Multicultural and Diverse Populations

Implications for Oncology and Palliative Care

Guadalupe Palos, Mi (Emma) Zhou, and Yanette Tactuk

Key Concepts

- The current demographic profile of the United States reflects the colorful tapestry of a multicultural nation that continues to increase in numbers and diversity.
- Palliative care in oncology represents a crucial phase of an individual's life, deeply affected by the complex dimensions of diversity and inequalities.
- Our social worker profession understands culture and ethnicity as interdependent social processes that affect and construct human interactions and behaviors.
- Social workers engaged in cancer and palliative care with multicultural groups must understand that life experiences and worldviews will differ between their patients, families, and even their own views.
- Oncology social workers who adapt their palliative care practices to the needs of our multicultural world will contribute to a higher quality of care for clients and families.

Keywords: culture, disparities, health inequities, palliative care, social work, worldview

Much of the richness of our nation's population evolves from our society's ethnic, cultural, and racial diversity. Regrettably, many of these multicultural groups experience a disproportionate burden of cancer, inadequate access to palliative care, and other disparities in health care. To close this gap, we social workers must first be aware of the differential treatment multicultural groups receive based on their diversity—in other words, ethnicity, religion,

Guadalupe Palos, Mi (Emma) Zhou, and Yanette Tactuk, *America's Growing Multicultural and Diverse Populations* In: *Oncology and Palliative Social Work*. Edited by: Susan Hedlund, Bryan Miller, Grace Christ, and Carolyn Messner, Oxford University Press. © Oxford University Press 2024. DOI: 10.1093/oso/9780197607299.003.0020 language, age, race, and other characteristics. We must also understand how the intersectionality of these dimensions creates a unique cultural identity for each client. It is almost impossible for a social worker to learn how these dimensions affect each client's perceptions, behaviors, and expectations about cancer, palliative care, or even death. Social workers who pause to reflect on these perspectives will be closer to developing culturally based interventions for diverse cultural groups.

This chapter discusses the effects of our nation's expanding diversity on oncology and palliative social work practice. We begin with a brief description of the demographics of our multicultural and at-risk populations. Next, we discuss social determinants contributing to unequal access to palliative care among certain groups. Then we explain how worldviews toward cancer and palliative care differ and sometimes clash between our patients, their families, and treatment providers, including social workers. Finally, we offer recommendations based on the framework of the intersectionality of diversity. This framework empowers social workers to adapt their interventions and models of practice to best serve populations facing unequal access to cancer, palliative, and end-of-life care. The chapter closes with remarks regarding priorities our society and practice must respond to over the coming decades.

Defining BIPOC and Minority Populations

In 2019, the National Institutes of Health (NIH) designated eight populations in the United States at risk for health disparities: American Indians/Alaska Natives, Asian Americans, Black people/African Americans, Hispanics/Latinos, Native Hawaiians and other Pacific Islanders, sexual and gender minorities, underserved rural populations, and socioeconomically disadvantaged populations (NIH, 2001). However, there is ample published evidence suggesting the elderly, disabled, sexual and gender minorities, and those with ethnicity, race, or tribal status also face these inequities when seeking palliative care (Haviland et al., 2021). Although some people are stepping away from it, many still use the acronym *BIPOC* (Black, Indigenous, and people of color) to capture many of the characteristics of these groups (Farzana, 2020). People in these groups also suffer from inequities in other parts of their lives due to political, economic, or power differentials. Thus, the definition of the term "*minority*" in this chapter applies to any group with few or no power positions in any given society.

One of the primary functions of the social work profession is to work with at-risk and multicultural communities, which encounter obstacles created by poverty, discrimination, and systematic or institutional racism. Social workers interact daily with people who face health inequities, including the at-risk minority groups the NIH identified. Because we live in such a diverse society, social workers will undoubtedly encounter beliefs, traditions, and behavior toward cancer, palliative care, and death that are unknown or unfamiliar to them even if they identify with one of the minority groups listed above.

The National Association of Social Workers' Definition of Multiculturalism

Inequities in cancer and palliative care, as well as access to health and other services, arise from poverty, marginalization, and systemic or institutional racism. In response to these injustices, the National Association of Social Workers (NASW) has developed a *Code of Ethics* that outlines core values rooted in the social work profession: service, social justice, integrity, competence, dignity, worth of the person, and the importance of human relations (NASW, 2021a). According to the *Code of Ethics*, multiculturalism is a philosophy that diverse cultural groups be recognized and given equal status in every society. According to NASW Standard 1.05, Cultural Awareness and Social Diversity (one of NASW's *Standards on Cultural Competence*) "social workers should continuously seek knowledge to improve their ability to meet the needs of people of diverse cultures and backgrounds" (NASW, 2021b). The union of these social work ethics/values and standards creates a roadmap to serve multicultural and at-risk populations as they face the daily life challenges, crises in their cancer journey, and preparation for death.

Changes in Current Demographics

Current demographic trends reflect the changing landscape of our nation's multicultural population groups. This review discusses three trends increasing the demand for multicultural palliative care. According to the 2020 census, there has been a 27% increase in people living in the United States who self-identify as multiracial. Demographic data from that year identified three groups with the highest prevalence, White (57.8%), Latino or Hispanic (18.7%), and Black or African American (12.1%) (U.S. Census Bureau, 2021).

Other growing groups include the American Indian and Alaska Native population (2.9%). Although White remains the most predominant race in terms of numbers, data indicates that by 2025, our nation will have no ethnic or racial majority.

In 2019, 57% of immigrants to the United States originated from ten countries. Although Mexico has been the largest source of immigrants, Mexican migration decreased from 30% in 2000 to 24% in 2019. Other countries of origin include China, India, the Philippines, El Salvador, Vietnam, Cuba, the Dominican Republic, Guatemala, and Korea. Census data from 2020 project that Asian and Hispanic immigration will continue to increase, with Asians having the highest number of immigrants. The countries from which populations come may change due to current political events (for example, the Ukraine-Russia war), which may contribute to an increasing number of immigrants seeking asylum or refugees fleeing their countries. Immigrants may be grouped as legal permanent residents, naturalized citizens, refugees, or undocumented persons (Budman, 2020; Echeverria-Estrada & Batalova, 2020; Zuckerman et al., 2011).

Another group experiencing a significant increase in numbers is persons 65 years or older, which constituted about 16.9% of the American population in 2020. By 2050, this population is projected to reach 22%. Interestingly, 19% of elderly adults in the United States are expected to be foreign-born by 2035. The number of older adults in the United States is rapidly increasing, particularly among those 85 years of age or older (USA Facts, 2022). Demographic shifts among the elderly will affect social workers who practice oncology and palliative care.

As shown in these demographic trends, multiculturalism refers not only to ethnicity or race but evolves from myriad unique characteristics of each person, thus allowing an individual to express their true self or cultural identity. A person's true self originates from multiple sources, including personal, cultural, social, religious, and economic characteristics. These features are often included in the determinants of health and inequities category. When social workers weave these determinants into their social work practice, they use a practice framework called the intersectionality of diversity to deliver cross-cultural care.

Worldviews of Patients, Providers, and Western Medicine Toward Palliative Care

We live in a multicultural society where one's worldview provides a framework for people to understand how to think or act in their world (Gray,

2011). Worldviews toward illness, treatments, dying, and death are complex and may often clash among patients, their families, and providers who follow the Western biomedical model of care. The biomedical model values individual autonomy, truth-telling, full disclosure, and privacy in patient-provider relationships. The nonbiomedical approach or in the context of this chapter, the "traditional" model of health, follows cultural, spiritual, familial, or religious values and practices to make decisions about palliative and end-of-life care. For instance, among some religious, ethnic, or cultural groups, there is a belief that telling a family member "bad news" is taboo because, "if you say it, it will happen" (Rising, 2015). Adherents of some religious groups believe that only God can heal illness and therefore, choose "to leave it in God's hands" rather than seek Western medicine's remedies (Rhodes et al., 2013).

Preparing the patient and family for death must be based on cultural, religious, and spiritual beliefs regarding after-death care, grieving and funerals, decisions for advance directives, disposition of the body, organ donations, and other unique needs and desires. These factors form one's worldview of the cancer experience—beginning at diagnosis, passing through treatment, follow-up, and palliative care, and ending in death. Social workers may encounter ethical dilemmas when there is discord among the worldviews of their clients, their health care providers, and the health care system. Thus, social workers must understand how each worldview shapes an individual's communication patterns, care expectations, mutual decision-making, and beliefs about suffering, bereavement, and dying.

Social Determinants Affecting Multicultural Groups

Numerous scholars have examined the impact of social determinants of health (SDOH) as barriers to palliative care (Gray et al., 2017; Haviland et al., 2021). SDOH refers to conditions in which people exist due to outside forces beyond their control. Figure 20.1 illustrates social, structural, and sociopolitical determinants that challenge or facilitate access to equitable, evidence-based palliative care. Determinants such as oppression, marginalization, and inequitable power are the root causes of health disparities. These factors influence a person's access to and the affordability and availability of resources needed to achieve equitable health care. Figure 20.1 also lists the NASW values contributing to the equitable distribution of resources required to achieve quality palliative care. Social workers' skills, training, and experience prepare them to consider the relationships between each element.

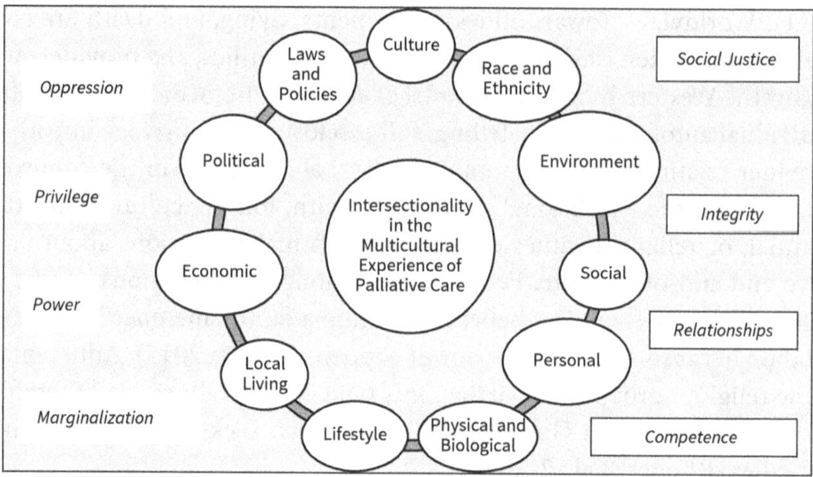

Figure 20.1 Determinants of disparities in cancer and palliative care.

The intersectionality of diversity framework is a crucial driver in modern social work values, principles, and practice. As noted earlier, the NASW *Code of Ethics* and *Standards on Cultural Competence* address the concepts of oppression, power inequalities, marginalization, privilege, and discrimination in identifying groups at risk of social injustices. Social workers' knowledge, skills, and training are valuable in guiding and counseling multicultural groups who may be unfamiliar with palliative care or vulnerable to inadequate palliative care.

Our nation's growing multicultural society requires social workers to use appropriate interventions for individuals with different worldviews, life experiences, languages, and notions of health care. These interventions are especially vital when patients and families have reached the stage in their cancer journey where they need palliative or end-of-life care. The challenging question for social workers is, How can I provide culturally based services to my clients and families with diverse backgrounds?

Cultural Humility and Cultural Competence—What's in a Name?

Social workers use the term "cultural humility" to define a process that will help us better understand the interaction of diversity with the social determinants within a sociopolitical context. The process comprises four basic principles: self-reflection and self-critique, respectful partnerships, lifelong learning, and institutional accountability. Practicing cultural humility requires looking at the intersectionality of the multiple and varied facets of each individual that embody diversity; this perspective also acknowledges the individuality of cultures and the impact of inequalities.

Cultural humility suggests that to provide services in a multicultural context, the social worker must reflect on their own cultural identity, biases, and values, which necessarily influence their personal and professional worldviews. Cultural humility is a lifelong process in which social workers enter with their clients, communities, colleagues, and themselves. In this approach, the social worker engages a client as an equal partner within the boundaries of social injustices.

Cultural humility differs from cultural competence in that it challenges social workers to examine and understand their own cultural identity and how it affects their counseling and service. This framework posits that cultural competence and multicultural counseling approaches may lead to stereotyping and generalizations and often does not consider issues of social justice or the intersecting dimensions of diversity (Tervalon & Murray-García, 1998). Cultural humility allows social workers to recognize power imbalances within the counseling relationship, communities, and society. Nonetheless, cultural humility, cultural competence, or multicultural counseling can be incorporated into social practice alone or together to deliver optimal care to multicultural groups. Each social worker must decide which approach(es) best serves their clients and their practice. Social workers can also explore their cultural sensitivity by asking, How does my own cultural identity influence my social work practice?

Interventions and Practice Models for Multicultural Populations

Palliative care social workers depend on their knowledge, skills, and methods that focus on cancer, multiculturalism, and social justice to combat inequalities and provide competent services in multicultural environments. The social work profession uses different interventions and practice models to plan an individual's approach to treatment. A basic framework that fits into any intervention or practice model includes practice goals; needs assessment and intervention focus; strategies, skills, and programs; and service delivery.

Table 20.1 presents a matrix of social work interventions and practice models to use with the multicultural groups discussed in this chapter.

Table 20.1 Matrix of Social Work Practice Interventions and Models for At-Risk Multicultural Groups

At-Risk Subgroups within Multicultural Groups	Undocumented Immigrants	Refugees & Asylum Seekers	LGBTQ+ People	Violence & Sexual Abuse	Human Trafficking	Cognitive and Physical Disabilities	Homeless	Incarcerated	Children & Adolescents, Elderly Abuse	Veterans
Model(s)	**Social Work Interventions**									
Individual and Family Counseling										
Supportive Counseling										
Narrative										
Trauma										
Systems										
Strengths										
Case Management										
Integrative										
Empowerment										

At-Risk Subgroups within Multicultural Groups	Undocumented Immigrants	Refugees & Asylum Seekers	LGBTQ+ People	Violence & Sexual Abuse	Human Trafficking	Cognitive and Physical Disabilities	Homeless	Incarcerated	Children & Adolescents, Elderly Abuse	Veterans
Conflict										
Feminist										
Anti-Oppression										
Family Therapy and Interventions										
Cognitive Behavioral Therapy										
Solution Focused										
Rational Emotive Behavioral										
Task-Centered										

The content in this table provides a profile of subgroups of individuals who often are "shadows" within the racial, ethnic, and cultural groups in the United States. The model(s) column presents practice models that may be appropriate for multicultural counseling. Social workers can choose to use models alone or in combination depending on the needs of their culturally diverse clients. The shading in each row suggests examples of models to use with a specific at-risk group. For example, a social worker could combine interventions from narrative, individual, and supportive models of practice to address the needs of women in both vignettes.

However, people of color or diverse cultural heritages may have also experienced trauma, violence, conflict, racism, discrimination, and other unique circumstances. Combining different interventions may be necessary to empower members of groups who have dealt with or are dealing both with such situations and their need for palliative care. For example, a social worker can use a combination of approaches to address trauma, oppression, power differential, privilege, and marginalization while also assisting the client with equitable access to services such as palliative care and addressing end-of-life concerns. Clinical vignettes about two women diagnosed with cancer who voiced unique needs based on their personal, cultural, religious, and structural determinants provide some scenarios through which to examine the intersectional framework and cultural humility (Boxes 20.1 and 20.2).

Box 20.1 Vignette 1: An Undocumented Immigrant Woman Diagnosed With Metastatic Breast Cancer

A young woman notices a lump in her breast shortly after the delivery of her son. This woman is non-English speaking, is undocumented, and does not have insurance. She is a stay-at-home wife and mother with few friends and is socially isolated from family and friends who remain in Mexico. This woman fears her undocumented status will prevent her from accessing the emergency Medicaid she will need to receive treatment and further care. The patient tells the social worker that her husband is supportive but works long hours at a stressful job, and she does not want to worry him. She also shares her belief that her husband will be unable to understand her experience because it is a "women's cancer." The social worker knows of a local community organization that provides health care services to clients who are refugees or undocumented. The social worker helps the woman complete the papers needed to receive emergency Medicaid for a mammogram and biopsy at a local public safety net hospital. Her results confirm a breast cancer diagnosis with metastasis to the lymph nodes in her neck. One of her main fears is that she will die alone. The woman wishes to return to her country. She would like to be with her family and friends as she prepares for her pending death. What strategies can the social worker use to support and respect her decision to return to her country?

Figure 20.2 provides an example of a plan of action for Vignette 1. This vignette calls for a social worker's insight, skills, and experience with basic cross-cultural approaches. For example, a cross-cultural approach would

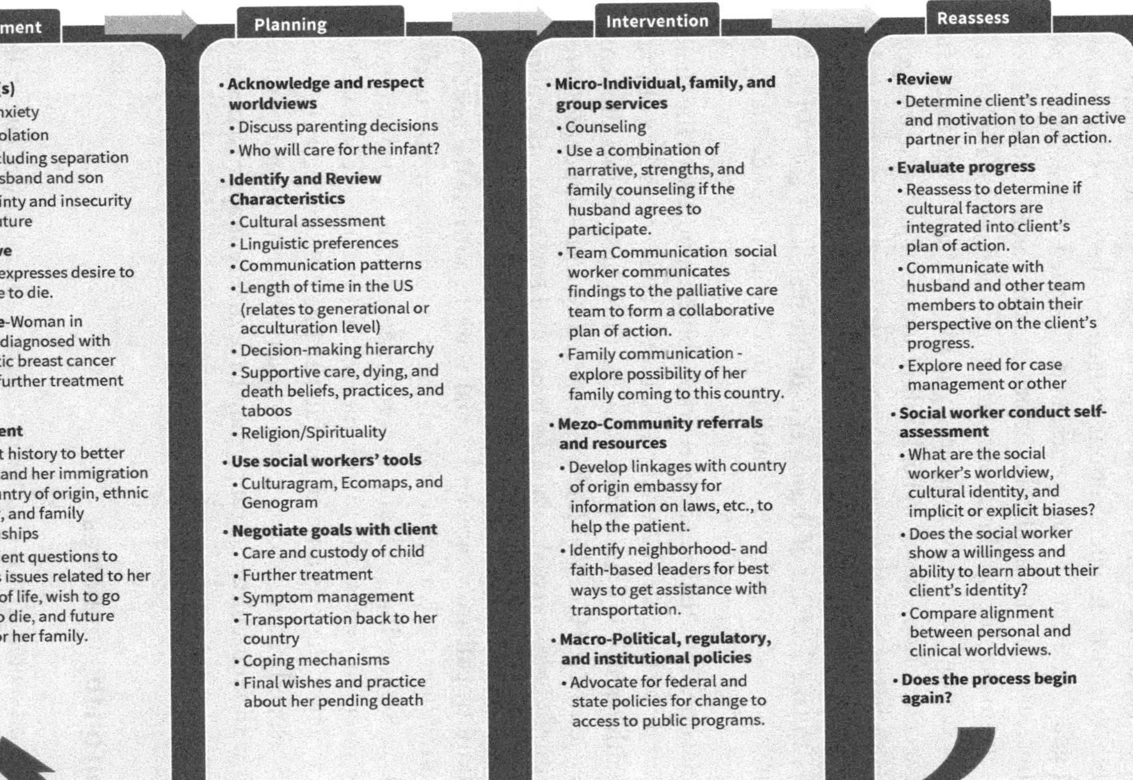

Figure 20.2 Example of social work intervention for an undocumented immigrant needing palliative care services.

consist of the following steps: determine the need for an interpreter, schedule the service before the interview with the client, establish rapport and engagement, conduct a biopsychological assessment, negotiate and plan goals with the patient and their family members (based on the client's expectations and preferences), provide interventions triaged by the client's immediate needs and goals, evaluate the outcomes, and if needed, renegotiate goals, interventions, and models, and begin the process once again. Other important questions to ask during clinic visits or family conferences are What is your country of origin and how long have you lived in the United States (to determine acculturation status)? What kinds of social support systems (generational, faith-based, neighborhood) do you have? What are your attitudes toward advance directives and does your religion contain spiritual taboos or practices to take account of during end-of-life planning? and What are your communication preferences regarding privacy and confidentiality of diagnosis?

Additional questions that can be used to establish rapport with the client and their family include the following: What is your understanding of your current health status? Whom would you like to include in this phase of your cancer journey? Have you had any experience with supportive care? and What things help you make your decisions and communication about care? Figure 20.2 maps out an approach that incorporates principles of cultural humility, palliative care, and social work to address the needs of the woman in Vignette 1. Examples of elements to address in the assessment include identifying mutually agreed interventions and outcomes, integrating interventions at the micro, mezzo, and macro levels, and determining whether there is a need for further intervention or a new action plan. Seasoned palliative care social workers with established practice in working with multicultural groups may have different approaches and interventions.

Reflection on the Vignettes

The vignettes presented in this chapter reflect the vulnerability of culturally diverse cancer patients who encounter inequities in their access to palliative care. Issues related to spirituality, advocacy, self-determination, emotional needs, and holistic care were integrated into approaches to address the patient's needs. The vignettes also underscore the need for multilevel interventions (micro, mezzo, and macro) to address inequities in delivering palliative care.

Box 20.2 Vignette 2: To Share or Not to Share

A 56-year-old Mandarin-speaking female patient receiving treatment for her diagnosis of recurrent ovarian cancer reaches out to the oncology social worker she trusts and respects. During their visit, she becomes tearful and anxious. She explains that when she was diagnosed with ovarian cancer, she was determined to fight and beat it. After completing the last chemotherapy treatment, she was happy and relieved and believed she could return to her routine. Sadly, her recent scan showed a recurrence of the disease, meaning she would need to begin a new treatment. The woman fears telling her friends about her diagnosis due to cultural stigmas and negative beliefs associated with cancer. She shares her sense of isolation with the social worker and longs for help but is unsure what type of action would be helpful to her. What type of a cross-cultural approach can you use to address the patient's sense of isolation and cultural beliefs regarding the stigma associated with cancer?

Guiding Best Practices for the Future

The current climate of rapid change and evolving uncertainty will affect social workers' practice nationally and globally. Social workers are uniquely situated and trained to strive for social justice and thus become change agents for society's powerless populations. Ongoing transitions in America's demographic landscape will continue to call for social workers to adapt their practice and advocate for patients and families with diverse cultural backgrounds who need palliative care.

Our profession's core values and competencies support the principle that equal access to palliative care is a fundamental human right. Substantial reform is underway in how social workers deliver multicultural palliative care and is helping ensure that equitable care reaches all groups. Figure 20.3 illustrates areas that can transform future social work education, practice, and research. For example, academic curriculums and field placements can focus on palliative care settings, including community and in-home settings. Regulations and guidelines for the social work profession can make education in multiculturalism mandatory for licensure and renewal.

Research in these areas will help form evidence-based practice for social workers. For instance, descriptive studies focusing on cross-cultural differences in patients' and caregivers' attitudes toward palliative and end-of-life care would contribute to the science of multicultural palliative care. Randomized clinical trials comparing the efficacy of models and interventions

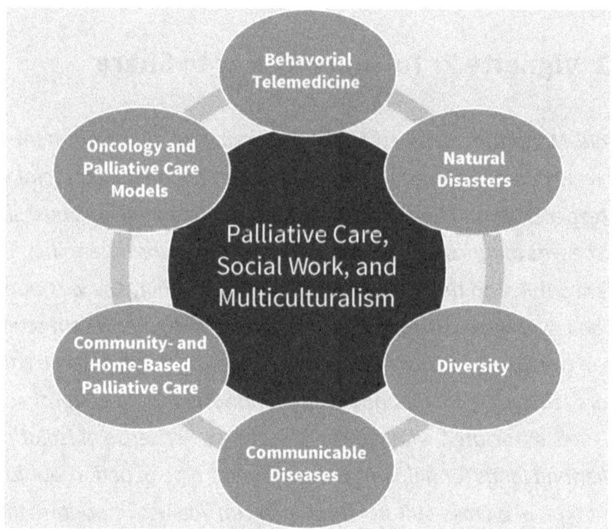

Figure 20.3 Future priorities in oncology and palliative care social work with multicultural groups.

among multicultural groups would be beneficial in shaping future palliative care practice. The future of social work offers exciting opportunities for ground-breaking expansion in our practice, exploration of our cultural heritage, conducting innovative research studies, and redesigning the curriculum. Social workers' unique skills, knowledge, and experience prepare us to be essential team members and leaders in the future direction of palliative care in our profession.

Learning Experience

- Read Vignette 2 and develop your appropriate cultural action plan based on your experience, knowledge, attitudes, and skills.
- Social workers can learn about their biases, stereotypes, and values by taking the Implicit Bias Test. The link to this exercise is included in the resource section.

Pearls

- The quest for cultural humility or competency becomes a lifelong adventure that provides challenges and opportunities for palliative care social workers.

- Trust and open communication with individuals, families, and communities of diverse backgrounds and cultural heritages begins with acceptance, genuineness, reflection, empathy, and other engagement skills embedded in social work values and principles.
- Oncology social workers must educate themselves about the multicultural values, practices, and taboos of patients and their families regarding cancer and palliative care to deliver effective interventions.
- Cultural humility is an approach that social workers can explore and integrate into social work across settings and diverse groups.

Pitfalls

- Using terms such as *people of color, minority, underserved,* or *BIPOC* may lead to assumptions or reinforce implicit biases about cancer patients and their families.
- Social workers' efforts to provide culturally and linguistically tailored palliative care services may be hindered by complex factors evolving from barriers to patients, providers, and health care systems.
- In America, it is common to categorize multicultural populations into broad ethnic groups without considering regional, tribal, linguistic, or generational differences and their meaning or impact on a person's life experience, contributing to inequities and racism.
- Multiculturalism tends to be viewed as fixed or stable when, in fact, culture continues as a dynamic process across an individual's life.

Additional Resources

Books and Publications

Altilio, T., & Otis-Green, S. (Eds.). (2011). *Oxford textbook of palliative social work*. Oxford University Press. https://global.oup.com/academic/product/the-oxford-textbook-of-palliative-social-work-9780197537855?cc=us&lang=en&

National Academies of Sciences, Engineering, and Medicine. (2017). *Communities in action: Pathways to health equity*. National Academies Press. https://www.nap.edu/catalog/24624/communities-in-action-pathways-to-health-equity

National Association for Social Workers. *Standards and indicators for cultural competence in social work practice*. https://www.socialworkers.org/LinkClick.aspx?fileticket=7dVckZooikjnmzhdcED##CAYUmk%3d&portalid=0

Websites

Association of Oncology Social Work: https://aosw.org/
Race IAT—Project Implicit: https://implicit.harvard.edu/implicit/user/agg/blindspot/indexrk.htm
Implicit Association Test (IAT): https://implicit.harvard.edu/implicit/takeatest.html
The IAT is a self-assessment to determine your attitudes or beliefs about topics. The site will also ask you (optionally) to report your attitudes or beliefs about these topics and provide some information about yourself.
National Library of Medicine. *Improving cultural competence: Core competencies for counselors and other clinical staff.* https://www.ncbi.nlm.nih.gov/books/NBK248422/
Substance Abuse and Mental Health Services Administration. *Improving cultural competence.* Treatment Improvement Protocol (Series No. 59). https://www.ncbi.nlm.nih.gov/books/NBK248428/
Uses Sue's (2001) multidimensional model for developing cultural competence. The chapters target specific racial, ethnic, and cultural considerations along with the core elements of cultural competence highlighted in the model.
Georgetown University National Center on Cultural Competency: https://nccc.georgetown.edu/
Provides national leadership and contributes to the knowledge of cultural and linguistic competency within systems and organizations.

References

Budman, A. (2020). *Key findings about U.S.* immigration. Retrieved from Pew Research Center website: https://www.pewresearch.org/fact-tank/2020/08/20/key-findings-about-u-s-immigrants/
Echeverria-Estrada, C., & Batalova, J. (2020, January 15). *Chinese immigrants in the United States.* Migration Policy Institute. https://www.migrationpolicy.org/article/chinese-immigrants-united-states-2018
Farzana, N. (2020). *Raising multiracial children: Tools for nurturing identity in a radicalized world.* North Atlantic.
Gray, A. J. (2011). Worldviews. *International Psychiatry, 8*(3), 58–60. https://www.ncbi.nlm.nih.gov/pubmed/31508085
Gray, N. A., Boucher, N. A., Kuchibhatla, M., & Johnson, K. S. (2017). Hospice access for undocumented immigrants. *JAMA Internal Medicine, 177*(4), 579. https://doi.org/10.1001/jamainternmed.2016.8870
Haviland, K., Burrows Walters, C., & Newman, S. (2021). Barriers to palliative care in sexual and gender minority patients with cancer: A scoping review of the literature. *Health and Social Care in the Community, 29*(2), 305–318. https://doi.org/10.1111/hsc.13126
National Association of Social Workers. (2021a). *Code of Ethics of the National Association of Social Workers.* NASW Press.
National Association of Social Workers. (2021b). *Standards and Indicators for Cultural Competence in Social Work Practice.* NASW Press.
National Institutes of Health. (2001). *Minority health and health disparities.* Retrieved from https://nimhd.nih.gov/about/overview/

Rhodes, R. L., Batchelor, K., Lee, S. C., & Halm, E. A. (2013). Barriers to end-of-life care for African Americans from the providers' perspective: Opportunity for intervention development. *American Journal of Hospice and Palliative Medicine, 32*(2), 137–143. https://doi.org/10.1111/hsc.1312610.1177/1049909113507127

Rising, M. L. (2015). Truth telling as an element of culturally competent care at the end of life. *Journal of Transcultural Nursing, 28*(1), 48–55. https://doi.org/10.1177/1043659615606203

Sue, D. W. (2001). Multidimensional facets of cultural competence. *Counseling Psychologist, 29*(6), 790–821.

Tervalon, M., & Murray-García, J. (1998). Cultural humility versus cultural competence: A critical distinction in defining physician training outcomes in multicultural education. *Journal of Health Care for the Poor and Underserved, 9*(2), 117–125. https://doi.org/10.1353/hpu.2010.0233

U.S. Census Bureau. (2021). *2020 census illuminates racial and ethnic composition of the country.* Retrieved from https://www.census.gov/library/stories/2021/08/improved-race-ethnicity-measures-reveal-united-states-population-much-more-multiracial.html

USA Facts. (2022). *Our changing population: United States.* Retrieved from https://usafacts.org/data/topics/people-society/population-and-demographics/our-changing-population?utm_source=google&utm_medium=cpc&utm_campaign=&msclkid=02c372d2324710388f2a100d328490fc

Zuckerman, S., Waidmann, T. A., & Lawton, E. (2011, October). Undocumented immigrants, left out of health reform, likely to continue to grow as share of the uninsured. *Health Affairs, 30*(10), 1997–2004. https://doi.org/10.1377/hlthaff.2011.0604

SECTION IV
PROFESSIONAL ISSUES

Eucharia Borden

COVID-19 has had a profound impact on lives and livelihoods, health systems, and economies around the world, presenting not only an unprecedented global health crisis but also unmatched challenges in the field of oncology and palliative social work. Policies and protocols meant to keep staff, patients, and families safe from the disease have greatly changed the way providers approach health care delivery. There exists a rich and important opportunity for health care institutions to implement strategies to support the workforce in new and innovative ways. COVID-19 also brought to the forefront of public health long-standing underlying social, economic, and structural inequities within health care. Social workers have a responsibility to step into leadership in collaborative practice and education to contribute to enhancing care for patients, families, and communities.

Given the complexities of our health care systems and the acute psychosocial issues that affect our patients, the need to refocus on leadership development has never been greater. Though their roles in the health field vary depending on the setting, oncology and palliative social workers are change agents by training. Credentialing and evidence-based certifications provide the basis of competency standards and elevate the social work profession. Increased participation from social workers at the organizational level and in policy creation could create a paradigm shift not only in cancer care delivery but within the overall health care system.

The authors in this section, which covers Chapters 21 through 28, discuss various professional issues that social workers face in providing oncology and palliative care. Topics such as ethics, leadership development, mentorship, credentialing, the impact of the COVID-19 pandemic, and culturally competent care are explored in depth. Chapter 21 discusses the intersection of clinical care, organizational structures, policies, and processes in the dynamic ethical landscape in oncology and palliative care. Chapter 22 addresses the ways that the COVID-19 pandemic has imposed stressors on the health care workforce. Factors contributing to staff burnout are presented along with a discussion about institutional responses and innovative strategies for optimal support. Chapter 23 delves into professional social work development and sustainability, which spans education, advocacy, research, leadership, and attention to self-care. Central to Chapter 24 is the importance of credentialing, continuing education, and maintaining certification. In the evolving health care landscape, remaining familiar with relevant research, techniques, and theories is critical. Chapter 25 explores the ever-evolving digital age and the potential implications, opportunities, and challenges associated with the various types of technology available in the provision of cancer care, sharing support, and accessing information and education. Chapter 26 focuses on social work leadership development at the macro, mezzo, and micro levels of practice. A critical area of focus in this chapter is the need for leadership training among diverse communities, such as people of color, and lesbian, gay, bisexual, transgender, queer, and intersex people (LGBTQI). Chapter 27 discusses the importance of social work leadership in interprofessional collaboration. Interprofessional collaborative practice (IPCP) and associated challenges are presented as critical areas for quality health care improvements. In Chapter 28, concepts such as pain, human suffering, and end of life are explored through illustrations of Chinese, Indian, and Muslim religious perspectives. International oncology and palliative care social work is explored in the delivery of patient-centered, culturally competent care.

21

Ethical and Legal Issues in Oncology and Palliative Care Social Work

Lori Eckel, Phylicia L. Woods, and Kathryn M. Smolinski

Key Concepts

- Ethical issues arise in oncology and palliative care at the clinician, organizational, and policy levels that affect social work practice.
- Social workers can effectively address ethical challenges to alleviate stress among patients, families, and health care teams.
- Social workers have the responsibility and training to address ethical issues at all practice levels using systems perspectives, relationship-building skills, communication, and advocacy.
- Social work practice is informed by institutional context and influenced by broader policy issues.

Keywords: clinical practice, ethics, law, organization, policy

The landscape of health care is inherently morally, ethically, and socially complex. The intersection of clinical care and organizational structures, policies, and processes highlights the dynamic ethical landscape in oncology and palliative care. The patient experience, treatment decisions, clinical outcomes, staffing, and conflicts in values all unfold within the ethical climate of the organization and broader health care policy. In addition to the impact on patients and their treatment, health care workers also can experience negative ramifications from the ethical climate in which they practice, namely, the factors that contribute to distress, compassion fatigue, and burnout. The well-being and availability of health care workers has specific and direct implications for care delivery and the patient experience. The National Association of Social Workers (NASW) *Code of Ethics* (2021) calls on social workers to engage as advocates and agents of social change both in clinical encounters and at the organizational and policy level (Figure 21.1).

Lori Eckel, Phylicia L. Woods, and Kathryn M. Smolinski, *Ethical and Legal Issues in Oncology and Palliative Care Social Work*
In: *Oncology and Palliative Social Work*. Edited by: Susan Hedlund, Bryan Miller, Grace Christ, and Carolyn Messner,
Oxford University Press. © Oxford University Press 2024. DOI: 10.1093/oso/9780197607299.003.0021

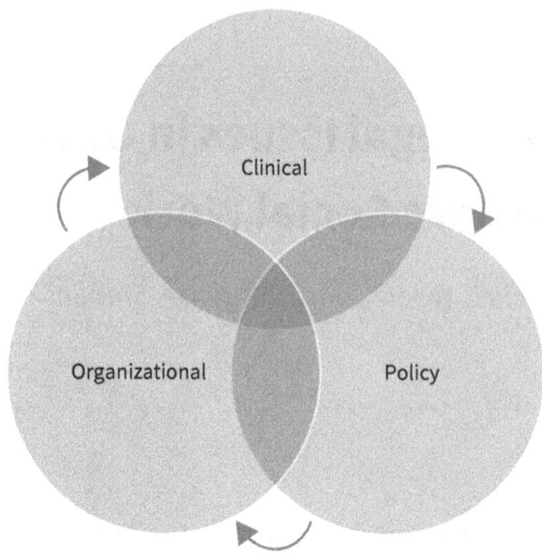

Figure 21.1 Ethical issues influence and action.

Biomedical Ethical Principles and Theory

Several ethical theories inform health care decision-making policy and practice. One cornerstone theory of medical ethics since 1977 views health care decision-making through biomedical principles and actions that violate or support such principles. This theory provides a framework within which to understand the ethical situations that social workers encounter at the micro, mezzo, and macro levels. The common principles of respect for autonomy, beneficence, nonmaleficence, and justice provide theoretical and practical guidance to oncology and palliative care social workers in decision-making situations (Beauchamp & Childress, 2019). These principles can frame the reasoning behind choices in treatment preferences and surrogate decision-making that are made in advance of or in critical moments when the time and circumstances in which to make critical decisions may not be ideal.

Ethical Issues at the Clinician Level

Respect for Autonomy

The NASW *Code of Ethics* (2021) values the inherent worth and dignity of everyone. Patients' autonomy is respected when patients have choices, are *allowed* to make health decisions, and can voice their preferences in advance. Advance directives such as medical powers of attorney and living wills were codified into law in 1990 under the Patient Self-Determination Act (which was included as an amendment to a previous bill), which honors patient autonomy to voice and document preferences in advance and have them followed in situations of incapacity (Omnibus Budget Reconciliation Act of 1990, Pub. L. No. 101-508 104 Stat. 1388). Laws were then enacted at the state level to ensure these rights were protected. Social workers in oncology and palliative care should be familiar with the laws in the state where they practice. While laws can help inform what actions and documents are legal, they may not always dictate the specific steps in care situations. What is legally permissible in a treatment situation may not always be considered ethically permissible (Box 21.1).

Box 21.1 Ethical Principles

- Autonomy—*The moral right of individuals to choose and follow their own life plan and actions; the obligation to respect individual's choices based on values and beliefs.*
- Beneficence—*The duty to bring about improvements in physical or psychological health that medicine can achieve; to be of benefit.*
- Nonmaleficence—*"Do no harm"; intervene to prevent further injury or reduce its risk.*
- Justice—*Fairness in the distribution of risks and benefits among all; guard against discrimination.* (Beauchamp & Childress, 2019)

To mitigate or avoid ethical situations in which patients and providers may be at odds, social workers can maintain open lines of communication between the patients and health care team members. Social workers can introduce advance care planning, discuss and document the patients' treatment preferences and values, and then review these during treatment. Facilitating the completion of advance care planning documents supports the normalization of this process as part of the treatment plan. When these documents need to be used, such as when patients are incapacitated and decisions must be made, surrogate decision-makers (those tasked with speaking on behalf of the patient) can feel the weight of this responsibility. Social workers can assess the surrogate's understanding of the disease and treatment, help them explore their feelings about the decision-making process, and facilitate meetings between the team and the surrogates.

Open, honest, and consistent communication about treatment choices, side effects, and outcomes can help social workers avoid ethical conflicts. Telling the truth when communicating allows patients to make the most informed decisions. Sometimes, providers may shy away from discussing a prognosis because they fear the patient might "lose hope" or "give up." Oncology social workers report feeling moral distress (knowing the right action to take but feeling constrained to do so) especially in direct-care situations involving decision-making with patients and families; this distress can increase when they "witness health care providers giving false hope to a patient or family" (Guan et al., 2021, p. e953). Besides the degradation of trust between the team and the patient, it can be unethical to withhold such information because of the practical consequences for patients and their families.

Understanding the treatment trajectory allows patients to prepare for their future by considering taking leave from work, drafting estate-planning documents, or considering or deciding on who will raise their minor children in the event of severe illness or death. Withholding or glossing over such discussions does not honor patients' abilities to make informed decisions about their future. When asked to participate in deceiving or telling less than the whole truth to patients or their families, social workers in one study experienced distress and many sought supports from supervisors or colleagues. These formal and informal conversations proved invaluable to social workers (Dennis et al., 2014).

Box 21.2

The social worker is working with a patient who is divorced and in treatment for advanced cancer. The patient completed an advance directive 10 years ago when still married that lists her former spouse as the health care agent. However, today, the patient has an acrimonious relationship with the former spouse. The patient's adult children are struggling with mental health and addiction, and one is deployed in the military; neither is involved nor supportive. The patient identifies a sister as best positioned to serve as a health care surrogate. The social worker helps the patient update the advance directive.

Beneficence and Nonmaleficence

Ethical issues can arise when the principle of respect for autonomy is juxtaposed with the principles of beneficence and nonmaleficence. Providers want to promote health, cure disease, minimize symptoms, and achieve other goals of medicine. Sometimes, such goals may or may not be attainable given the gravity of a cancer diagnosis or its progression. To avoid harm and maximize benefit, providers will suggest treatment options that work toward a particular goal. Conflicts emerge when the goal is unclear or contested by the patient or the people within their support system request a treatment the team does not see as beneficial. Perhaps the patient misunderstood the information? Perhaps the goal was unclear or unachievable? When there is a treatment impasse, other people within the hospital or health care facility can offer resources. Members who sit on an ethics committee (if one exists), staff who work in a pastoral care or risk management department, or patient and family services workers may all aid in fostering a comprehensive review of the ethical situation and seeking resolution.

Justice

The principle of justice focuses on the fair distribution of benefits, risks, and costs across the patient population and influences policy and procedures in cancer settings, especially those that affect treatment protocols, bed availability, or other operational decisions (Beauchamp & Childress, 2019). We can view this principle in terms of social justice (a fundamental tenet of social work practice), considering how many patients lack access to affordable legal assistance when confronted with the myriad issues that arise in oncology and palliative care settings. The types of legal issues that individuals diagnosed with cancer may face range from housing to work to end-of-life care (Box 21.2). Successfully solving the issues social determinants of health present—for example, lack of access to affordable and comprehensive health care, unstable housing, denied employee or public benefits, or lack of legal documents that may protect patients' rights—has been shown to improve well-being (Bednar & Antoniadis, 2018).

Connecting patients to legal services can help address the challenges to income, denied benefits, and worries over financial and medical decision-making a cancer diagnosis can elicit. Social workers can harness legal advocates through medical-legal partnerships (MLPs) that bring lawyers onto the medical team, integrating legal interventions alongside medical and psychosocial treatments. These partnerships can be designed with collaboration of social workers, medical administration, law school clinics, legal aid organizations, bar associations, or pro bono departments within law firms. MLPs are established to serve individuals with lower incomes who could not otherwise afford a lawyer; commonly, these individuals are the same clients with whom social workers are already working on analogous issues (Bednar & Antoniadis,

2018). Creative partnerships such as MLPs can improve outcomes at the patient, institutional, and societal levels.

Ethical Issues at the Organizational Level

Screening and Prevention

Many health care institutions have mission-driven goals to care for the most vulnerable. However, there can be a mismatch between mission and vision with actual care delivery and outcomes. Structural barriers to cancer screening and prevention—lack of access to transportation, lower health literacy, and an inability to negotiate requesting provider referrals or scheduling—contribute to health disparities for those who are nonwhite, less educated, financially or geographically disadvantaged, unhoused, or with lower English proficiency (American Cancer Society Cancer Action Network, 2021). The lack of culturally specific or language-specific information, a sense that they are not represented culturally among the workforce assisting them, and historical mistrust can contribute to delays in cancer screening or lack of participation. Although health disparities are not new, responses to the problem can vary widely. Larger public health challenges such as the COVID-19 pandemic have only highlighted the growing disparities; for example, health care practitioners believe that COVID-related delays in cancer screening will cause an increase in cancer in the overall population over the next few years and escalate the cancer disparity in historically marginalized and underserved populations (Carethers et al., 2020). While some organizations are engaging in community partnerships that address social determinants of health or culturally specific services, the burden of bridging the divide often weighs more heavily on patients than on institutions. Social workers can act on the principles of justice, beneficence, and nonmaleficence by speaking up about and speaking out against these barriers and advocating within organizations to reconsider approaches to screening and prevention.

Cancer-Directed Treatment

Even when diagnosed and addressed to the best of a social worker's or institution's ability, structural barriers in cancer care can persist. While a range of clinical indicators guide the options and treatment trajectory for patients diagnosed with cancer, the range of treatments offered or initiated may be influenced by factors beyond clinical indications. The intention to provide patient-centered medical treatment for all can be thwarted by the financial reality of a patient's ability to pay. Health insurance, whether private or public, does not guarantee access to all potential medical treatments. Burdensome (pre)authorization processes, copayments, and network-based coverage highlight the functional rationing of care and raise ethical questions related to the principle of justice.

Pain Management

Along with the financial roadblocks to equitable access to cancer-related treatment, patients may also encounter organizational barriers to or limits on accessing cancer-related pain management. The health care entity and the payor's well-intended beneficence-based efforts to curb unintended opioid-related deaths have created safeguards that can functionally contribute to pain or suffering for patients living with (and dying from) serious illness. The gatekeeping of pain relief grows only more complex for cancer survivors. The transition from active cancer treatment to survivorship can reveal the ways in which health care delivery is siloed, leaving patients with cancer-related chronic pain-management needs either unmet or not easily met by the structure of the system. By tracking examples of barriers to care, social workers can leverage an organizational response across departments to support more continuity in care (Box 21.3).

Box 21.3

The social worker has worked with a patient who recently completed cancer treatment and entered survivorship but continues to experience pain related to treatment. The oncologist only prescribes opioids for patients in active treatment and is no longer willing to refill medications. The primary care clinic policy limits prescribing to short-term low-dose opioids only. No pain-management program is available, and palliative care has a long wait for new patients. The social worker asks leaders to convene representatives from oncology, palliative care, and primary care to address gaps in and barriers to care for the patient.

Psychosocial Support Services

An essential part of cancer care includes psychosocial care. To meet accreditation requirements, cancer centers must have psychosocial support services available. These services may include distress screening, classes, support groups, or counseling. The ethical lens of justice and fairness ideally would direct and guide the delivery of these services to account for myriad cultural, language, scheduling, transportation, or childcare needs; however, not all institutions are able to provide accessible or culturally responsive services. The disconnect between organizational mission, vision, or values with program structures or resourced services highlights the ethical tensions that arise for social workers tasked with delivering such services. Social workers can be active agents in program development that centers the needs of patients who are most historically underserved.

Access to Palliative Care in Oncology

Varied models of palliative care delivery exist in oncology. Many cancer centers have integrated specialty palliative care services while others collaborate and consult with palliative care providers outside the cancer center. A patient's access to specialty palliative care services may not necessarily reflect their need for palliative care but rather the availability of services or the discretion of referring providers. The American Society of Clinical Oncology (ASCO) detailed a vision for access to palliative care over a decade ago that advocates for structural and policy changes; however, 2020 data reveal continued inadequate access (Ferris et al., 2009).

Providers of palliative care services are often faced with demands that exceed available resources, raising ethical questions about distributive justice, prioritization, and allocation in the context of competing needs among patients and institutional stakeholders. Weighing level of quality against access to services creates hierarchies related to perceived urgency, evaluation of suffering, or obligations to institutional or clinical stakeholders, such as referring providers or productivity measures. Ambiguity and lack of transparency about referral pathways, decision-making processes, or access to palliative care may reflect implicit or explicit bias; that such barriers to palliative care still exist suggests a need for more clarity about minimal standards in palliative care service delivery (Philip et al., 2019). Institutions, clinicians, and patients all benefit when the ethics around balancing service demands with available resources are clear. Professional society statements, such as the vision ASCO set forth, suggest more steps are necessary to expand access to palliative care services through education and policy, such as standardized tools for referrals. Social workers can advocate for or collaboratively develop such tools or standards (Box 21.4).

Box 21.4

The social worker has been frustrated with the long waits for patients to access palliative care. They notice in the monthly social work newsletter legislative action to increase the palliative care workforce. The social worker writes a letter to Congress in support of PCHETA and convinces other social workers to do the same.

Ethical Climate

How an organization deals with ethical issues—the perception of those dealings as well as the ethical actions or behaviors of health care workers within the organization—all contribute to the ethical environment of the organization (Pugh, 2015). The ethical climate of an organization is defined by the degree of alignment between mission and values and organizational culture, policies, and practices (Mills, 2013). The ways in which organizations respond to problems such as staffing, workload, burnout, compassion fatigue, or moral distress may both reflect and affect the ethical climate of the organization.

Burnout, Compassion Fatigue, and Moral Distress

Social workers often find themselves and their colleagues wrestling with uncomfortable feelings about point-of-care decisions. Moral distress commonly arises when a patient (or family member) insists on or declines a medical treatment in opposition to the view of the medical team (Guan et al., 2021). For example, an individual with advanced cancer may desire that the team attempt resuscitation and maximum life support when providers believe this causes unnecessary harm or suffering. When providers are troubled at the prospect of delivering such interventions yet want to respect the patient's autonomy over their treatment, an ethical dilemma arises. Social workers may be in the crosshairs of such a dilemma, finding that their professional values are incongruent with those of other health professionals or at odds with institutional priorities or processes. While many health organizations aim to improve patients' well-being, these same institutions can unwittingly or even intentionally compromise health care workers' well-being by restricting or undermining their experience of compassion in care (Kreitzer et al., 2019).

Professional and Ethical Responsibility

Social workers have a professional and ethical responsibility to engage in activities that contribute to their own well-being, resilience, or sustainability in practice. Skill development that facilitates the social worker's ability to anchor in strengths, set boundaries, manage emotions and/or thought patterns, and find meaning can support sustainability in practice. While necessary to professional practice, individuals should not bear the full responsibility of well-being in the workplace. Health care organizations must proactively contribute to the well-being of social workers and other health care professionals by enabling control, structuring rewards, building community, promoting fairness, recognizing values, and calibrating workloads (Back et al., 2016).

Ethical Issues at the Policy Level

Oncology and palliative care social workers are keenly aware of the challenges of a fragmented health care system and understand the importance of coordinated care while keeping patient preferences at the core of decision-making. There is a growing need for more social workers to engage in macro policy development (Reisch, 2017). Social workers need to address the legal issues affecting those living with cancer by thoughtfully contributing to the construction of new policies as well as amending existing policies that create undue barriers to care.

Advocacy

History of Social Work Advocacy

To fully meet the needs of individuals and communities, social work pioneers recognized the value of advocacy. These trailblazers realized that long-term policy changes required their involvement in the development of legislation and policies that promote social justice, advance human rights, and improve well-being. Social workers have successfully organized labor unions, advocated for child-labor laws, and helped establish Medicare and Medicaid. These contributions have changed our world in a positive way.

Social workers can offer critical input on key policies under national discussion, such as increasing access to palliative care. Imagine what monumental changes might unfold if the full weight of the social work profession lobbied and educated local, state, and federal policymakers on the importance of incorporating into legislation both patient perspectives and evidence-based practices. While the availability of palliative care services is growing in states, federal legislative and regulatory action is needed to increase access to these services.

Since 2013, advocacy organizations like the Association of Oncology Social Workers (AOSW), American Cancer Society Cancer Action Network, and American Academy of Hospice and Palliative Medicine have lobbied the U.S. Congress in support of the Palliative Care Hospice Education and Training Act (PCHETA). This bipartisan bill seeks to increase the availability and quality of care by establishing workforce training programs, creating a public awareness campaign about the benefits of palliative care, and enhancing research in the field. For several years, PCHETA has been introduced and failed in both chambers of Congress. If passed, the law would make significant investments into the palliative care workforce.

Ways to Engage in Advocacy

Despite holding tremendous promise and having significant support from members of Congress, palliative and oncology social workers must leverage their collective weight to assist PCHETA in becoming law. Practitioners could participate in organized activities to raise awareness for a robust palliative care workforce and increased access to palliative care services. Specifically, lobby days, e-action alerts, and letter-writing campaigns are ways social workers can engage in advocacy to garner support of lawmakers to move PCHETA and other critical policies forward (DeRigne et al., 2014).

- *Lobby days*—Events where social workers, patients, and constituents travel to state capitols or the nation's capital to meet with legislators and staff to urge action on current legislation.
- *Letter-writing campaigns*—Collectively, letters to policymakers articulating a groups' position on an existing bill and/or personal connections to a policy issue being debated.

- *E-action alerts*—Messaging by organizations, professional societies, or academic institutions to a network of people to take action on a legislative, regulatory, or political issue.

Each of these advocacy methods can be used to urge elected officials to act on specific policy issues. Additionally, social workers can join professional societies or nonprofit organizations such as AOSW or NASW that have advocacy arms as a foray into legislative advocacy.

Ethical and Legal Issues in Advocacy

Patient voices are critical and should be at the core of policy decision-making. Personal stories can influence legislative advocacy by sharing patients' lived experiences, concerns, challenges, and feelings while living with cancer. Social workers must be mindful of ethical and legal issues that could arise while advocating, particularly when using professional experiences or asking patients to tell their stories. Social workers have a duty to the patients and communities they serve to maintain trust and confidentiality, stay within professional boundaries, and always respect the patient's right to decide when engaging in political action. Should social workers choose to use a patient story while advocating, the onus is on the social worker to ask the patient for permission, respect the patient's decision on what can or cannot be shared, and maintain confidentiality. Moreover, it is important to keep the lines of communication open and ensure that patients never feel pressured to participate in meetings, write their own letters, or permit the social worker to share their stories with legislators.

Guiding Best Practices for the Future

Fierce dedication to enhancing the well-being of individuals, families, and communities positions social workers to be leaders in creating balanced policies that dismantle social inequalities and health inequities. The NASW *Code of Ethics* encourages social workers to promote social justice and change. Leaders in the profession have inspired monumental changes in public health and social policies. Our nation is at an inflection point in health care, and the unique perspectives and expertise of social work practitioners are more indispensable than ever (Reisch, 2017). Increased participation from social workers at the organizational level and in policy creation could create a paradigm shift not only in cancer care delivery but within the overall health care system. The profession should embrace its roots in advocacy and begin to engage more in policy development and implementation.

Pearls

- Oncology and palliative care social work practice may reflect a variety of roles—clinician, advocate, educator, collaborator, and leader.
- Social workers can play a part in mitigating moral distress and addressing ethical dilemmas.
- Social workers can influence and transform policies to positively benefit people, organizations, communities, and society.
- Social and political action evoke the principles of social work practice.

Pitfalls

- Complexity in navigating ethical dilemmas requires broad scope of knowledge—moral reasoning, various professional codes and obligations, policy, and law amid broader societal structural inequity—"it's a lot to chew on."
- Oncology patients may not have easy access to affordable legal resources.
- Policy practice happens incrementally; it takes time to learn and practice amid other pressing demands, which can create barriers to action.
- Social workers may encounter barriers to getting a "seat at the table" around decision-making for broader organizational issues.

Additional Resources

Association of Oncology Social Work: https://aosw.org/publications-media/advocacy/ (Advocacy efforts.)

The Hastings Center: https://www.thehastingscenter.org (Produces publications on ethical issues in health, science, and technology that inform policy, practice, and public understanding of bioethics.)

American Journal of Bioethics: https://bioethicstoday.org

References

American Cancer Society Cancer Action Network. (2021, April 8). *Disparities in cancer screening and early detection.* Retrieved from https://www.fightcancer.org/policy-resources/disparities-cancer-screening-early-detection

Back, A. L., Steinhauser, K. E., Kamal, A. H., & Jackson, V. A. (2016). Building resilience for palliative care clinicians: An approach to burnout prevention based on individual skills and workplace factors. *Journal of Pain and Symptom Management, 52*(2), 284–291. https://doi.org/10.1016/j.jpainsymman.2016.02.002

Beauchamp, T. L., & Childress, J. F. (2019). *Principles of biomedical ethics.* Oxford University Press.

Bednar, T., & Antoniadis, D. (2018). Medical-legal partnerships in cancer care. In P. Hopewood & M. J. Milroy (Eds.), *Quality cancer care* (pp. 161–197). Springer.

Carethers, J. M., Sengupta, R., Blakey, R., Ribas, A., & D'Souza, G. (2020). Disparities in cancer prevention in the COVID-19 era. *Cancer Prevention Research, 13*(11), 893–896. https://doi.org/10.1158/1940-6207.CAPR-20-0447

Dennis, M. K., Washington, K. T., & Koenig, T. L. (2014). Ethical dilemmas faced by hospice social workers. *Social Work in Health Care, 53*(10), 950–968. https://doi.org/10.1080/00981389.2014.950402

DeRigne, L., Rosenwald, M., & Naranjo, F. A. (2014). Legislative advocacy and social work education: Models and new strategies. *Journal of Policy Practice, 13*(4), 316–327. https://doi.org/10.1080/15588742.2014.929071

Ferris, F. D., Bruera, E., Cherny, N., Cummings, C., Currow, D., Dudgeon, D., JanJan, N., Strasser, F., von Gunten, C. F., & Von Roenn, J. H. (2009). Palliative cancer care a decade later: Accomplishments, the need, next steps—from the American Society of Clinical Oncology. *Journal of Clinical Oncology, 27*(18), 3052–3058. https://doi.org/10.1200/JCO.2008.20.1558

Guan, T., Nelson, K., Otis-Green, S., Rayton, M., Schapmire, T., Wiener, L., & Zebrack, B. (2021). Moral distress among oncology social workers. *JCO Oncology Practice, 17*(7), e947–e957. https://doi.org/10.1200/OP.21.00276

Kreitzer, L., Brintnell, S. E., & Austin, W. (2019). Institutional barriers to healthy workplace environments: From the voices of social workers experiencing compassion fatigue. *British Journal of Social Work, 50*(7), 1942–1960. https://doi.org/10.1093/bjsw/bcz147

Mills, A. E. (2013). Ethics and the healthcare organization. In G. Filerman, A. E. Mills, & P. Schyve (Eds.), *Managerial ethics in healthcare: A new perspective* (pp. 19–50). Health Administration Press.

National Association of Social Workers. (2021). *Code of ethics.* Retrieved from https://www.socialworkers.org/About/Ethics/Code-of-Ethics/Code-of-Ethics-English

Omnibus Budget Reconciliation Act of 1990, Pub. L. No. 101-508 104 Stat. 1388. (1990).

Philip, J., Russell, B., Collins, A., Brand, C., Le, B., Hudson, P., & Sundararajan, V. (2019). The ethics of prioritizing access to palliative care: A qualitative study. *American Journal of Hospice and Palliative Medicine, 36*(7), 577–582. https://doi.org/10.1177/1049909119833333

Pugh, G. L. (2015). Perceptions of the hospital ethical environment among hospital social workers in the United States. *Social Work in Health Care, 54*(3), 252–268. https://doi.org/10.1080/00981389.2015.1005271

Reisch, M. (2017). Why macro practice matters. *Human service organizations: Management, leadership & governance, 41*(1), 6–9. https://doi.org/10.1080/23303131.2016.1179537

22 Living and Working Through Pandemics, Disasters, and Other Traumatic Events

Impact on Professionals

Susan Hedlund, Bryan Miller, and Leena Nehru

> While we might feel small, separate, & all alone,
> Our people have never been more closely tethered.
> The question isn't *if* we can weather this unknown,
> But *how* we will weather this unknown together.
>
> **(Gorman, 2021, p. 174)**

Key Concepts

- Disaster preparedness, response, and recovery-related research, theories, and models have evolved over the past several decades.
- Burnout is an occupational hazard that reached new critical levels for health care professionals during the COVID-19 pandemic.
- Interventions to mitigate and address compassion fatigue and burnout needs to be multilevel and multifaceted, with attention to those most at risk.
- Oncology and palliative social workers are poised to take a leadership role in assisting organizations in recognizing and addressing inequities, compassion fatigue, staff burnout, and institutional resilience strategies.
- The COVID-19 pandemic presents new challenges as well as opportunities for research to provide guidance for optimal models of support for health care professionals.

Keywords: burnout, compassion fatigue, crisis, disaster response, disparities, pandemic, resilience, staff support, stressor

Susan Hedlund, Bryan Miller, and Leena Nehru, *Living and Working Through Pandemics, Disasters, and Other Traumatic Events*
In: *Oncology and Palliative Social Work*. Edited by: Susan Hedlund, Bryan Miller, Grace Christ, and Carolyn Messner,
Oxford University Press. DOI: 10.1093/oso/9780197607299.003.0022

History of Postdisaster Response and Recovery

In the last 50 years, the number of disasters has increased more than fourfold, in part influenced by climate change (Walton et al., 2021). Defined as a situation or event that overwhelms local capacity, a disaster necessitates national or international external assistance. Disaster settings are full of potentially traumatic stressors—extreme or severe events that are so powerful, harmful, and threatening that they may demand extraordinary coping efforts (Meichenbaum, 2012). Many individuals who have been exposed to traumatic stressors suffer negative psychological consequences, ranging from mild anxiety to clinical disorders such as panic disorder, major depression, substance abuse, or post-traumatic stress disorder (PTSD). Behavioral health specialists are embedded within teams of the Red Cross and Red Crescent, as well as national disaster medical assistance teams to assist both those who have experienced the disaster and the first responders who deploy to these crises.

The World Health Organization considers severe acute respiratory syndrome coronavirus 2 (SARS-CoV-2), the virus that has caused the most recent outbreak of a coronavirus disease (COVID-19), a disaster. Unlike disasters that are single events in time (e.g., fires, floods, earthquakes, hurricanes), the COVID-19 pandemic had been going on for over 24 months with no clear end in sight, as of this writing. The health care workforce, 50% of which was already "burned out" before COVID (National Academies of Sciences, Engineering, and Medicine, 2019), faced unprecedented stressors since the pandemic began. Early on, the lack of personal protective equipment (PPE) and transmission risks to health care worker's families caused great distress. As time passed, the distress of restrictive visitation policies, caring for dying patients without family members available, increased staffing shortages, and more recently, conflicts over vaccination, took their toll. This chapter addresses the impacts of the pandemic and other disasters on professionals working in health care settings.

Features Unique to the COVID-19 Pandemic

COVID-19 had a profound impact on lives and livelihoods, health systems, and economies around the world. As of May 13, 2022, there were more than 517 million confirmed cases of COVID-19 worldwide, which had resulted in over 6.2 million deaths and an estimated total death toll—associated directly or indirectly with the pandemic—of 15 million (Cennimo et al., 2022). Pandemics, natural disasters (e.g., tornados, hurricanes, and earthquakes), and other traumatic events (i.e., 9/11 terrorist attacks, workplace violence, and living in war zones) each have unique features and differentiate themselves in a variety of ways. Montano and Savitt (2020) note that COVID-19 does not fit neatly into the current classification of hazard events, which most scholars argue fall into one of three categories: emergencies, disasters, and catastrophes (paras. 4–5). COVID-19's impacts include not only the limits on resource sharing that may also occur in geographically limited disasters but also a unique expanse of illness and death, widespread economic impacts, long duration, and strains on health and governance systems (Montano & Savitt, 2020). Although epidemiologists expect COVID-19 eventually to move into an endemic phase, it remains an ongoing global threat as new variants continue to emerge.

Impact on Communities of Color

The COVID-19 pandemic brought to the forefront of public health long-standing underlying social, economic, and structural inequities within health care. Cumulative data show stark disparities in COVID-19 case rates and mortality for Black, Hispanic, and American Indian and Alaska Native people, who are more at risk of getting sick and dying from the disease than White people. Additionally, overall data for Asian populations may mask underlying disparities among diverse subgroups (Artiga et al., 2021).

Access and Care Issues

Many challenges with access and care issues were documented during the pandemic in the United States. Reduced access to elective procedures and delaying preventive care, with fear of contagion, limited appointment availability, information gaps, supply shortages, and the impacts of unemployment (and subsequent loss of health insurance coverage and income) contributed to overall limited access to services and compounded problems in a fragmented United States health care system. Fair access to medical and behavioral health care for vulnerable patient populations during and after the crisis conditions of the COVID-19 pandemic remains a valid concern. Health care systems must be careful to not further marginalize structurally disadvantaged populations, which include patients from communities of color and those with chronic medical conditions, persons with disabilities, and patients with socially stigmatized conditions, such as major mental illness

(American Medical Association [AMA], 2020). Preventing health care disparities includes making careful decisions about allocating scarce resources. Policymakers, insurers, and health systems expanded telehealth options to maintain and increase access during the pandemic, though there have been service and payment parity issues. Furthermore, patients in rural and remote communities—which often comprise poorer and historically marginalized populations—face unique access and care vulnerabilities, including fewer health care professionals and hospital beds per capita, increased rates of underlying medical conditions, and limited access to technologies to allow for telemedicine (Erwin et al., 2020).

Staff Shortages

Staff shortages have been a key challenge during the COVID-19 pandemic (and other disasters). At peak phases of the pandemic, some hospital systems and facilities were overwhelmed with patient surge; some had to use military medical teams for health care personnel staffing assistance. Critical workforce shortages have been attributed to health care workers becoming ill, complying with isolation/quarantine requirements, coping with family concerns and obligations, reducing work hours (voluntarily or involuntarily), and/or leaving the field altogether.

The Threat to Health Care Workers' Health

The COVID-19 pandemic presented several occupational and domestic stressors to health care personnel, including initial uncertainty about transmissibility factors, delays in testing and diagnosis, shifting recommendations regarding PPE, triage of scarce resources, provision of ineffectual care, exposure to high patient morbidity and mortality, and the inability to allow therapeutic family presence at the patient bedside, among other difficult realities (Hines et al., 2021). Health care personnel are affected by distress like that of the general population (e.g., effects of lockdown and containment, risk of personal or families' and friends' illnesses, uncertainty about pandemic duration), plus they can experience "frontline"-specific factors, such as extended workloads, feelings of powerlessness, and concerns about the suffering and potential poor outcomes of their patients. High levels of uncertainty and insecurity constitute a risk to their mental health (Robert et al., 2020). Racial and ethnic minority groups are disproportionately represented in essential work settings, including health care facilities, and thus have more chances to be exposed to COVID-19 due to close contact with the public or other workers, being unable to work from home, and working when sick due to lack of paid sick days (CDC, 2020). Furthermore, many health care personnel have contracted (or will contract) COVID-19, with some becoming very ill and some dying from the disease (Walton et al., 2020).

Vaccine Divisiveness

Since the onset of the pandemic, pharmaceutical companies have been rapidly developing novel COVID-19 vaccines and therapeutics, which have provided important medical countermeasures for mitigating disease-related hospitalizations and deaths (Borio et al., 2022). Initial prioritization of COVID-19 vaccine allocation in the United States included health care workers, though there has been vaccine hesitancy among a portion of eligible individuals with potential contributing factors including concerns about safety, side effects, and overall effectiveness. COVID-19 vaccine acceptance and public distrust also are shaped by racial and social inequality, political polarization, and other factors, such as the newness of the vaccines, the speed with which they were developed, and their initial availability by Emergency Use Authorization without full U.S. Food and Drug Administration approval (Hoffman et al., 2021). Group-thinking behavior (us versus them) among those who are vaccinated and those who remain unvaccinated may further lead to workplace tension and divisiveness. In addition to being steeped in ethical and legal concerns, potential vaccine mandates (whether employer mandated or government imposed) can affect health care workers' autonomy, employment status, and economic security and lead to workforce shortages.

Institutional Responses

Government and institutional mandates, policies, and processes rapidly evolved during the COVID-19 pandemic in response to the scientific guidance and best practices that emerged. Included among these are modeling for staffing during surges at facilities, addressing health care resource challenges (e.g., availability of PPE, intensive care unit beds, ventilators), stay-at-home orders, staff illness or exposure, childcare and school closures, and vaccine roll-out, among others. Cancer centers implemented COVID-19 screening of patients and staff and established visitor guidelines and restrictions, as well as return-to-work guidelines for staff who may exhibit symptoms or have members within their household who are symptomatic or test positive for COVID-19. Telemedicine services have expanded rapidly, with workplace implementation including both in-person care and hybrid models. Early pandemic survey data from three national professional social work organizations showed that 20% of respondents reported a reduction in work hours, and two-thirds indicated a temporary shift to working from home (Zebrack et al., 2021). Many health care institutions also adopted mandatory COVID-19 vaccination policies for staff, with exemptions for medical or religious reasons.

Disaster Management Plans

Disaster management plans facilitate preparedness in case of a disaster. They include identifying who does what and a chain of leadership, plans for disaster recovery sites, operational assumptions, resource demands, and prioritization. The intention is to reduce the harmful effects of a disaster and to integrate and coordinate across multiple systems (Federal Emergency Management Agency, 2021). As the COVID crisis unfolded, most health systems were taxed, with many facilities experiencing shortages of available beds, full intensive care units, and increasing staffing crises. Many cancer centers had already developed guidelines for cancer and symptom-directed treatment that helped them manage and triage cancer care during the pandemic. They included ethical principles and classifications for cancer and symptom-directed treatment and symptom management (generally, prioritized as A, B, and C), and outlined processes for patient appeals in case of delayed or limited treatment. A multidisciplinary panel of physicians, ethicists, social workers, nurses, and a patient representative developed and oversaw the implementation of these guidelines. While not all cancer centers had this, several in Canada and the United States developed these guidelines (Hedlund and Blanke, 2020). While without question, cancer surgeries and treatments have been delayed because of the pandemic and the overwhelmed health care systems, most have not had to implement their disaster management triage systems at the extreme.

Crisis Standards of Care and Health Care Workers' Moral Distress

Disease outbreaks, other natural disasters, and mass-casualty events have pushed health care and public health systems to identify and refine emergency preparedness protocols for disaster response. Ethical guidance, alongside legal and medical frameworks, are increasingly common components of disaster response plans. One systematic review of the literature suggested that crisis standards of care should include ethical justifications for triage, duty to provide care, concepts of duty to plan, utilitarianism, moral distress, professional norms, reciprocity, allocation criteria, equity, duty to steward resources, social utility, and social worth (Leider et al., 2017).

Although public health preparedness efforts have paid increasing attention to crisis standards of care (CSC) in recent years, U.S. facilities have rarely implemented CSC plans, although some components are common (e.g., medical professionals in emergency departments regularly implement triage procedures). Conversely, countries outside the United States more commonly implement CSCs within a natural disaster or humanitarian crisis response and may offer important insights into ethics and disaster response for US-based practitioners. As noted by the American Public Health Association, for ethical guidance to be useful, it must be practical and implementable. The Task Force for Mass Critical Care noted in an influential 2014 consensus paper that public and private entities have a "duty to plan," and that "failure to do so places the frontline worker in the untenable position of making weighty, life-altering decisions without the opportunity to consult others or fully consider the ethical consequences of various decisions" (Ornelas et al., 2014).

An article published in 2020 in the *Journal of the American Medical Association* suggests that among states with crisis standards of care guidelines, most deprioritized some patients with cancer during resource allocation, and one-fourth categorically excluded them (AMA, 2021; Hantel et al., 2021). The authors concluded that predictions of a second wave of COVID-19 infection, the U.S. Food and Drug Administration's emergency-use authorization of remdesivir, and ongoing shortages of PPE make the need for equitable CSC paramount, and that oncology populations need to be carefully considered, given their baseline vulnerability (AMA, 2021).

The concept of prioritizing, limiting, and/or rationing care is one that creates great discomfort for medical professionals in the United States. It adds to the experience of moral distress—a situation where a medical professional believes they know the "correct course of action," however, that action is at odds with the decisions or priorities of others. Knowing that our ability to treat cancer patients with potentially lifesaving treatments is denied due to lack of beds or the need to prioritize other patients can create tremendous suffering on the part of the medical clinician. Traditional medical ethics values personal autonomy; however, amid a public health crisis, attempting to do the most good for the greatest number of people edges autonomy out. Most health care providers in the United States find this concept unfamiliar and uncomfortable. The moral distress of this exhausted workforce must be acknowledged and addressed in proactive ways by our health systems (Lake et al., 2022).

Models for Staff Support

Much literature has evolved over the course of the pandemic that addresses the distress of both the general population and health care professionals. When "stay at home" orders were initially implemented, society shared in collective grief as people faced loss of normalcy, safety, and connection (Berinato, 2020). Prior research has shown that if the social and emotional impacts of a mass trauma are left unaddressed, they can inflict long-lasting damages to people's sense of meaning, justice, and order. Trauma affects not only individuals but also entire communities (Hobfoll et al., 2014).

As noted by Maunder and colleagues (Maunder et al., 2021), among health care workers (and many other essential workers) the COVID-19 pandemic created a cycle of understaffing alongside difficult work conditions. Robust interventions to bolster individuals, improve work environments, and address health system drivers of burnout are important to support hospital-based health care workers. Those most at risk are nurses, intensive care unit and emergency department staff, women, and residents and trainees. As noted, people of color are also at greater risk. The Centers for Disease Control and Prevention found that as of July 2020, more than half (53%) of confirmed COVID-19 cases among health care workers were among people of color, including 26% who were Black, 12% who were Hispanic, and 9% who were Asian (Artiga et al., 2022).

There is an urgent need for institutionally integrated approaches to prevent burnout and support the mental health of health care workers during the COVID-19 pandemic and on an ongoing basis hereafter. Mass trauma intervention practices generally have adopted providing psychological first aid, including promoting a sense of safety, restoring calm, enhancing self-efficacy, cultivating connection, and instilling hope. Although different approaches to supporting health care workers during a pandemic have been explored, the optimal approach remains unclear (Pollock et al., 2020).

The Princess Margaret Cancer Centre (a tertiary teaching hospital) developed and implemented one exemplary model of staff support called CREATE: Compassion, REsilience, And TEam building. CREATE is a proactive team-based support intervention delivered at the point of care by psychosocial coaches to multidisciplinary and frontline oncology teams. It incorporates peer support, validation of emotional responses and normalization of traumatic reactions, problem-solving, and mutual instruction on effective coping within an instructional context of an institutional framework that includes foundational safety measures and mental health supports for all staff (Shapiro et al., 2021). According to Shapiro and colleagues, "the unique strengths of CREATE are that it is a proactive model, it is embedded into the workflows of health care teams, and it is tailored to immediate psychosocial needs and post-pandemic distress" (Shapiro et al., 2021, p. 3). The embedded team supports the building of resilience among their health care workers. The rapid mobilization of CREATE within weeks after the COVID-19 pandemic declaration conveyed a meaningful message that the institution values health care workers and is committed to their well-being.

Now more than ever, it is important for health care systems and health care organizations to create and ensure an infrastructure and resources to support physicians, nurses, and all health care team members. The AMA recommends 17 steps that health care organizations can take to effectively care for health care workers during times of crises and suggests that focusing on becoming a resilient organization is more essential than focusing on individual resilience (AMA, 2021). Suggestions include workload distribution, online resources, institutional policies that ensure that paid time off and sick days remain unaffected, and that no out-of-pocket expenses occur for employees with COVID-19–related illnesses. Other suggestions include providing meals, childcare, and pet-care resources as well as assuring access to PPE (Walton et al., 2020).

The Intensive Care Society (United Kingdom) offers several helpful ways of thinking about maintaining staff mental health before, during, and after the COVID-19 pandemic. They suggest that hospitals should think about where their organization is in relationship to phases of the pandemic, be cognizant of the issues and impacts these will have for them, and take note of recommended approaches. Organizationally, they suggest that leaders understand the needs of their workforce and establish whether any members of their team are more vulnerable than others, including those with existing needs or current mental health difficulties; those who have caregiving responsibilities at home; and those who have survived a stress or trauma experience. Individual health care workers strategies include enhancing self-compassion, mindfulness, grounding, balancing home and work, limiting exposure to social media, enhancing social connection, and adopting healthy living strategies (Tomlin et al., 2020).

Guiding Best Practices for the Future

Strategies for guiding best practices for the future will require ongoing education of clinical staff education along the spectrum of disaster care, including prevention programs to promote workplace support and health care staff resiliency. There is much that hospitals and health care providers can do to help staff manage the mental health burden of working during a disaster like the COVID-19 pandemic. Early experiences from China and Europe suggest that health care staff will likely experience negative mental health outcomes due to the pandemic and their employment. Evidence also suggests that—as is true with any trauma—the potential for post-traumatic growth exists, given proactive support, community cohesion, and institutional leadership. There exists a rich and important opportunity for health care institutions to implement strategies to support the workforce in new and innovative ways.

Additionally, the COVID-19 pandemic has awakened all health care workers but especially oncology and palliative social workers to the enormous health disparities that have existed for vulnerable populations for decades. The pandemic has disproportionately affected people of color, those living in poverty, and those who lack adequate access to health care. These are often people who rely on lower paying jobs, who lack paid time off, and who rely on public transportation to meet basic needs. The health care systems must prioritize outreach and access to health care for these more vulnerable populations. Creating partnerships within communities of color and agencies who work with the most vulnerable should be priorities for health care systems moving forward. Numerous professional organizations are prioritizing strategies of outreach and health equity. Together, social workers must share our collective energy and wisdom to change the landscape of access to health care nationally, while also prioritizing the health and well-being of the health care workforce.

Pearls

- COVID-19 has imposed enormous stresses on the health care workforce.
- Innovative system-level strategies are required to support the health care workforce.
- Understanding the mental-health needs of the health care workforce will be essential as we recover from the pandemic.

Pitfalls

- Strategies that suggest individuals prioritize "self-care" without providing them the means by which to do so are insufficient to support the health care workforce.
- Research findings across event types—emergencies, disasters, and catastrophes—are categorically different.
- Further research is needed to discover and implement innovative models of staff support.

Additional Resources

American Hospital Association. *COVID-19: Stress and coping resources.* https://www.aha.org/behavioralhealth/covid-19-stress-and-coping-resources

American Medical Association. *Caring for health care workers during crisis: Creating a resilient organization.* https://www.ama-assn.org/system/files/2020-05/caring-for-health-care-workers-covid-19.pdf

U.S. Department of Health & Human Services Assistant Secretary for Preparedness and Response. *Technical resources, assistance center, and information exchange* (TRACIE). https://asprtracie.hhs.gov/

Washington State Department of Public Health. *COVID-19 behavioral health group impact reference guide.* https://doh.wa.gov/sites/default/files/legacy/Documents/1600/coronavirus//BHG-COVID19BehavioralHealthGroupImpactReferenceGuide.pdf

References

American Medical Association. (2020, April 8). *Access and health equity during a pandemic.* https://www.ama-assn.org/delivering-care/ethics/access-and-health-equity-during-pandemic

American Medical Association. (2021, October 11). *Caring for our caregivers during COVID-19.* https://www.ama-assn.org/delivering-care/public-health/caring-our-caregivers-during-covid-19

Artiga, S., Hill, L., & Haldar, S. (2022, August 22). *COVID-19 Cases and deaths by race/ethnicity: Current data and changes over time.* Kaiser Family Foundation. https://www.kff.org/racial-equity-and-health-policy/issue-brief/covid-19-cases-and-deaths-by-race-ethnicity-current-data-and-changes-over-time/#

Berinato, S. (2020, March 23). That discomfort you're feeling is grief. *Harvard Business Review.* https://hbr.org/2020/03/that-discomfort-you're-feeling-is-grief

Borio, L. L., Bright, R. A., & Emanuel, E. J. (2022). A national strategy for COVID-19 medical countermeasures: Vaccines and therapeutics. *Journal of the American Medical Association, 327*(3), 215–216. https://doi.org/10.1001/jama.2021.24165

Cennimo, D. J., Bergmen, S. J., Olsen, K. M., Windle, M. L., Bronze, M. S., & Miller, M. M. (2022, June 3). Coronavirus disease 2019 (COVID-19). *Medscape*. https://emedicine.medscape.com/article/2500114-overview

Centers for Disease Control and Prevention. (2020, December 12). *Risk of exposure to COVID-19 racial and ethnic health disparities*. www.cdc.gov/coronavirus/2019-ncov/community/health-equity/racial-ethnic-disparities/increased-risk-exposure.html

Erwin, C., Aultman, J., Harter, T., Illes, J., & Kogan, C. (2020). Rural and remote communities: Unique ethical issues in the COVID-19 pandemic. *American Journal of Bioethics*, *20*(7), 117–120. https://doi.org/10.1080/15265161.2020.1764139

Federal Emergency Management Agency. (2021). *Developing and maintaining emergency operations plans: Comprehensive preparedness guide (CPG) 101, Version 3.0*. https://www.fema.gov/sites/default/files/documents/fema_cpg-101-v3-developing-maintaining-eops.pdf

Gorman, A. (2021). *The miracle of morning: Call us what we carry*. Viking.

Hantel, A., Marron, J. M., Casey, M., Kurtz, S., Magnavita, E., & Abel, G. A. (2021). U.S. state government crisis standards of care guidelines: Implications for patients with cancer. *JAMA Oncology*, *7*(2), 199–205. https://doi.org/10.1001/jamaoncol.2020.6159

Hedlund, S., & Blanke, C. (2020). *Guidelines for treatment of patients with cancer during the COVID-19 pandemic*. Knight Cancer Institute, Oregon Health & Sciences University.

Hines, S. E., Chin, K. H., Glick, D. R., & Wickwire, E. M. (2021). Trends in moral injury, distress, and resilience factors among health care workers at the beginning of the COVID-19 pandemic. *International Journal of Environmental Research and Public Health*, *18*(2), 488. https://doi.org/10.3390/ijerph18020488

Hobfoll, S. E., Watson, P., Bell, C. C., Bryant, R. A., Brymer, M. J., Friedman, M. J., Friedman, M., Gersons, B. P., deJong, J. T., Layne, C. M., Maguen, S., Neria, Y., Norwood, A. E., Pynoos, R. S., Reissman, D., Ruzek, J. I., Shalev, A. Y., Soloman, Z., Steinberg, A. M., & Ursano, R. J. (2014). Five essential elements of immediate and mid-term mass trauma interventions: Empirical evidence. *Psychiatry*, *70*(4), 283–315. https://doi.org/10.1521/psyc.2007.70.4.283

Hoffman, D., Stewart, A., Breznay, J., Simpson, K., & Crane, J. (2021, October 18). Vaccine hesitancy narratives. *Voices in Bioethics*, *7*. https://doi.org/10.52214/vib.v7i.8789

Lake, E. T., Narva, A. M., Holland, S., Smith, J. G., Cramer, E., Rosenbaum, K., French, R., Clark, R., & Rogowski, J. A. (2022). Hospital nurses' moral distress and mental health during COVID-19. *Journal of Advanced Nursing*, *78*(3), 799–809. https://doi.org/10.1111/jan.15013

Leider, J. P., DeBruin, D., Reynolds, N., Koch, A., & Seaberg, J. (2017). Ethical guidance for disaster response, specifically around crisis standards of care: A systematic review. *American Journal of Public Health*, *107*(9), e1–e9. https://doi.org/10.2105/AJPH.2017.303882

Maunder, R. G., Heeney, N. D., Strudwick, G., Shin, H. D., O'Nell, B., Young, N., Jeffs, L. P., Barrett, K., Bodmer, N. S., Born, K. B., Hopkins, J., Juni, P., Perkhun, A., Price, D. J., Razak, F., Mushquash, C. J., & Mah, L. (2021). Burnout in hospital-based health care workers during COVID-19. *Science briefs of the Ontario COVID-19 Science Advisory Table*. https://doi.org/10.47326/ocsat.2021.02.46.1.0

Meichenbaum, D. (2012). *Roadmap to resilience: A guide for military, trauma victims, and their families*. Institute Press.

Montano, S., & Savitt, A. (2020, September 10). *Not all disasters are disasters: Pandemic categorization and its consequences*. Social Science Research Council. https://items.ssrc.org/covid-19-and-the-social-sciences/disaster-studies/not-all-disasters-are-disasters-pandemic-categorization-and-its-consequences/

National Academies of Sciences, Engineering, and Medicine. (2019). *Taking action against clinician burnout: A systems approach to professional well-being*. National Academies Press. https://doi.org/10.17226/25521

Ornelas, J., Dichter, J. R., Devereaux, A. V., Kissoon, N., Livinski, A., Christian, M. D., & Task Force for Mass Critical Care. (2014). Methodology: Care of the critically ill and injured during pandemics and disasters: CHEST consensus statement. *Chest*, *146*(4 Suppl.), 35S–41S. https://doi.org/10.1378/chest.14-0746

Pollock, A., Campbell, P., Cheyne, J., Cowie, J., Davis, B., McCallum, J., McGill, K., Elders, A., Hagen, S., McClurg, D., Torrens, C., & Maxwell, M. (2020). Interventions to support the resilience and mental health of frontline health and social care professionals during and after a disease outbreak, epidemic, or pandemic: A mixed methods systematic review. *Cochrane Database of Systematic Reviews*, *11*(11), CD013779. https://doi.org/10.1002/14651858.CD013779

Robert, R., Kentish-Barnes, N., Boyer, A., Laurent, A., Azoulay, E., & Reignier, J. (2020). Ethical dilemmas due to the COVID-19 pandemic. *Annals of Intensive Care*, *10*(1), 84. https://doi.org/10.1186/s13613-020-00702-7

Shapiro, G. K., Schulz-Quach, C., Mathew, A., Mosher, P., Rodin, G., de Vries, F., Hales, S., Korenblum, C., Black, S., Beck, L., Miller, K., Morita, J., Li, M., & Elliott, M. (2021, March 12). An institutional model for health care workers' mental health during COVID-19. *NEJM Catalyst*. https://doi.org/10.1056/CAT.20.0684

Tomlin, J., Dalgleish-Warburton, B., & Lamph, G. (2020) Psychosocial support for health care workers during the COVID-19 pandemic. *Frontiers in Psychology*, *11*, 1960. https://doi.org/10.3389/fpsyg.2020.01960

Walton, M., Murray, E., & Christian, M. D. (2020). Mental health care for medical staff and affiliated health care workers during the COVID-19 pandemic. *European Heart Journal: Acute Cardiovascular Care*, *9*(3), 241–247. https://doi.org/10.1177/2048872620922795

Walton, D., Arrighi, J., van Aalst, M., & Claudet, M. (2021). *The compound impact of extreme weather events and COVID-19: An update of the number of people affected and a look at the humanitarian implications in selected contexts*. International Federation of Red Cross and Red Crescent Societies.

Zebrack, B., Grignon, M., Guan, T., Long, D., Miller, N., Nelson, K., Otis-Green, S., Rayton, M., Schapmire, T., & Wiener, L. (2021). Six months in: COVID-19 and its impact on oncology social work practice. *Journal of Psychosocial Oncology*, *39*(3), 461–468. https://doi.org/10.1080/07347332.2021.1893421

23
Professional Social Work Development and Sustainability

Alison Snow and Heather Honoré Goltz

Key Concepts

- Oncology social work represents a unique field of study and professional practice that requires a wide array of content knowledge and competencies in oncologic diseases, treatments, disease/treatment trajectories, interventions, and appropriate resources, and awareness of the practical and psychosocial implications of cancer for patients and their families.
- Oncology social workers are trained in Council on Social Work Education–accredited programs and adhere to the National Association of Social Work's *Code of Ethics*; their scope of practice and practice standards are guided by the Association of Oncology Social Work *Scope and Standards of Practice.*
- Sustainment in oncology social work involves education, advocacy, research, leadership, and attention to self-care.
- Continuing education is essential for professional development, the career trajectory, professional mobility, and sustainment in oncology social work.

Keywords: advocacy, mentorship, oncology social work competencies, professional development, social work education, supervision, sustainability

Oncology social workers (OSWs) are skilled clinicians who have received academic and professional training to provide screening, biopsychosocial-spiritual assessments, and interventions across the cancer continuum. They work within health care settings, including academic medical centers, community hospitals, private practice, and community-based organizations. Just as social workers are the primary mental and behavioral health clinicians in most health care settings (Heisler, 2018; Whitaker et al., 2006), OSWs

Alison Snow and Heather Honoré Goltz, *Professional Social Work Development and Sustainability* In: *Oncology and Palliative Social Work*. Edited by: Susan Hedlund, Bryan Miller, Grace Christ, and Carolyn Messner, Oxford University Press.
 DOI: 10.1093/oso/9780197607299.003.0023

are integral members of the interdisciplinary team and have essential clinical roles and responsibilities such as those associated with accreditation-mandated cancer survivorship and distress management programs and services (Deshields et al., 2021). Within collaborative cancer care, OSWs bring their person-centered and strengths perspectives, grounded in a social and economic justice framework, to address the psychosocial impact of cancer among patients and their support systems.

OSWs are health care professionals with specific expertise in assisting patients, caregivers, and families with emotional and practical concerns, including addressing the often-negative influence of social determinants of health on access to care and oncologic treatment and outcomes (Association of Oncology Social Work [AOSW], n.d.). They are also experts in community- and oncology-specific resources, often connecting patients and families to these invaluable services and advocating for development or expansion of institutional or community programs and resources. OSWs assist the oncology team with understanding and problem-solving issues including, but not limited to, barriers to care, treatment decision-making, suicide risk assessment, discharge planning, adjustment to survivorship, and end-of-life planning. Because of their cross-cultural knowledge and linguistic and cultural awareness and competence, OSWs are particularly vital to institutional efforts to provide quality cancer care to minoritized patients and those who are non-English-speaking or have limited proficiency in English, socioeconomically disadvantaged, or medically underserved.

This chapter describes the emerging landscape in social work education; opportunities for developing OSW competencies; and resources for ongoing professional development through continuing education, research, mentorship, and supervision. We address advocacy for systems change, including job flexibility and compensation, both of which are integral to sustaining the OSW profession, which has been perhaps irreparably changed by the intersecting pandemics of COVID-19 and pernicious racism. Finally, the chapter discusses the important issue of self-care as it relates to professional sustainability.

Academic Training Programs

In 2022, the U.S. Bureau of Labor Statistics (n.d.) estimated that 26% of social workers are employed as health care social workers, inclusive of OSWs. Employment expansion in this area is projected to grow by 13% between the years 2020 and 2030, buoyed by increases in older adult and minoritized populations and their corresponding health and supportive care needs. Older adults who are immigrants, those with lower health literacy or English language proficiency, and/or racial/ethnic and gender/sexual minorities experience greater disparities in access to health care and guidelines-concordant treatment—this is particularly true among those with cancer diagnoses. There has been a corresponding increase in enrollments in social work education programs as organizations and communities recognize the need for a highly competent professional workforce whose training reflects the 21st-century needs of these populations.

Social work education is both values- and competency-based (Council on Social Work Education [CSWE], 2022). Social workers can complete three successively more specialized levels of education—baccalaureate, master's, and doctoral. Successful completion of programmatic requirements, including a field practicum, leads to achieving a bachelor of social work degree (BSW) and/or master of social work degree (MSW). The BSW is a generalist, nonclinical degree, providing entry-level social workers with competencies needed to address the psychosocial, financial, practical, or instrumental needs of traditionally underrepresented and minoritized individuals, families, or groups, as well as their service organizations and communities. In addition to field experiences, MSW degrees provide competencies necessary for clinical and nonclinical work assessing, evaluating, and intervening within these same systems of practice. An increasing number of MSW programs offer concentrations or certificates in health care, health/integrative health, and aging/gerontology. However, as discussed later in this chapter, very few offer trainings in oncology social work, particularly in specialized knowledge areas such as palliative or end-of-life care, or in essential practice behaviors such as interprofessional communication, collaboration, and intervention.

While BSW-level social workers may be eligible for licensure in a number of states after graduating from a CSWE-accredited program, the MSW is considered the terminal degree for the profession (CSWE, 2022; National Association of Social Workers [NASW], 2016). In most states, earning a MSW from a CSWE-accredited program is the minimum academic preparation necessary to become eligible for licensure to practice as a health care social worker (NASW, 2016) or OSWs (AOSW, n.d.). Comparatively fewer students enroll in programs of study leading to the research-focused doctorate (PhD) or advanced practice doctor of social work (DSW); this level does not convey eligibility for licensure.

Along with overall increasing enrollments in social work education, a recent CSWE survey of accredited programs identified long-standing differences in the sex and race/ethnicity of new graduates (2018). BSW- and MSW-level social work education continues to be heavily female (both

>83%). Approximately one-half of BSW (50.9%) and MSW (48.4%) graduates report diverse racial/ethnic identities, with increasing numbers of Black and Hispanic/Latinx graduates. However, gains in social work education have not been uniform, as fewer than 5% of MSW graduates report Asian, Native Hawaiian/Pacific Islander, or American Indian/Alaska Native race/ethnicity.

While social work programs are becoming more responsive to the needs of a growing and more diverse health care workforce, their graduates are encountering additional barriers to social work careers due to widespread issues in licensure and credentialing. In August 2022, the Association of Social Work Boards released its long-anticipated report on exam pass rates over the past decade. Although results indicated higher first-time and eventual pass rates for women and younger test takers on the clinical and master's exams, substantial differences also emerged depending on test takers' race/ethnicity and primary language. For example, the eventual pass rate for test takers reporting White race was over 90% for both the clinical and master's exams versus those reporting Asian (79.7% and 75.5%), Hispanic/Latino (76.6% and 71.2%), Black (57% and 51.9%), and Native American/Indigenous (73.5% and 72.2%). Test takers whose primary language was not English also fared much worse on the clinical and master's exams (70% and 63.2%). In response to this report, several social work organizations, including CSWE, NASW, and the Social Work and Hospice Care Network (SWHPN), issued statements calling for investigation into implicit bias in the exam and reaffirming commitment to antiracism, diversity, equity, and inclusion (ADEI) by opening searches for alternate credentialing providers for continuing education and removing requirements concerning pass rates from accreditation standards.

Ongoing disparities in exam pass rates may have long-standing implications for the OSW profession, as MSW degrees from CSWE-accredited programs and masters or clinical-level licensure are required for practice. Yet, little is known about the actual racial/ethnic composition of MSW graduates who pursue careers specializing in oncology. A 2020 survey of AOSW membership revealed that approximately 86.4% of participants identified as White/Caucasian; 7.5% Asian/Asian American, Native Hawaiian/Pacific Islander, or American Indian/Alaska Native; 5.4% Black/African American; and 4.6% Hispanic/Latino. Participants in a study of AOSW members conducted during this same period reported their sample as 89.5% White, 3.4% Black/African American, 2.4% Asian, and 3% "other" (Perlmutter et al., 2021). If representative of the wider membership, these figures represent only modest increases in members from underrepresented populations since its 2016 membership survey. Thus, while the social work profession is improving in terms of overall diversity of social workers entering the profession and perhaps entering OSW career paths, inequities persist in the ability of those from minoritized races/ethnicities to move from trainee to professional status.

Accreditation and Standards of Practice

The CSWE (2022) defines competent preparation and sets the educational policies and accreditation standards (EPAS) for competency-based education in social work. In this capacity, it serves as the accrediting body for over 850 BSW and MSW degree-granting programs. CSWE does not accredit doctoral degree programs in social work, as these are not considered terminal degrees for practice.

Social work trainees benefit from a professional values- and competency-based education that equally considers the explicit curriculum (academic courses, field practicum, and degree plans) and explicit curriculum (the learning environment, inclusive of faculty role modeling and mentoring). CSWE-accredited programs are required to develop curricula that consider the multidimensional nature of competence—the knowledge, skills, values, and cognitive and affective processes (critical thinking and affective response)—and the competencies and related professional behaviors necessary for professional practice.

Consistent with the NASW *Code of Ethics* (2021) and professional values, the CSWE EPAS call attention to historical and contemporary issues of power, privilege, intersectionality, and social and economic justice within social institutions and the wider society. The newly released 2022 CSWE EPAS outlines competencies related to ethical and professional behavior; engaging in research/evaluation and policy practice; and engaging, assessing, intervening, and evaluating practice with various clients and stakeholders. To strengthen professional competence in ADEI throughout the workforce, social work students will also receive competence preparation in promoting and protecting human rights and social, racial, economic, and environmental justice, as well as engaging ADEI in practice.

While the 2022 CSWE EPAS shapes the landscape of social work education, other standards guide the scopes of practice for health care/medical social workers and OSWs. For example, the NASW offers generalized *Standards for Practice in Health Care Settings* (2016) and the more specialized *Standards for Palliative and End of Life Care* (2004). These standards primarily target social workers in health care or broadly defined palliative/end-of-life care settings; integrate the NASW *Code of Ethics*, particularly values related to self-determination, the inherent worth and dignity of persons, and cultural competency; and provide guidance on quality care and advocacy on behalf of patients and their families, integration of best practices in direct services, interdisciplinary teamwork, professional development, supervision and leadership, and participation in research/evaluation and policy.

The AOSW *Scope and Standards of Practice*, which is also the foundation of the independently administered OSW certification credential, provide targeted and comprehensive guidance for the OSW profession (AOSW, n.d.; Board of Oncology Social Work [BOSW], n.d.) and are supported by two recent nationwide studies analyzing competencies and practice behaviors (Perlmutter et al., 2021; Zebrack et al., 2022). OSWs play a central role in many cancer organizations' Commission on Cancer–mandated distress screening and survivorship initiatives. They also perform a variety of direct and indirect biopsychosocial-spiritual care functions as part of interdisciplinary cancer care teams. In doing so, OSWs use the full spectrum of competencies acquired through the MSW combined with the unique competencies gained through OSW-specific activities (e.g., supervision and mentoring, continuing education activities, practice experience focused on cancer care, inclusive of palliative and end of life) necessary to facilitate access to care, coping, and improved quality of life and outcomes among patients throughout the cancer continuum, as well as their caregivers, families, survivors, and communities.

Mentorship, Supervision, and Other Professional Development Activities

Mentorship provided by an experienced social worker enhances the mentee's professional well-being, promotes resilience, and provides opportunities for professional growth (Gardner et al., 2015; Toh et al., 2018). Toh and colleagues (2018) describe mentoring as a crucial source of support for those working in fields with an elevated risk of compassion fatigue and burnout. Several national organizations offer continuing education and mentorship (see Tables 23.1 and 23.2). OSWs can also find formal and informal mentoring opportunities outside the larger organizations. Given its implicit role within the mentoring process, informal mentoring has been understudied in the literature in comparison to formal mentorship. Especially in a field with such a high rate of burnout, having a mentor offers OSWs individualized support, which both enhances professional well-being and promotes resilience. The benefits of informal and formal mentoring are reciprocal, with mentors reporting higher levels of career success, satisfaction, commitment to work, and personal growth (Toh et al., 2018).

Table 23.1 Opportunities for Developing OSW Competencies: Professional Organizations that Offer National Conferences/Continuing Education and Mentorship

Professional Organization	Website	Annual Conference	Continuing Education/ Webinars	Mentorship Opportunities
Association of Oncology Social Work (AOSW)	www.aosw.org	✓	✓	✓
American Psychosocial Oncology Society (APOS)	www.apos-society.org	✓	✓	✓
Association of Pediatric Oncology Social work (APOSW)	www.aposw.org	✓	✓	
Society for Social Work Leadership in Healthcare (SSWLHC)	secure.sswhlc.org	✓	✓	✓
Social Work Hospice & Palliative Care Network (SWHPN)	www.swhpn.org	✓	✓	✓
Society for Social Work and Research (SSWR)	Secure.sswr.org	✓	✓	✓

Table 23.2 Opportunities for Developing OSW Competencies: Fellowships/Internships/ Mentoring

Program Name	Opportunity for Professional Development	Mentoring Opportunity	Certification
New York University Silver School of Social Work Zelda Foster Studies	MSW Fellowship in Palliative and End-of-Life Care	✓	
New York University Silver School of Social Work Zelda Foster Studies	Post Master's Leadership Fellowship in Palliative and End-of-Life Care	✓	
New York University Silver School of Social Work Zelda Foster Studies	Post Master's Certificate Program in Palliative and End-of-Life Care		✓
University of Pennsylvania Social Policy & Practice	Post Master's Advanced Certificate in Oncology Social Work Program		✓
Smith College School of Social Work	Palliative and End-of-Life Care Certificate Program	✓	✓

Formal mentoring is beneficial since it provides an avenue for building and enhancing social networks and establishing norms, values, and skills, while supporting a mentee's career goals (Gardner et al., 2015). In the context of OSW, mentoring can offer mentees a sense of competence by providing an opportunity for reflection and a space to process emotional reactions. Processing emotional responses with a mentor can prevent frustration and burnout (Erickson & Grove, 2007). Workforce development programs across Europe and the United States are integrating mentorship components into their curricula. These programs have developed to meet the needs of the next generation of OSWs in response to a workforce shortage and to meet the needs of an aging society (Gardner et al., 2015). Securing a mentor can be done through a professional organization, through an employer (informal or formal), or through a formalized training program.

OSWs can also be administrators or clinical supervisors, providing supervision to address the training needs of workers and to meet state licensing requirements. Professional supervision includes the development of competence, knowledge, and ethical practice (e.g., assisting new employees with health care but not oncology experience acculturate to working in a cancer center). Supervision can be facilitated in individual, group, or peer formats as most social workers obtain their specialty level skills on the job. Social work supervision is a fundamental element of practice and allows for case discussion, reflection, support, training, and professional development. The goal of supervisory sessions is to improve performance and job satisfaction (Kennedy et al., 2015). However, Zebrack and colleagues (2008) reported that 30% of OSW supervisors indicated that they had little to no competence in this area, a finding that indicates the need for more training opportunities for OSW supervisors. OSWs in health care settings are often supervised by non-social-work professionals and work in multidisciplinary departments, which reduces their ability to obtain supervision from experienced social workers or have access to OSW mentors.

Repetitive losses experienced during daily practice often lead to OSWs experiencing compassion fatigue and burnout. Joubert and colleagues (2013) found that when supervision focused on clinical practice with patients and families with links to professional social work theories and frameworks, OSWs experienced less burnout. Additionally, they reported that attention to helping OSWs manage the emotional impact of the work as well as assistance managing caseloads and organizational challenges within the health care system were important emphases of supervision. Tsesmelis Piccolino (2022) recommends incorporating the concept of vicarious resilience into supervision as a way to support OSW practitioners and offset the risk of compassion fatigue. Vicarious resilience can also help OSWs find meaning and purpose in their work and thereby influence sustainment in the field (Tsesmelis Piccolino, 2022).

Supervision during COVID-19 rapidly evolved to focus on helping supervisees navigate a world in which uncertainty, risk, and anxiety exploded for not only cancer patients and families (who already faced fear and uncertainty due to the diagnosis) but also social workers practicing in health care settings. Many supervisory sessions switched to virtual or telephonic sessions. Supervisors had to adjust the focus of supervision to assist OSWs to work with ambiguity, endure risks associated with their professional environment, and accept change, while simultaneously remaining resilient and patient focused. They also had to actively reflect on and assess their cultural self-awareness and at times, enhance their cross-cultural knowledge to provide culturally competent supervision to a diverse OSW workforce wrestling with COVID-19, societal and institutional racism, discrimination, and other personal and professional challenges (Box 23.1).

Box 23.1 Case Example of OSW Supervisory Relationship Focused on Professional Development and Sustainability

Ava is a 30-year-old Chinese female. She was working as an inpatient social worker at a hospital in New York City covering the Asian Services team and assisting patients with discharges. Fluent in Mandarin and Cantonese, Ava graduated from New York University School of Social Work and completed focused learning in palliative care. She was seeking to continue to care for the Chinese patient population in a different setting. A seasoned oncology social work manager recruited Ava to join the outpatient oncology social work team to help them better reach a large population of Chinese cancer patients in need of supportive services programming. Ava's professional goals were to continue to care for the vulnerable, immigrant patient population with a focus on the unique needs of Chinese-immigrant cancer patients. She developed a support program, which includes monthly support groups and quarterly celebratory events in recognition of major Chinese holidays. She also continued to expand her community outreach work with local agencies through joining both the diversity committee and community advisory board at the cancer center where she worked. She conducted research by tracking her own interventions and working with a statistician to analyze the data. With mentorship she learned how to write a manuscript for publication and how to submit an abstract after joining AOSW. She then presented her work at the national AOSW conference and two local social work departmental grand rounds. Even though COVID-19 and xenophobia created challenges for Ava living far from her family during a grim time, she persevered and has continued to make an impact on the community with impressive attendance at her monthly group meetings. Additionally, she works on presentations with other medical professionals and brings speakers to educate the community on various important topics relevant to them. Ava's dedication coupled with support from her supervisor to pursue professional opportunities to assist the Chinese-immigrant community has resulted in programmatic growth and demonstrated success. Her supervisor nominated her for recognition through a 40 under 40 in Cancer award, for which she was selected. The award reflects her professional achievements.

Ava's case example demonstrates the importance of supervision and mentorship in oncology social work and how this relationship can result in the achievement of professional goals, lead to career advancement, and influence practice at micro, mezzo, and macro levels.

Committees and Professional Organizations

Seeking and accepting opportunities to participate in various committees both within and outside one's primary workplace offers numerous opportunities for growth and engagement in the field. As stated in the case example, Ava joined institutional committees as well as AOSW. Through committee work, social workers can demonstrate the value they bring to the interdisciplinary team as well as develop an understanding of the larger context within which they are working. Accepting opportunities that provide growth and continued learning, such as committee work, can also be an avenue to assuming leadership roles. Participation in the institutional cancer committee (the committee focuses on keeping/obtaining accreditation from the American College of Surgeons Commission on Cancer) is another opportunity for OSWs working in a cancer center to take a leadership role. Regardless of employment setting, professional organizations such as AOSW, APOS, and SWHPN provide opportunities for OSWs to join committees, access continuing education, and network.

Psychosocial Oncology Research

Ava's experience illustrates the multiple ways that OSWs use research to assess the unmet needs of patients and groups, develop culturally and linguistically appropriate evidence-based programs, evaluate the effectiveness of interventions, disseminate research/evaluation findings, engage communities and stakeholders, and advocate for needed resources. It also highlights research as an integral component of professional development and sustainability in oncology social work. Research is a required part of the MSW curriculum; however, social workers often graduate without training in how to conduct research in practice settings. The field is challenged in finding support from funders of cancer research such as the National Cancer Institute and the American Cancer Society (ACS). ACS recently eliminated their health professional training grants for oncology social workers, which they began funding in 1989, and in 2020, they suspended both the master's and doctoral training grants in oncology social work. These grants were extremely beneficial in the training and recruitment for the next generation of oncology social work professional and researcher and the impact of their elimination remains to be seen.

OSW research has made numerous contributions to the field despite challenges in finding support from major funders of cancer research required to establish a solid knowledge base. Also lacking are postdoctoral opportunities (Oktay & Zebrack, 2018). In 1994, AOSW created the Social Work Oncology Research Group, which aims to promote relevant research and to support AOSW practitioners who are interested in strengthening the research component of their jobs or are interested in learning more about research.

Advocacy

As we see from Ava's experience, advocacy is essential for both effective OSW practice and the profession's sustainability. Social workers need to remain up-to-date on recent changes in social work education standards and the NASW *Code of Ethics* (e.g., use of technology and social media), as well as policy and regulatory issues influencing professional practice. In addition to advocating within their organizations for awareness of the profession and its programs and services, OSWs must advocate for interprofessional collaboration, co-operation, and approaches to cancer care delivery. Furthermore, OSWs need to advocate for appropriate and equitable reimbursement for their services (Zebrack et al., 2008), particularly as they relate to programs/services required for Joint Commission and Centers for Medicare and Medicaid Services Accreditation.

Advocacy is also necessary with major funders and donors, especially as relates to patient-centered opportunities and the community programs and services that were reduced or eliminated during the COVID-19 pandemic.

Recent findings from Zebrack and colleagues (2021) underscore the importance of advocacy for legislative policies that support interstate licensure and telehealth communication, since many OSWs pivoted to HIPAA-compliant virtual platforms because of COVID-19. However, many OSWs need to practice with patient populations residing across their licensure jurisdictions. Reimbursement is sorely needed for telehealth visits, advance directive/goals of care discussions, survivorship care plans, and other areas of OSW practice to ensure patient access to high-quality cancer care. Of note, in 2022, more than a dozen state social work boards have signed onto draft legislation for an interstate licensure compact that if adopted would set and enforce licensing standards for telehealth and promote continuity of care across member jurisdictions (NASW, 2022).

Self-Care

In order for OSWs to stay motivated and engaged in their work, they must attend to self-care and prevent burnout. COVID-19 heightened the importance of self-care. OSWs on the front line of the pandemic faced additional challenges to their psychological well-being (Seng et al., 2021). Given OSWs' deep connections with patients and families, the work often involves repetitive loss. Simultaneously, OSWs like Ava may be navigating unique challenges associated with their life stage and psychosocial or financial situation. Thus, it is imperative for OSWs to practice and supervisors to encourage self-care. Strategies include speaking with a therapist, mindful meditation, writing/journaling, and seeking support from colleagues. The OSW's institution might also offer employee wellness programs (Crowe, 2015; Kearney et al., 2009). The benefits of self-care include decreased burnout, compassion fatigue, and moral distress (Crowe, 2015). By learning and implementing self-care skills, OSWs can gain personal and professional well-being, job engagement, compassion satisfaction, and resilience (Kearney et al., 2009).

Compensation

Sustainment of OSWs in the profession also considers compensation and benefits. In 2022, median annual salaries for health care social workers were approximately $61,000, compared to $78,070 for registered nurses and $99,330 for psychologists employed in hospitals (U.S. Bureau of Labor Statistics, n.d.). While OSW median salaries ($60,001–$70,000) are higher than those of their health care social work peers, a recent nationwide study reported that almost 40% of OSWs have current student loan debt (Guan et al., 2022). The latter is a particularly problematic barrier to attracting and sustaining diversity among OSWs, as those who are first-generation college students and those identifying as members of minoritized populations are more likely to acquire student loan debt and carry higher loan balances.

Social workers must be paid competitively for the work they do. This requires both managers and supervisors to advocate for salary increases within their work settings and professional organizations like NASW and AOSW to push for competitive salaries nationwide. Social workers should also consider employment opportunities that provide both tangible and intangible benefits. For example, some social work positions offer union benefits, including but not limited to job stability, lower out-of-pocket prescription costs, regular salary increases, and even pensions. Additional benefits may include access to funding for professional development or conference registration or travel, books and journal subscriptions, reimbursement for licensure- and certification-related fees, and free supervision necessary for the licensed clinical social worker (LCSW) credential.

Community Engagement and Social Determinants of Health

OSW demonstration of community involvement through leadership or oncology-related educational presentations in the community are part of the core criteria the BOSW has determined necessary for certification. Participation in community cancer prevention and screening programs are additional opportunities for OSWs to build on their clinical work and engage more broadly in macro practice. These opportunities also help sustain OSWs, offering ways for OSWs to expand beyond direct practice and develop new skills.

Social determinants of health (SDOH) are "the conditions in which people are born, grow, work, live and age, and the wider set of forces and systems shaping the conditions of daily life" (World Health Organization, n.d.). SDOH refers to social, economic, and political structures that influence health outcomes, including access to healthy food, safe housing, and supportive social networks. Efforts to understand community concerns, attitudes, and beliefs about cancer and its treatment and environmental determinants informs the social work practitioner, strengthens the understanding of social variables, and broadens the practice base of social work (McClintock et al., 2005). With the biopsychosocial and person-in-environment frameworks, OSWs are well positioned to assume an increasingly prominent role in community engagement and related macro-level activities necessary for improving SDOH.

Guiding Best Practices for the Future

OSWs can find opportunities for professional development through professional associations such as AOSW, APOS, and Society for Social Work Leadership in Healthcare (SSWLHC) (Table 23.1). These organizations offer social workers opportunities for networking, continuing education, and leadership using a variety of delivery formats and focusing on differing practice experience levels. Pre-COVID-19, professional development trainings were primarily offered using in-person or hybrid delivery formats. However, in addition to ushering in enhanced safety protocols and codes of conduct, the pandemic has raised awareness of inequities in OSWs' personal and professional circumstances and daylighted substantial racial/ethnic barriers in accessing institutional resources for professional development.

The initial pandemic lockdown forced widespread cancellations of many professional meetings and trainings. Given the profession's need for ongoing professional development, the lockdown spawned profession-wide concerns related to OSWs' ability to deliver continuing education and complete trainings necessary for social work licensure and OSW certification. One positive development the pandemic fostered was the OSW profession's pivot from a primary reliance on traditional educational approaches and formats to more contemporary approaches. As a result, organizations such as AOSW leveraged public health and safety guidance, curriculum/instruction developers, and meeting administrators to offer fully online webinars and conferences.

Leadership development is another key factor in professional sustainability. OSWs can seek out a variety of leadership opportunities, including developing new initiatives, speaking to community audiences or fellow professionals, serving on committees, writing grants, or publishing in professional journals. Not only is the health care system in a state of disruption with recent changes due to the COVID-19 pandemic but also shifts in work settings are applying internal and external stressors to the OSW profession. Professional sustainment is critically important for individual OSWs and the larger OSW community. The OSW profession needs the next generation of leaders to have the vision and competencies necessary to preserve the unique roles and functions of OSWs in oncology settings.

Pearls

- OSWs should advocate for and assist in the development of academic training programs that acknowledge the critical need for ADEI and remove barriers to training a diverse workforce prepared to build a more inclusive environment so that all stakeholders feel comfortable and valued.
- Working professionals should perform an assessment of national, local, and institutional trends in compensation and utilize advocacy and policy practice skills to gain competitive salaries and other employment benefits.
- Participation in committees and professional organizations is an opportunity for professional growth and leadership.
- OSWs are encouraged to seek continuing education opportunities to advance their knowledge in conducting research, a critical area for professional sustainability. Social work is grounded in the skills of process and outcomes and therefore, OSWs can make a significant contribution to the oncology literature.
- Graduate students and working professionals should be taught ways to incorporate self-care into practice.

Pitfalls

- OSWs have an elevated risk for burnout and should be aware of resources available to them to address compassion fatigue and secondary trauma.
- Changes in social work education, licensure, and credentialing (e.g., EPAS, OSW-C, interstate licensure compact) will force OSWs to leverage new competencies in practice and can create interprofessional conflict that will need to be navigated.
- Despite OSWs vital contributions, salaries lag behind those of other helping professions.
- OSWs need to advocate for their role on national institutional committees and boards that set policies and standards as they have an immediate and direct impact on our profession.

- The overall profession of social work is recruiting and training learners from diverse backgrounds, as demonstrated in recent CSWE reports and the published literature; however, these trends do not appear to be manifesting in diversification of the OSW workforce.

Additional Resources

Altilio, T., Otis-Green, S., & Cagle, J. (Eds.). (2022). *The Oxford textbook of palliative social work*. Oxford University Press.

Association of Oncology Social Work. (n.d.). *Scope and standards of practice*. Retrieved February 1, 2022, from https://aosw.org/publications-media/scope-of-practice/

Board of Oncology Social Work. (n.d.). *Certified Oncology Social Worker (OSW-C) initial certification requirements through December 31, 2022*. Retrieved February 1, 2022, from https://oswcert.org/oncology-social-work-certification-osw-c-requirements/

Breitbart, W., Butow, P., Jacobsen, P., Lam, W., Lazenby, M., & Loscalzo, M. (Eds.). (2021). *Psycho-oncology* (4th ed.). Oxford University Press.

Christ, G., Messner, C., & Behar, L. (Eds.). (2015). *Handbook of oncology social work: Psychosocial care for people with cancer*. Oxford University Press.

Council on Social Work Education. (2022). *2022 Educational policies and accreditation standards (EPAS)*. Council on Social Work Education.

Halpern, J. J. (2020). *Core curriculum for palliative and hospice social work*. Social Work Hospice and Palliative Care Network.

National Association of Social Workers. (2016). *NASW standards for social work practice in health care settings*. https://www.socialworkers.org/LinkClick.aspx?fileticket=fFnsRHX-4HE%3d&portalid=0

Websites

American Psychosocial Oncology Society: www.apos-society.org
Association of Pediatric Oncology Social Work: www.aposw.org
Association of Community Cancer Centers: www.accc-cancer.org
Association of Oncology Social Work: www.aosw.org
American Society of Preventive Oncology: www.aspo.org
Board of Oncology Social Work Certification: www.oswcert.org
Cancer*Care*: www.cancercare.org
Cancer.Net: www.cancer.net
Cancer Support Community: www.cancersupportcommunity.org
National Association of Social Workers: www.socialworkers.org
Social Work Hospice and Palliative Care Network: www.swhpn.org
Society for Social Work and Research: secure.sswr.org

References

Association of Oncology Social Work. (2020). *Membership survey*. [Unpublished raw data].

Association of Oncology Social Work. (n.d.). *Scope and standards of practice*. Retrieved February 1, 2022, from https://aosw.org/publications-media/scope-of-practice/

Association of Social Work Boards. (2022). *2022 ASWB* exam *pass rate analysis: Final report*. https://www.aswb.org/wp-content/uploads/2022/07/2022-ASWB-Exam-Pass-Rate-Analysis.pdf

Board of Oncology Social Work. (n.d.). *Certified Oncology Social Worker (OSW-C) initial certification requirements through December 31, 2022*. Retrieved February 1, 2022, from https://oswcert.org/oncology-social-work-certification-osw-c-requirements/

Council on Social Work Education. (2022). *2022* Educational *policy and accreditation standards for baccalaureate and master's social work programs*. https://www.cswe.org/getmedia/94471c42-13b8-493b-9041-b30f48533d64/2022-EPAS.pdf

Crowe, C. (2015). Burnout and self-care considerations for oncology professionals. *Journal of Pain Management, 8*(3), 191–195.

Deshields, T. L., Wells-Di Gregorio, S. Flowers, S. R., Irwin, K. E., Nipp, R., Padgett, L., & Zebrack, B. (2021). Addressing distress management challenges: Recommendations from the consensus panel of the American Psychosocial Oncology Society and the Association of Oncology Social Work. *CA: A Cancer Journal for Clinicians, 71*(5), 407–436. https://doi.org/10.3322/caac.21672

Erickson, R. J., & Grove, W. J. C. (2007, October 31). Why emotions matter: Age, agitation, and burnout among registered nurses. *Online Journal of Issues in Nursing, 13*(1). https://doi.org/10.3912/OJIN.Vol13No01PPT01

Gardner, D. S., Gerbino, S., Walls, J. W., Chachkes, E., & Doherty, M. J. (2015). Mentoring the next generation of social workers in palliative and end-of-life care: The Zelda Foster studies program. *Journal of Social Work in End-of-Life and Palliative Care, 11*(2), 107–131. https://doi.org/10.1080/15524256.2015.1074142

Guan, T., Zebrack, B., Otis-Green, S., & DesJardin, G. (2022, August 5). Salary and student loan debt for oncology social workers: Findings from the oncology social work competencies, opportunities, roles, and expertise (CORE) survey. *Journal of Psychosocial Oncology, 41*(2), 196–209. https://doi.org/10.1080/07347332.2022.2101906

Heisler, E. J. (2018, April 20). The mental health workforce: A primer. *Congressional Research Service*, 7–5700. https://fas.org/sgp/crs/misc/R43255.pdf

Joubert, L., Hocking, A., & Hampson, R. (2013). Social work in oncology—Managing vicarious trauma—The positive impact of professional supervision. *Social Work Health Care, 52*(2–3), 296–310. https://doi.org/10.1080/00981389.2012.737902

Kearney, M. K., Weininger, R. B., Vachon, M. L. S., Harrison, R. L., & Mount, B. M. (2009). Self-care of physicians caring for patients at the end of life: "Being connected . . . A key to my survival." *Journal of the American Medical Association, 301*(11), 1155–1164. https://doi.org/10.1001/jama.2009.352

Kennedy, V., Smolinski, K., Colon, Y., & Zabora, J. (2015). Educating and training professional social workers. In J. Holland, W. Breitbart, P. Jacobson, M. Loscalzo, R. McCorkle, & P. Butow (Eds.), *Psycho-oncology* (3rd ed., pp. 689–694). Oxford University Press. https://doi.org/10.1093/med/9780199363315.001.0001

McClintock, M. K., Conzen, S. D., Gehlert, S., Masi, C., & Olopade, F. (2005). Mammary cancer and social interactions: Identifying multiple environments that regulate gene expression throughout the life span. *Journals of Gerontology*, Series B, *60*(1), 32–41. https://doi.org/10.1093/geronb/60.special_issue_1.32

National Association of Social Workers. (2004). *Standards for palliative and end-of-life care.* https://www.socialworkers.org/LinkClick.aspx?fileticket=xBMd58VwEhk%3d&portalid=0

National Association of Social Workers. (2016). *NASW standards for social work practice in health care settings.* https://www.socialworkers.org/LinkClick.aspx?fileticket=fFnsRHX-4HE%3d&portalid=0

National Association of Social Workers. (2021). *Code of ethics.* https://www.socialworkers.org/About/Ethics/Code-of-Ethics/Code-of-Ethics-English

National Association of Social Workers (2022). *Interstate Licensure Compact.* https://www.socialworkers.org/Advocacy/Interstate-Licensure-Compact-for-Social-Work

Oktay, J. S., & Zebrack, B. (2018, June 25). Oncology social work research. *Encyclopedia of Social Work.* https://doi.org/10.1093/acrefore/9780199975839.013.1268

Perlmutter, E. Y., Herron, F. B., Rohan, E. A., & Thomas, E. (2021). Oncology social work practice behaviors: A national survey of AOSW members. *Journal of Psychosocial Oncology, 40*(2), 137–151. https://doi.org/10.1080/07347332.2021.1942386

Seng, B. K., Subramaniam, M., Chung, Y. J., Syed Ahmad, S. A. M., & Chong, S. A. (2021). Resilience and stress in frontline social workers during the COVID-19 pandemic in Singapore. *Asian Social Work and Policy Review, 15*(3), 234–243. https://doi.org/10.1111/aswp.12237

Toh, Y. P., Karthik, R., Teo, C. C., Suppiah, S., Cheung, S. L., & Krishna, L. (2018). Toward mentoring in palliative social work: A narrative review of mentoring programs in social work. *American Journal of Hospice and Palliative Medicine, 35*(3), 523–531. https://doi.org/10.1177/1049909117715216

Tsesmelis Piccolino, S. (2022). Vicarious resilience: Traversing the path from client to clinician through a search for meaning. *Social Work in Health Care, 61*(6–8), 1–15. https://doi.org/10.1080/00981389.2022.2134274

U.S. Bureau of Labor Statistics, Department of Labor. (n.d.). *Occupational outlook handbook.* Retrieved August 15, 2022, from https://www.bls.gov/ooh/

Whitaker, T., Weismiller, T., Clark, E., & Wilson, M. (2006). Assuring the sufficiency of a frontline workforce: A national study of licensed social workers. In National Association of Social Workers, *Social work services in health care settings* [Special report]. Retrieved from https://www.socialworkers.org/LinkClick.aspx?fileticket=OilZ7p_EEnE%3D&portalid=0

Zebrack, B., Grignon, M., Guan, T., Long, D., Miller, N., Nelson, K., Otis-Green, S., Rayton, M., Schapmire, T., & Wiener, L. (2021). Six months in: COVID-19 and its impact on oncology social work practice. *Journal of Psychosocial Oncology, 39*(3), 461–468. https://doi.org/10.1080/07347332.2021.1893421

Zebrack, B., Schapmire, T., Otis-Green, S., Nelson, K., Miller, N., Donna, D., & Grignon, M. (2022). Establishing core competencies, opportunities, roles, and expertise for oncology social work. *Journal of Social Work, 22*(4), 1085–1104. https://doi.org/10.1177/14680173211051

Zebrack, B., Walsh, K., Burg, M. A., Maramaldi, P., & Lim, J.-W. (2008). Oncology social worker competencies and implications for education and training. *Social Work in Health Care, 47*(4), 355–375. https://doi.org/10.1080/00981380802173954

World Health Organization. (n.d.). *About social determinants of health.* Retrieved January 10, 2022, from https://www.who.int/social_determinants/sdh_definition/en/

24 The Increasing Role of Credentialing, Certification, and Continuing Education

Brittany Nwachuku, Jennifer Bires, and Vickie Leff

Key Concepts

- Certification encourages and recognizes professional achievement and in turn, advances the social work profession.
- Certification is the official recognition of a social work professional's expertise, clinical judgment, and achievement, and relies on verification of competency through examination.
- Continuing education (CE) is specialized training in the topic areas that social workers want and need to learn to best serve their clients and organizations.
- The National Association of Social Work (NASW) is the largest membership organization of professional social workers that enhances professional growth and development of its members.
- The Association of Oncology Social Work (AOSW) is a social work organization dedicated to the enhancement of psychosocial services to people with cancer, their families, and caregivers.
- Social Work Hospice and Palliative Network (SWHPN) is a social work organization that promotes advancement of knowledge and best practices for hospice and palliative care social workers to ensure that all patients and families facing serious illness can access expert social work services.

Keywords: antiracist, certification, continuing education, COVID-19, decolonization, evidence based, job analysis, pandemic

The profession of social work has an established history in health-related fields, and today medical social workers (e.g., oncology and palliative social workers) serve at nearly every site where physical and mental health needs

Brittany Nwachuku, Jennifer Bires, and Vickie Leff, *The Increasing Role of Credentialing, Certification, and Continuing Education* In: *Oncology and Palliative Social Work.* Edited by: Susan Hedlund, Bryan Miller, Grace Christ, and Carolyn Messner, Oxford University Press. DOI: 10.1093/oso/9780197607299.003.0024 are being met (McCormick et al., 2014). Social workers have provided essential psychosocial services as a part of palliative and serious illness care for decades. Oncology and palliative social workers position themselves in medical centers, hospitals, clinics, nursing homes, home health agencies, and hospices. Though their roles in the health field vary depending on the setting, oncology and palliative social workers are change agents by training. Zebrack et al. (2008) concluded that "oncology social workers are the primary providers of psychosocial services in major oncology treatment centers and community health care settings throughout the world, both because of their knowledge about cancer and its psychosocial impact, and because of their practice versatility" (p. 355). Moreover, oncology and palliative social workers often help patients make health-promoting behavior changes, provide patient advocacy and education, service provision, and referral, understand end-of-life care and standards of ethical decision-making, and offer psychosocial counseling. However, "the field has experienced a difficult time with clarifying, documenting, explaining and justifying their role on the interdisciplinary team," even though social workers make up the largest group of licensed mental health providers in the United States (Head et al., 2019, p. 16; Substance Abuse and Mental Health Services Administration, 2020).

In 2018, the National Consensus Project for Quality Palliative Care developed the standards of practice and core competencies for the generalist social worker in palliative care (Glajchen et al., 2018). These consensus-derived core competencies set the stage for further research into advanced practice skills (Ferrell et al., 2018). As many health social workers encounter situations dealing with serious illness, it is important to identify the foundational skills needed to provide best care for patients and families. Social workers who specialize in serious illness care, however, need more specific certifications to objectively validate their advanced practice skills.

The process involved in earning an Oncology Social Work Certificate was the first developed in the oncology, palliative care, and end-of-life field. In 2000, the AOSW sent a survey to members, of whom 83% supported a specialty accreditation for oncology social workers with 93% of respondents reporting that the field of oncology social work required special skills (Viatones et al., 2015). Soon thereafter, AOSW developed the certification process to recognize oncology social workers with experience and expertise and elevate the profession. The AOSW certificate has become the preferred credential for the positions of psychosocial services coordinator and survivorship program coordinator for the American Society of Clinical Oncology's Commission on Cancer. The Board of Oncology Social Work (n.d.) mission states that the organization is "to ensure excellence in psychosocial care to oncology patients, families, caregivers and their communities." Oncology social workers certified by BOSW must demonstrate:

- excellence in oncology-specific social work practice
- ongoing oncology-specific education and training
- ongoing professional oncology work employment
- ongoing professional and community engagement

The initial application requires:

- MSW
- a minimum of 6,240 hours of paid post-MSW experience in oncology, palliative care, and/or end-of-life care within the most recent 5-year period
- active state-issued social work license
- proof of two oncology-related community and/or leadership activities
- three letters of recommendation

Renewal occurs every 2 years and requires:

- current employment of no fewer than 20 hours in oncology, palliative care, and/or end-of-life care
- active state-issued social work license
- 20 CE units (CEUs) specific to oncology, palliative care, and/or end-of-life care
- proof of continued involvement in two community and/or leadership activities

The Advanced Certified Hospice and Palliative Social Work (ACHP-SW) certification is a portfolio certification created in 2008. This certification is available through the NASW developed with support from the National Hospice and Palliative Care Organization (NASW, 2004). Eligibility requirements include:

- MSW from a graduate program accredited by the Council on Social Work Education
- 20 or more CEUs related specifically to hospice and palliative care
- documentation of at least 2 years of supervised social work experience in hospice and palliative care
- active state-issued social work license

- adherence to NASW *Code of Ethics* (2021) and NASW *Standards for Palliative and End-of-Life Care* (2004)

Development of the Advanced Palliative & Hospice Social Work Certification Program (APHSW-C) began as an effort to further clarify and identify the roles, skills, and tasks social workers specializing in serious illness use, with the goal of creating a scientifically sound and evidence-based certification exam. This certification was created to further differentiate the growing field of palliative care. An initial application requires:

- MSW or BSW
- 2 years post-MSW experience in serious illness care in the past 5 years
- 3 years supervised BSW experience in serious illness care in the past 5 years
- active state-issued social work license
- adherence to the NASW *Code of Ethics* (2021)
- successful passing of the APHSW-C exam
- recertification every 4 years requires 40 CEUs

In 2017, the SWHPN began to develop the first nationwide job analysis of hospice and palliative social workers. A Gordon & Betty Moore Grant funded the research, completed in 2018. The result of the survey was the creation of an in-depth outline of the role of the social worker, which was then used to develop an evidenced-based certification exam for those who wanted to receive specialty certification in the field.

The SWHPN survey used historical and current data on the role of social work to help identify primary roles and competencies (Head et al., 2019). The goal was to determine the most important tasks related to this specialty care. Hundreds of social workers from around the United States participated. A 10-person advisory committee, with a wide range of experience, oversaw the research. The committee worked closely with PSI Services, a company with more than 70 years of experience conducting job analysis, developing tests, and delivering testing services. The committee developed the detailed content outline, listing the content in outline format that became the guide for test development.

The APHSW-C used the survey results to identify four major areas of practice: assessment and reevaluation; planning and intervention; death, grief, and bereavement; and professionalism. These categories make up the outline of the 175-question APHSW-C exam. Having an objectively, psychometrically sound certification program for social workers in serious illness care has elevated the field, increased awareness of the expert skills of the social worker, and opened possibilities for reimbursement of social work services. Currently, there are about 680 APHSW-certified social workers.

Separate from academic credentials and professional certification, social work licensing is what is required to practice social work in a state. Each state has its own laws; state licensure confirms that the licensee has completed a BSW or MSW, undergone several years of supervision, logged a certain number of clinical practice hours, and passed an exam. "Social work licensure protects the public by ensuring that social workers possess the proper education and training to provide ethical and competent services. Each state's regulatory board grants social workers their licenses, so criteria for licensure and levels of licensure vary by location" (Social Work Guide, 2020).

Oncology and palliative social workers practice in rapidly changing and complex environments and workplaces (often with diminishing financial resources) where they face an increase in evidence-based practice requirements within an ever-shifting information landscape (Biggerstaff, 2000). To address these challenges, social workers need to engage in "lifelong learning"—continuing education (CE)—to stay abreast on current practices that promote quality care. In this chapter, we conceptualize CE as "an ongoing process of education and development that continues throughout the professional career" (McCormick et al., 2014, p. 345).

In many states, CE has become accepted as a requirement for renewal of a license to practice social work. This training requirement is in keeping with the general goals of professional credentialing, which is done for the dual purpose of establishing professional practice guidelines and protecting the public by training social workers to practice ethically (Biggerstaff, 2000). The NASW has developed a curriculum model to "equip community-based mental health practitioners to assist with cancer-related issues" (Zebrack et al., 2008, p. 360). In addition, the AOSW set out to formally assess oncology social workers' roles, functions, scopes of practice, and levels of competence in key areas of practice, as well as their perceptions of professional development and training needs.

Credentialing and Certification

Credentialing encourages and recognizes professional achievement and in turn, advances the profession of social work. Evidence-based certification is a professional's official recognition of expertise, clinical judgment, and achievement, and relies on verification of competency through examination (Head et al., 2019. The APHSW-C exam is an objective measure of competence. Evidence- and exam-based advanced practice certification verifies the expert skill level social workers bring to the field; academic programs preparing social workers for practice can use the exam to guide curriculum development. Commitment to updating the job description every 5 to 7 years maintains the quality and applicability of the APHSW-C, assuring the public of these expert skills.

Social work certification programs help identify content and criteria for social workers and ensure continuing education relevant to the changing and growing field of palliative care. We know that social workers who choose to specialize in oncology, palliative, or hospice care face more complex and challenging situations in their practice. Objective validation of these skills (based on a consensus of advanced practice parameters) both reassures patients and families that they are receiving high-quality services and validates the social worker as an equal member of the serious illness team. Both overlap and differences exist among social work specialties surrounding cancer care. Offering a variety of types of certifications allows agencies to choose which requirements will constitute specific job descriptions. Many agencies have added attaining the APHSW-C and OSW-C into their clinical ladder, rewarding the advanced certificate with higher pay and more responsibilities.

A handful of course-based certificate programs exist for advanced serious illness care, including palliative and oncology social work. These are primarily based in educational centers and involve anywhere from 8 hours to 12 months of coursework led by subject matter experts. Participants who complete the course receive a certificate indicating they have taken and passed the course. Examples of relevant certificate courses include the Online Post-Master's Certificate Program from NYU School of Social Work. This certificate program is part of NYU Silver's Zelda Foster Studies Program in Palliative and End-of-Life Care (PELC), which encompasses a range of initiatives designed to develop and mentor PELC social work leaders at all stages of their careers (NYU Silver School of Social Work, 2022). The California State University's Shirley Haynes Institute for Palliative Care offers an online Post-MSW Palliative Care Social Work Certificate Program to MSWs that prepares "social workers with the additional knowledge and skills they need to work effectively on a palliative care team in a hospital, hospice or other setting. Three course levels totaling 180 classroom hours comprise the program, each building upon the last" (California State University, 2013). The Smith College School of Social Work offers a Palliative and End-of-Life Care Certificate, which provides "an opportunity for social workers to deepen clinical and leadership skills in palliative care and participate in relational ways of learning in a community of colleagues with an outstanding faculty of leaders in the field" (Smith College, n.d.). Specific to oncology, the University of Pennsylvania's Advanced Certificate of Oncology Social Work Practice is designed for current health care social workers to "gain superior knowledge and skills for work with individuals, families, and communities impacted by cancer" (University of Pennsylvania, n.d.).

Continuing Education

Researchers indicate several implications for the CE requirements for both oncology and palliative social workers (McCormick et al., 2014; Mitchell, 2012; Zebrack et al., 2008). Today, oncology social workers must be knowledgeable about the numerous factors that influence the delivery and receipt of cancer care in the United States and around the world (Zebrack et al., 2008). A critical component for oncology and palliative social work CE is careful attention to the plight and psychosocial needs of vulnerable, oppressed, and disadvantaged populations. Social workers must be attuned to the realities of how downturns in the American economy, inequitable health care policies, variable unemployment and foreclosure rates, and persistent socioeconomic disadvantages create pathways for the proliferation of health disparities among these populations (Mitchell, 2012). It is critically important that oncology and palliative social workers be well trained for the challenges they face in modern health care practice. Social workers must be aware of the realities of the differential burdens borne by disadvantaged clients and familiar with evidence-informed strategies to advocate for and intervene effectively on behalf of such clients. This requires the development of programs and treatment models to determine which programs and interventions are most effective for client populations. Therefore, Zebrack et al. (2008) recommend that CE emphasize "grant-writing, fundraising, new language acquisition, program development, and community organization to facilitate the integration and movement of social workers into communities where the patients live, work, and seek services" (p. 370).

Oncology and Palliative Social Work During COVID-19

Finally, COVID-19 has wreaked havoc in the lives of individuals, families, communities, and societies and in the process, intensified existing vulnerabilities, oppression, and inequities among patient populations. Oncology and palliative social workers play an essential role in serving and protecting the most vulnerable of people, including those affected by cancer. The NASW states that social workers should "enhance human well-being and help meet the basic human needs of all people, with particular attention to the needs and empowerment of people who are vulnerable, oppressed, and living in poverty" (NASW, 2017, para. 1). The disruption in services the COVID-19 pandemic caused has negatively affected the ability of people with cancer and other serious illnesses to access adequate care. In responding to the pandemic, oncology and palliative care social workers were on the front lines of providing psychosocial services to those in need. This includes providing adequate social support for the general population and fellow medical professionals, advocating for social inclusion for the most vulnerable, elevating awareness about the pandemic and the science that surrounds it, and implementing mental health support and community-based strategies to support resilience and psychologically vulnerable individuals and groups (Afomachukwu, 2021). While this is not a complete description of how oncology and palliative care social workers responded in that time of crisis, COVID-19 has undoubtedly changed not only the way all humans live but how social workers provide psychosocial care. Continuing education for oncology and palliative social workers should promote access to prevention and control strategies for the most at-risk populations and investigate the systemic causes of ongoing inequitable access to health care and social work services. In addition, CE programs should discuss how organizations and individuals are coping and review global and local responses to the range of the pandemic's potential health and economic impacts (Vivian & Heesoon, 2020).

Guiding Best Practices for the Future

Given the challenges that oncology and palliative social workers face in delivering quality care to ever more diverse cancer populations, it makes sense that they would benefit from credentialing, certification, and CE requirements that prepare them to assist in reducing health disparities and promoting cultural competence, humility, and antiracist oncology practice. Mitchell (2012) concludes that this education should critically analyze the intersection of race, culture, gender, socioeconomic status, and similar nonmedical factors that contribute to psychosocial disparities and develop interventions to address such disparities in their practice. However, addressing injustice is predicated on accepting that injustice exists. Kendi (2019) defines antiracism as being able to perceive all races as equal. He further implies that to be antiracist, one must "deracialize behavior, or remove the tattooed stereotype from every racialized body" (p. 105). Credentialing, certification, and CE requirements for both oncology and palliative social workers should prioritize antiracism, promote conversation around the historical complexities of race, gender, and unequal social power, and challenge racial socialization. Doing so can help social workers (re)educate themselves about the racial and gender stereotypes and beliefs they implicitly or explicitly hold that can result in negative patterns of thinking, feelings, and behaviors toward other people (Singh, 2019). In addition, CE curriculum should create space for discussion around the concept of intersectionality and how the emergence of multiple identities further perpetuates injustice for marginalized populations in cancer care. Social identities can include one's race, gender, sexual orientation, religious beliefs, and socioeconomic status as it pertains to one's care (Crenshaw, 1991). Bringing these core concepts into the requirements for credentialing, certification, and CE can help social workers understand more clearly the complexities among and within various social groups, how their upbringing has influenced their own perceptions, and how acknowledging these experiences can have a positive effect on the relationships they build with others (Leary, 2005). Although open and respectful discussions around these concepts is important, social workers must also *act* to decolonize patient education to include content that illustrates human diversity through a wide array of resources. Singh et al. (2020) state that "decolonization is centered on examining the concepts of power and access to opportunities while critically questioning and disrupting the systems and structures that maintain inequities" (p. 262). When patient education centers around decolonization, one can prioritize the voices of underrepresented populations (Singh et al., 2020). This can also be key in allowing cancer patients from underrepresented populations to feel seen, heard, and represented within oncology practice settings.

As discussed in this chapter, oncology and palliative social workers serve at the core of psychosocial care in serious illness. These individuals provide advocacy and clinical services to their patient populations and work collaboratively with other health professionals on interdisciplinary teams. Oncology and palliative social workers' most important service is "to assess patient, and family care needs, and provide interventions that help clients work towards solutions, solutions that address their physical, intra-psychic, interpersonal, and environmental problems" (Fobair et al., 2009, p. 155). Due to the specialized skills and training needed to fulfill this role, social workers must remain abreast of the credentialing, certification, and CE requirements in their respective states. By obtaining proper certification and credentials, oncology and palliative social workers can effectively highlight their array of skills and experience. In addition to having the credentials and general skills overall to succeed in the field, designations such as ACHP-SW, APHSW-C, and BOSW show competence in the field of oncology and allow practitioners to abide by principles and values centered on the NASW *Code of Ethics* (2021).

This chapter detailed how the field of oncology and palliative social work is constantly advancing. Maintaining familiarity—through CE—with current and rapidly growing research, techniques, and theories helps oncology and palliative social workers retain skills, acquire new knowledge, and provide quality care to their client populations. All social workers must be aware of the CE process—from licensure and license renewal to developing specialized expertise to completing CEUs, as well as the conditions for maintaining credentialing and certification requirements.

Pearls

- Credentialing and evidence-based certifications provide the basis of competency standards and elevate the social work profession.
- Access to education in oncology and palliative care social work has grown significantly over the last 10 years.
- Continuing education for oncology and palliative social workers should focus on their specific role in reducing health disparities, promoting cultural competence, humility, and antiracist oncology practice.

Pitfalls

- Lack of research in oncology social work.
- Continuing education enhances the credentials and certifications of oncology and palliative social workers; it does not replace them.
- Lack of institutional financial support for advanced practice certifications.

Additional Resources

Advanced Palliative Care and Hospice Social Work Certification: https://aphsw-c.org/
Association of Oncology Social Workers: https://aosw.org
Board of Oncology Social Work: https://oswcert.org/
National Association of Social Workers: https://www.socialworkers.org
Social Work, Hospice and Palliative Care Network: https://www.swhpn.org/

References

Afomachukwu, O. (2021). Role of the social worker in the outbreak of pandemics: A case of COVID-19. *Cogent Psychology*, *8*(1), 1. https://doi.org/10.1080/23311908.2021.1939537

Biggerstaff, M. A. (2000). A critique of the model state social work practice act. *Social Work*, *45*(2), 105–115. https://doi.org/10.1093/sw/45.2.105

Board of Oncology Social Work. (n.d.). *Our mission*. Retrieved January 15, 2022, from https://oswcert.org/

California State University. (2013, July 9). *OSU institute offers first online post MSW certificate in palliative care*. Shiley Haynes Institute for Palliative Care. Retrieved January 17, 2022, from https://csupalliativecare.org/postmswannounced/

Crenshaw, K. (1991). Mapping the margins: Intersectionality, identity, and violence against women of color. *Stanford Law Review*, *43*(6), 1241–1300.

Ferrell, B., Twaddle, M., Melnick, A., & Meier, D. (2018). National consensus project clinical practice guidelines for quality palliative care guidelines, 4th edition. *Journal of Palliative Medicine*, *21*(12), 1684–1689. https://doi.org/10.1089/jpm.2018.0431

Fobair, P., Stearns, N. N., Christ, G., Dozier-Hall, D., Newman, N. W., Zabora, J., Schnipper, H. H., Kennedy, V., Loscalzo, M., Stensland, S. M., Hedlund, S., Lauria, M. M., Fife, M., Herschl, J., Marcusen, C. P., Vaitones, V., Brintzenhofeszoc, K., Walsh, K., Lawson, K., & Desonier, M. (2009). Historical threads in the development of oncology social work. *Journal of Psychosocial Oncology*, *27*(2), 155–215. https://doi.org/10.1080/07347330902775301

Glajchen, M., Berkman, C., Otis-Green, S., Stein, G., Sedgwick, T., Bern-Klug, M., Christ, G., Csikai, E., Downes, D., Gerbino, S., Head, B., Parker-Oliver, D., Waldrop, D., & Portenoy, R. (2018). Defining core competencies for generalist-level palliative social work. *Journal of Pain and Symptom Management*, *56*(6), 886–892. https://doi.org/10.1016/j.jpainsymman.2018.09.002

Head, B., Peters, B., Middleton, A., Friedman, C., & Gunman, N. (2019). Results of a nationwide hospice and palliative care social work job analysis. *Journal of Social Work End of Life Palliative Care*, *15*(1), 16–33. https://doi.org/10.1080/15524256.2019.1577326

Kendi, I. X. (2019). *How to be an antiracist*. One World.

Leary, J. (2005). *Post traumatic slave syndrome: America's legacy of enduring injury and healing*. Uptone.

McCormick, A. J., Stowell-Weiss, P., Carson, J., Tebo, G., Hanson, I., & Quesada, B. (2014). Continuing education in ethical decision making using case studies from medical social work. *Social Work in Health Care*, *53*(4), 344–363. https://doi.org/10.1080/00981389.2014.884042

Mitchell, J. (2012). Integrating education on addressing health disparities into the graduate social work curriculum. *Journal of Teaching in Social Work*, *32*(5), 471–486. https://doi.org/10.1080/08841233.2012.725458

National Association of Social Workers. (2004). *Standards for palliative and end-of-life care*. https://www.socialworkers.org/LinkClick.aspx?fileticket=xBMd58VwEhk%3d&portalid=0

National Association of Social Workers. (2017). *Code of ethics*. https://www.socialworkers.org/About/Ethics/Code-of-Ethics/Code-of-Ethics-English

National Association of Social Workers. (2021). *Code of ethics*. https://www.socialworkers.org/About/Ethics/Code-of-Ethics/Code-of-Ethics-English

NYU Silver School of Social Work. (n.d.). Zelda Foster Studies Program in Palliative and End-of-Life Care [Review]. *Zelda Foster Studies*. Retrieved December 23, 2022, from https://socialwork.nyu.edu/faculty-and-research/faculty-initiatives/zelda-foster-studies.html

Singh, A. A. (2019). *The racial healing handbook: Practical activities to help you challenge privilege, confront systemic racism, and engage in collective healing*. New Harbinger.

Singh, A. A., Appling, B., & Trepal, H. (2020). Using the multicultural and social justice counseling competencies to decolonize counseling practice: The important roles of theory, power, and action. *Journal of Counseling and Development*, *98*(3), 261–271. https://doi.org/10.1002/jcad.12321

Smith College. (n.d.). *Palliative and end-of-life care certificate*. Smith College School for Social Work. Retrieved January 17, 2022, from https://ssw.smith.edu/palliative/apply

Social Work Guide. (2020, October 12). *Social work licensing guide*. https://www.socialworkguide.org/licensure/

Substance Abuse and Mental Health Services Administration. (2020). *Clinical support system for serious mental illness (CSS-SMI)*. https://www.samhsa.gov/clinical-support-system-serious-mental-illness-css-smi

University of Pennsylvania. (n.d.). *Advanced certificate in* oncology *social work practice*. School of Social Policy and Practice. Retrieved January 17, 2022, from https://www.sp2.upenn.edu/program/advanced-certificate-in-oncology-social-work-practice/

Viatones, V., Schutte, J., & Mattison, D. (2015). OSW-C: The importance of certification for oncology social workers. In *Handbook of Oncology Social Work* (pp. 757–762). Oxford University Press.

Vivian, M., & HeeSoon, L. (2020). Social work values in action during COVID-19. *Journal of Gerontological Social Work*, *63*(6–7), 565–569. https://https://doi.org/10.1080/01634372.2020.1769792

Zebrack, B., Walsh, K., Burg, M. A., Maramaldi, P., & Lim, J. (2008). Oncology social worker competencies and implications for education and training. *Social Work in Health Care*, *47*(4), 355–375. https://doi.org/10.1080/00981380802173954

25

How Technology Is Transforming Oncology and Palliative Care

Opportunities and Challenges

Michael Wong, A. J. Cincotta-Eichenfield, Carolyn Messner, and Sunita Jadhav

Key Concepts

- New technological possibilities may bolster medical care in oncology.
- New technologies may support educational care in oncology.
- New technologies may strengthen supportive care in oncology.

Keywords: adaptation, care, digitality, education, psychosocial support, technology, virtual

All aspects of the foundational tasks of the patient/physician encounter—from taking the patient's history through physical exams, laboratory tests, imaging, diagnosis, planning, and treatment—are undergoing technological transformation. Virtual doctor/patient visits (commonly referred to as telehealth or telemedicine) have increased due to the pandemic. Virtual physical examinations are complemented by blood and tissue testing, noninvasive monitoring, and body imaging to adhere to mandated treatment algorithms and pathways. The entire medical and palliative care knowledge base has become readily available via technological advancements, and practitioners are presently both spectators and avid participants in the tectonic shifting of oncology and palliative care. While many technological advancements are a welcome outcome of both the pre- and COVID eras, oncology and palliative social workers must keep a close eye on ensuring that the entire cancer care team attends to the human side of cancer and maintains the importance of the relationships among the doctor, health care team, patient, and caregivers.

Michael Wong, A. J. Cincotta-Eichenfield, Carolyn Messner, and Sunita Jadhav, *How Technology Is Transforming Oncology and Palliative Care* In: *Oncology and Palliative Social Work*. Edited by: Susan Hedlund, Bryan Miller, Grace Christ, and Carolyn Messner, Oxford University Press. © Oxford University Press 2024. DOI: 10.1093/oso/9780197607299.003.0025

The ever-evolving digital age has rendered possible new pathways for oncological support. Magnified in importance during the COVID-19 pandemic, digital connections around cancer-specific topics and communications persist beyond what was physically or medically possible within the walls of hospitals, discussion groups, or other physical spaces. Whether through formalized professional support offerings, friendships forged on social media, or the proliferation of new media initiatives like podcasts and other creative content, digital interconnectedness has become embedded in the illness world and made space for focused, hyperspecific, and accelerated sharing of medical, social, emotional, and experiential knowledge.

People living with cancer and their caregivers have a difficult time understanding their type of cancer, its treatment, side effects, and pain management. Technology enables patients and their loved ones to access state-of-the-art information from cancer organizations offering telephone consultation, webcasts, and podcasts with thoughtful and compassionate leaders in oncology and palliative care. Organizations partnering with the communications industry can now provide virtual information that is accessible anytime, anywhere. These programs demonstrate the positive impact of digital media on patient/caregiver learning and create an increased ability to generate informed questions of health care teams.

The Impact of Technology and Telehealth on Medical Oncology and Palliative Care

The rapid rise and ready acceptance of information technology has disrupted the physician–patient relationship, which affects expectations, performance, and outcomes for all. The COVID-19 pandemic has accelerated and cemented these into some form of permanency. Although the situation remains in flux, one can be certain that there will be no return to the way things were done prepandemic. This chapter touches on the most impactful of these changes—telehealth. Although telehealth existed in some forms before COVID, new technologies have kindled, supported, and allowed its further evolution. Additionally, shifts in societal standards fostered a receptive environment for its rapid and universal acceptance.

The Rapid Emergence of Telehealth

Although there are many definitions of the term *telehealth*, an expanded definition encompasses virtual physician visits in the context of the surrounding "electronic" environment and support systems. As society moved to the routine use of personal smart devices and the acceptance of a connected digital social media life, the stage was set for the explosive emergence of telehealth. In a 2021 study, almost 9 in 10 individuals in the United States reported using the Internet. A survey representing nearly 237 million adults in the United States annually showed that 27.4% used technology to interact with the health care system, an increase of 12.5% between 2011 and 2018 (Mahajan et al., 2021).

The Telehealth Encounter

Although the telehealth encounter is highly individualized to practice and patient, the central component consists of a remote encounter between the physician and the patient, connected via electronic means facilitated by software. A specific example of such an encounter would be a doctor appointment booked on the patient's web-based portal initiated by the physician within the institution's/clinic's electronic medical record (EMR) system. The patient receives and accepts a notification that the appointment has begun on their smart device, after which the doctor and patient can speak and see each other on their respective devices. In addition to the appointment itself, doctors can order and review investigations, imaging, and lab tests within this electronic environment.

The Significant Impact of Telehealth in the Health Care Enterprise

Consulting firm McKinsey & Company published a 2021 report which found that use of telehealth has increased 38 times over the pre-COVID-19 baseline. Indeed, in "April 2020, overall telehealth utilization for office visits and outpatient care was 78 times higher than in February 2020" (McKinsey & Company, 2021). They predicted that up to $250 billion of U.S. health care costs could potentially shift to virtual-centric care. A return to the pre-COVID way of practicing medicine and receiving medical care is unlikely. The McKinsey report also found that around 40% of surveyed consumers believed they will continue to use telehealth going forward (up from 11% of consumers using telehealth prior to COVID-19) and that 84% of physicians were offering virtual visits and 57% would prefer to continue doing so. Furthermore, the report tracked regulatory changes that enabled greater telehealth access during COVID-19, many of which have been made permanent.

The Pros and Cons of Telehealth

Some obvious advantages of telehealth are immediately apparent. For patients with access to the Internet and a computer or smartphone, no travel is required, the encounter can occur anywhere, and access to medical care is only a "click" away. These features are readily compatible with the safety protocols that health care practitioners and institutions established and implemented due to the COVID-19 pandemic. Telehealth can flatten disparities by extending care to those who are housebound or otherwise unable to travel; providing easier, cheaper, and less time-consuming access to patients who live farther from care facilities or who don't have access to reliable transportation; and increasing access to health care for underserved populations. For physicians, no clinical physical space is necessary, encounters can occur anywhere (home/office/clinic), and efficiency increases while cost decreases since less space and fewer personnel are required.

Closer inspection suggests that one set of disparities may have been exchanged for another. Telehealth favors the tech-savvy, which may create a barrier for either the young or the old. Certain races and ethnicities or those without English fluency may be excluded. Additionally, telehealth requires reliable Internet access and available smart devices, which may prevent financially or technologically disadvantaged people from accessing care through electronic means.

Providers also require a capable and secure EMR system with readily available information technology support. Meticulous attention to HIPAA compliance and the handling of sensitive medical information mandates ever-escalating, costly, top-level security features in response to increasingly sophisticated attempts to breach patient information and tighter regulatory requirements. The typical 15% reimbursement discount to providers for telehealth compared to in-person visits further sets the stage for a host of telehealth barriers.

The physician–patient relationship is the gravitational core of health care. It all starts there, and everything is pulled back into it. These encounters are emotional, and one might even argue that parts of the healing process can even be spiritual. Those that participate in telehealth have long felt that it diminishes these perhaps less tangible aspects of the physician–patient relationship. An article titled "I'm Not Feeling Like I'm Part of the Conversation" touches on this angst. Respondents to the study cited "concerns about errors in their care because of perceived difficulty completing the physical exam, perceptions that providers paid less attention to them, barriers to speaking up and asking questions, and difficulty establishing a provider-patient relationship" (Gordon et al., 2020, p. 1751). Ultimately, patients report feeling less involved during the visit, difficulty finding opportunities to speak, and rushed by the provider.

Specific Impact of Telehealth on Oncology and Palliative Care

Despite its many benefits, telehealth can fall short when it comes to providing quality palliative and hospice care. The patient population is often elderly or frail, not fluent in or lacking access to current technology, and had experienced a lifetime of face-to-face physician care. End-of-life care is highly focused on symptom control and requires patients to be able to transmit fear, sadness, and anxiety, which becomes harder to do in an electronic environment. Furthermore, touch can be therapeutic in such circumstances. While clinical results are important, patients and families are also aware of and can respond positively or negatively to the care team's personal attitudes, closeness, and psychological support. While these obstacles may appear unsurmountable to using telehealth in the palliative care and hospice contexts, best practices and quick reference tools can minimize some of the potential negatives and help practitioners find ways to use technology effectively (Webb et al., 2021).

New Media and Social Connectivity in Oncology—Vectors of Cancer Support in the Digital Age

New media, social media, and ever-emerging digital avenues have allowed for accelerated and hyperspecific online social interaction, connection, and engagement for people with cancer. From medical visits to peer dialogues and support groups, digital interconnectedness mirrors in-person paradigms but also transcends boundaries of physical possibility, enhancing illness-specificity, limiting health risks, and enabling social, emotional, and experiential information sharing. Online networks render new pathways for support, holding a unique utility for coping with the isolation and distress of cancer.

Oncology professionals and people with cancer have formed collaborative, multidisciplinary online communities to discuss changing diagnosis and treatment landscapes (Subbiah et al., 2019). Digital discourse expands support networks but also creates outlets for misinformation, and disreputable information can have a negative impact on decision-making processes, treatment outcomes, and more (Johnson et al., 2021). Alternatively, professionally moderated online groups; cancer-specific networks; and community-created media create a web of informational, social, and emotional content informed by lived experience and medical knowledge.

Sharing Support

Illness-narrative-based media, like podcasts and videos, provide emotional affirmation amid the solitude of illness. Audiences can define, refine, and reenvision their own experiences alongside recorded dialogues. Episodes preserve lived experience, emphasizing the value of emotional expressiveness throughout the illness journey. "I've always been very open about my illness because I think it's important to not stigmatize it," John, a patient and graphic novelist who creatively represents his illness in his work, shared.

> I grew up in the 1980s and 1990s, when HIV was rampant, and as a queer teenager, you pretty much were told "You're going to die young, you're going to get this disease, and you're going to die." So, I think when I was diagnosed with cancer, I had a more prepared notion of death. . . . It's important that people share their stories . . . because cancer is such an all-encompassing word. . . . Just the second you hear it, you think "death sentence." . . . At the time of my diagnosis, everything I read online, everything the doctors told me was [that I had] two to three years [to live]. But every two years that I've survived, there's been new forms of medication, new forms of radiation. Part of why I did a clinical trial was because it's my hope that . . . it's going to pass through the FDA and help hundreds of thousands of people who have neuroendocrine tumors. (Barnhart & John, 2021)

The positive power of narrative is multiplied online. Connectivity in cancer communities can help validate feelings, reduce social isolation, and foster supportive peer interactions (Lazard et al., 2021). "How am I going to get through this?" Se'Nita, a young adult with breast cancer, asked after her diagnosis.

> I ended up doing 16 rounds of chemo and . . . every week I went on social media and did an act of kindness challenge. So many people have participated. . . . That support helped me to keep my mind off everything that I was going through. People doing meal trains for me, people sending me gifts, and flowers—that just made my day, every day. . . . I don't know how to repay anyone, but thank you, It definitely kept me going. (Fortune & Se'Nita, 2021)

Digital Disparities

The pandemic has amplified the economic, occupational, and health inequalities woven into the fabric of the U.S. landscape, making the intersections of social support, health care information sharing, and digital technologies even more relevant and all the more notable when barriers in access systematically prevent certain populations from finding support. COVID-19 has disproportionately affected oncology populations, which have worse outcomes due to the disease than people without cancer (Wang et al., 2021). Black and Hispanic people with cancer used telehealth less frequently than White people with cancer and were more likely to be diagnosed with, hospitalized for, or die from COVID-19 (Guthrie, 2020; Wang et al., 2021). In speaking to concurrent crises for communities of color impacted by cancer and COVID-19, Rahsaan, a bereaved podcast guest, shared,

> Cancer, like many other illnesses, definitely shows the effects of systemic racism. We see inequity in the kinds of care people get, even in diagnosis and survival rates. Pancreatic cancer, specifically, is a disease that adversely affects Black and Brown people for a host of reasons. One, a lot of risk factors are highly correlated with things that come from generational poverty and systemic inequity.
>
> Now, we're having this reckoning with Black Lives Matter, and one thing I would like people to keep always at front of mind, is that it's not just about police brutality, it's everything from health care to food access to job access to housing access. Systemic racism runs rampant through every aspect of society, and that definitely includes cancer. . . . Take up that battle and help. If you are passionate about beating cancer, if you're passionate about Black lives, if you are passionate about making sure that everybody has a fair shake, I'd encourage you to advocate for pancreatic cancer research, to lobby your officials, to get involved in organizations like PANCAN [Pancreatic Cancer Action Network]. . . . There's a lot we all can do, because . . . there's so much that we unfortunately have been bogged down with in terms of the biases that affect who gets what health care. (Barnhart & Rahsaan, 2020)

The Use of Technology in Cancer Patient Education

The use of teleconferencing for cancer patient education started 30 years ago (Institute of Medicine, 2008, pp. 119–125; Glajchen & Moul, 1996). With newer technology of webinars and Zoom calls, these programs have transformed patient's, caregivers', and health care professionals' access to information from experts in oncology and palliative care on the telephone and online. The pandemic spurred a dramatic increase in the use of virtual technology. Online workshops, for example, are a wonderful complement to telehealth/telemedicine appointments. They are available for free in real time and are archived for free on many nonprofit cancer organizations as podcasts in the United States and internationally. As one workshop participant shared,

> I applaud these one-hour free simultaneous teleconference/webinars, which bring together expert speakers for these virtual informative workshops. The team of speakers articulated the importance of communicating treatment side effects without delay. They clearly explained the benefits of participating in clinical trials. It was a global call with a large number of participants showing the confidence in expert evidence-based information. Throughout COVID, these programs have been a lifeline to those of us living with cancer, caregivers, and health care professionals. Thank you!" (Anonymous workshop participant, June 20, 2022)

As Schreyer explained, "COVID is not simply a pandemic. It is more accurately described as part of a concatenation of interconnected biological and social systems and states, a syndetic" (Schreyer, 2021, pp. 184–185). It involves a pandemic, coupled with chronic health disease, like cancer, and a society with disparate access to health care, racism, and lack of social justice.

Cancer as a Dread Disease and Now COVID

When diagnosed with cancer, the first questions that occur to most are "Will I die?" "What is my type of cancer?" "I do not understand my type of cancer." "Where do I go for treatment and care?" "Will I suffer great pain?"

People's understandings of cancer are developed early in their lives, often formed by experiences with a family member, parent, sibling, uncle, aunt, or friend who had cancer and may have died. As a child or teen, we may have witnessed their suffering and assume our fate will be the same. Many people have no knowledge of the decades of innovations in cancer treatment that have occurred in the recent decades. A parallel process has developed with COVID, albeit much more quickly. Whereas just 2 years ago, COVID seemed like a potential death sentence, most everyone today has access to reliable, often free vaccines that have drastically reduced the average person's odds of dying from COVID.

The Role of Oncology and Palliative Social Workers in Organizing Patient Education Workshops

Who better than oncology and palliative social workers to organize virtual patient-education workshops? Social workers are trained in psychosocial awareness to the needs of patients and their caregivers to learn about cancer in a safe, nonthreatening manner not only with experts in oncology and palliative medicine but also with the full health care team (including oncology social workers, oncology nurses, oncology dietitians, and physical therapists). One might say that social workers are compassionate experts at bringing together the full interprofessional team and to fostering excellent communication among themselves and with patients and caregivers.

When designing a 1-hour teleconference or webcast specifically for adult cancer patients and their caregivers, best practice suggests using the first half-hour to for presentations by expert speakers and the second half-hour for questions and answers. The oncology and palliative social worker planning the workshop needs to clearly outline the topics each speaker will address, the agenda (including expectations about time), and guidelines for appropriate and respectful dialogue. Speakers are cautioned not to provide statistics of survivorship or mortality but to convey the information and tools that participants may use with their health care team to receive innovative care. As one provider explained, "the single biggest problem in communication is the illusion that it has taken place." The importance of choosing speakers wisely cannot be stressed enough—find experts who can use layman's language to discuss complex concepts and who are sensitive to social determinants of health, health care disparities, and social justice. Finding the best speakers requires research and care: obtain each speaker's resume/CV and bio sketch, listen to them on their institution's website or on other forms of social media, and interview each speaker. The quality of each workshop wholly depends on the speakers' ability not only to discuss the topics assigned to them in a clear and understandable manner but also to effectively field both telephone and online questions during the question-and-answer period (Hodorowski et al., 2015).

The Importance of Reaching Out to Diverse Communities

One of the greatest challenges of oncology and palliative care workshops is outreach and engagement of people who need access to information about their particular type of cancer, including rare cancers, the current standard of care, radiation therapy, new treatments, immunotherapy, targeted treatments, management of treatment side effects, symptoms discomfort, and pain. COVID and concerns about exposure to seasonal flu made in-person workshops for cancer patients risky at best and lethal at worst. Many nonprofit organizations moved cancer workshops to virtual platforms in March 2020 at the start of COVID-19. Recognizing the potential dangers of in-person workshops for cancer patients suggests the ongoing importance of doing so.

Many nonprofit organizations collaborate with other nonprofit organizations to get "the greatest penetration into the community" (J. Silver, personal communication, July 15, 2018) that one is trying to reach. A few examples include:

- Sisters Network® Inc.—A National African American Breast Cancer Survivorship Organization: http://www.sistersnetworkinc.org/
- Bladder Cancer Advocacy Network: www.bcan.org
- NORD®—National Organization of Rare Diseases: www.rarediseases.org
- International Waldenstrom's Macroglobulinemia Foundation: www.iwmf.org.

Sometimes, members of a specific community reach out to a nonprofit organization to help them hold virtual informational workshops about cancer. For example, the hearing-impaired community reached out to a nonprofit organization to request closed-captioning on their virtual patient-education workshops. The results were immediate and positive. As one cancer patient emailed after a closed-captioned workshop,

> The captioning was EXCELLENT! There is no way I could have ever understood those medical terms and clinical trials without captioning. Now I can look them up online and discuss with my oncologist. The captioning is beyond helpful. It can be lifesaving, as far as I'm concerned. I very much appreciate your efforts! I can find no fault and only benefit to adding captioning to the video replay. It should help many, many patients listening in (hearing impaired or not). (Anonymous, personal communication, October 2021)

Psychosocial Care in Cancer and the COVID-19 Pandemic: Highlights From a Tertiary Cancer Hospital in Mumbai

Despite lockdowns, diminished access to transportation, and fears of becoming ill during the COVID-19 pandemic, some cancer patients made the journey to Mumbai for cancer treatment and psychosocial care. The Indian health care system (like similar systems around the world) moved to a distance care model and enforced social distancing. However, oncology social workers, assisted by stakeholders and hospital administrators persisted in finding ways to help cancer patients access care in their country. One way they managed the challenges of social distancing and a lack of hospital rooms or medical offices was to use empty hotel rooms, school buildings, and government-provided units specially extended to support patients coming to Mumbai for cancer treatments.

The tertiary cancer care hospital in Mumbai, Tata Memorial Hospital, which is globally renowned for both superior medical treatment and psychosocial support, offered care to approximately 1,600 inpatient and outpatient cancer patients during the pandemic even during periods of complete lockdown and when many hospitals were closed to the public. These facilities carefully planned the clinical management of patients by scaling down surgeries, modifying treatment modalities, and prioritizing certain kinds of patients over others, which led to some difficult choices (Pramesh & Badwe, 2020).

Challenges and Interventions

While medical doctors and other health care team members struggled to find beds and provide care to cancer patients during COVID, oncology and palliative social workers helped patients with different challenges, such as finances and social support during a time when there was a hold on donations, outpatients were not allowed into hospitals to minimize disease transmission, and few health care workers were available to staff health care centers. Social workers used mobile phones to communicate with the approximately 1,000 cancer patients located in and around Mumbai. They also used technology to access hospital databases, confirm safety protocols, investigate whether a patient's basic needs were being met, and follow up with patients and caregivers on conformance with the treatment plan and whether the patient was suffering any side effects. Despite the elevated costs and shortages of forms of transportation, social workers in Mumbai arranged both local (typically an ambulance) and distant forms of transportation when patients in advance phases of illness desired to return home with loved ones. Hospitals and generous donors assumed much of the financial burden of this care. Hospitals collaborated with local municipalities to arrange free pick-up and drop-off service for COVID-positive patients, caregivers, and staff. Telephonic and video counseling facilitated by oncology social workers and translators allowed patients and caregivers to receive medical information and counseling in their mother tongue to reduce stress and anxiety. The continued availability of experts helped reduce uncertainty and increase positive outcomes for cancer patients amid the chaos and confusion of the pandemic.

On-the-Job Training

Virtual platforms helped support quality oncology care in India during the pandemic. Doctors and other medical practitioners were required to attend weekly three-hour-long continued medical education webinars to stay updated about COVID. Oncology social workers and volunteers received virtual training about COVID-specific government programs from which patients could benefit. Officials from government-supported insurance programs held online advocacy meetings with staff at institutions for vulnerable, destitute, geriatric, and socially isolated patients as well as orphans (Redondo et al., 2020). Virtual platforms served as optimal vehicles for staff training and information about accommodations during COVID. Online platforms encouraged online donations of money and other needed items.

Ethical and Professional Considerations in Mumbai

Helping patients in the developing country of India, Mumbai used technology and digital aids to ethically ensure that there was the right dissemination of information during a time when new information and guidelines on COVID were causing fear and concern among patients.

Accepting and Adapting to COVID and Cancer as a Way of Life in Mumbai

The COVID lockdown and lack of in-person consultation created a phase during which patients and caregivers began to come to terms with the idea of COVID becoming a pandemic in India (Box 25.1). They had to learn new social norms related to preventing its spread all the while dealing with their cancer diagnosis and treatment. Patients used new technologies to continue seeking treatment for their cancer despite COVID fears. Some patients booked online video consultations, some found creative means of virtually or physically accessing local cancer hospitals, and some even risked traveling to Mumbai, at

Tata Memorial Hospital, for treatment where they used tools to find housing and care. During the follow-up period, they adopted different forms of technology as a way to find community with fellow cancer patients, stay abreast of new medical developments and treatments, maintain connections with their health care team, and find coping strategies for living with their disease, whether active or in remission. Despite using technology to foster acceptance and adaptation to both COVID and cancer, however, palliative care and palliation became more challenging for patients, caregivers, doctors, and social workers, as online consultations are not as effective in helping patients express pain and sorrow, connect physically or emotionally with their care team, facilitate proper wound care or treatment delivery methods, and address psychosocial or financial concerns (Damani et al., 2020).

Box 25.1 A Narrative from the Pandemic

Munni, a 16-year-old adolescent girl in treatment for cancer hailed from rural India and was treated at Tata Memorial Hospital in Mumbai. Her COVID diagnosis, which isolated her from family, led to her crying inconsolably, resisting isolation, and pleading that her parents be allowed to be with her in the hospital. The treating consultant felt helpless to forgo the strict COVID guidelines. However, they were amazed the following morning to see a nurse without PPE helping rural folks in the isolation ward like Munni by connecting them with their families on video calls. The joy of helping and adapting is what the pandemic taught Munni and the world.

Autonomy at End of Life, Unfinished Business, Information, and Knowledge about Disease

Medical professionals often face a professional dilemma when trying to respect patient autonomy. Patients and loved ones can face difficult situations when a patient's determination over advance directives is strong and/or at odds with other people in their family or community in Mumbai. Members of the multiprofessional team at Tata Memorial Hospital play a crucial role in understanding a patient's views on end of life, identifying where gaps or differences exist between the patient and family, and facilitating communication about them (Pautex et al., 2010). The pandemic both increased the need for communications around end-of-life wishes and concerns and added to the limitations social workers faced in fostering this communication because of a lack of transportation and resources coupled with complete lockdown at various times meant that close relatives could not always reach Mumbai (Box 25.2).

Box 25.2

Chandra was a 74-year-old widower receiving treatment for oral cancer that was diagnosed a month before the first COVID lockdown in Mumbai. He refused help from his married daughter and chose palliation and hospice admission. Multiple counseling sessions with this patient, telephone discussion with his daughter and son-in-law, and the patient's creation of advance directives eased the path to autonomy.

Shobha was a 43-year-old, unmarried woman living alone; she had a married brother and sister in Mumbai. Her cervical cancer, which had infiltrated the rectum and urethra, required palliative surgery that resulted in permanent catheters and additional stomas, which were crippling and rendered her dependent on family in Mumbai. Wishing to die without further cuts, scars, or tubes, she refused more surgery and conferred with oncology social workers about hospice care. The oncology social workers, after hearing her concerns and receiving a thorough assessment of her prognosis from her care team honored her request and facilitated the hospice admission with prior consent from her sister and brother.

The use of technology and virtual tools to engage and empower people with cancer and caregivers has tremendously bolstered the way that medical care, psychosocial support, and patient education is delivered in the oncology sphere in Mumbai. Telehealth, virtual supportive counseling, digital media, online advocacy, and remote learning workshops, all magnified in importance during the ongoing COVID-19 pandemic, have solidified new avenues of support for those affected by cancer in uncertain times.

In Mumbai, for the networked systems of telehealth, digital media, remote education, and online support to be truly supportive and meet the needs of diverse oncology patient populations, oncology and palliative care social workers must consult patients about their comfort level with virtual systems of care and work to find ways to engage patients and caregivers in the process of finding a way that will be positive and meaningful for them. Also of key importance is understanding whether patients and caregivers have easy access to the digital resources at hand.

In the context of oncology care in India, cancer patients at a specialized hospital, Tata Memorial Hospital, were able to access continued cancer care during the COVID pandemic in large part due to the use of technological advancements. This case study reveals some useful ways other health care systems might accept and adapt to the changing digital landscape around cancer care that COVID has facilitated with outreach from Tata Memoria Hospital. On-the-job training for staff and virtual training for volunteers helped them add new technologies and processes to their toolboxes.

Members of multidisciplinary teams from Mumbai were able to offer high-quality care at a distance through virtual means. Patients from rural communities and caregivers based in Mumbai at Tata Memorial Hospital learned to use technology during periods when loved ones were isolated due to COVID for their needs. The pandemic forced many in rural regions in India to turn toward digital technology to access greater assistance in their oncology and COVID care.

Guiding Best Practices for the Future

- Respect the agency of diverse patient populations when presenting oncology, palliative care, and psychosocial oncology information to people living with cancer, their families, partners, and caregivers.
- Oncology professionals need to better understand pathways of virtual information sharing and create more uniform online channels for cancer-specific support and education.
- Regular revision of best practices is important in an ever-evolving digital oncology landscape.

Pearls

- Digital interactions allow for rapid illness-specific support and knowledge exchange.
- Technological tools can notify patients in advance about conduct, agenda, and expectations.
- Virtual platforms offer a portable space of adaptation, learning, and education for oncology professionals, people with cancer, COVID and their caregivers.
- Social workers need a strong ability to use digital tools to reflect the specific needs of diverse patient populations and present information in accessible ways.

Pitfalls

- Avoid assuming one size fits all in patient education and support.
- Cancer misinformation can be widespread online, leading to potential danger.

- Digital disparities are magnified in the shift toward virtual communications, support, and telehealth.
- Some patients are unable to find closure, unburden themselves, and feel as if they have "completed unfinished business" in virtual care contexts.

Additional Resources

American Cancer Society: www.cancer.org (800-227-2345)
American Society of Clinical Oncology: www.cancer.net
Cancer*Care*: www.cancercare.org; www.cancercare.org/connect; www.cancercare.org/podcasts
Cancer Support Community: www.cancersupportcommunity.org (888-793-9355)
National Comprehensive Cancer Network®, NCCN Guidelines for Patients: www.nccn.org/patients

References

Barnhart, R. & Rahsaan. (Host & Guest). (2020, November 9). On grief, on love, on power (No. 16) [Audio podcast episode]. In *Cancer Out Loud*. Cancer*Care*. https://podcasters.spotify.com/pod/show/canceroutloud/episodes/On-Grief--On-Love--On-Power-em4jjh/a-a3p6t1u

Barnhart, R. & John. (Host & Guest). (2021, March 22). Back to the drawing board (No. 21). [Audio podcast episode]. In *Cancer Out Loud*. Cancer*Care*. https://podcasters.spotify.com/pod/show/canceroutloud/episodes/Back-to-the-Drawing-Board-et0o2i/a-a5032q8

Damani, A., Ghoshal, A., Salins, N., Bhatnagar, S., Sanghavi, P. R., Viswanath, V., Ostwal, S., Chinchalkar, G., & Vallath, N. (2020). Approaches and best practices for managing cancer pain within the constraints of the COVID-19 pandemic in India. *Indian Journal of Palliative Care*, *26*, S106–S115. https://doi.org/10.4103/IJPC.IJPC_216_20

Fortune, S. & Se'Nita. (Host & Guest). (2021, October 25). I decided that I was going to tell my story (No. 34) [Audio podcast episode]. In *Cancer Out Loud*. CancerCare. https://podcasters.spotify.com/pod/show/canceroutloud/episodes/34--I-Decided-That-I-Was-Going-to-Tell-My-Story-e195gl9/a-a6ohl88

Glajchen, M., & Moul, J. W. (1996). Teleconferencing as a method of educating men about managing advanced prostate cancer and pain. *Journal of Psychosocial Oncology*, *14*, 73–87. https://doi.org/10.1300/J077v14n02_05

Gordon, H. S., Solanki, P., Bokhour, B. G., & Gopal, R. K. (2020). "I'm not feeling like I'm part of the conversation": Patients' perspectives on communicating in clinical video telehealth visits. *Journal of General Internal Medicine*, *35*(6), 1751–1758. https://doi.org/10.1007/s11606-020-05673-w

Guthrie, G. (2020, October 5). The impact of COVID-19 on Black and Hispanic people with cancer. *Cancer.net*. https://www.cancer.net/blog/2020-10/impact-covid-19-black-and-hispanic-people-with-cancer-research-2020-quality-care-symposium

Hodorowski, J. K., Messner, C., & Kornhauser, C. (2015). The importance of patient education. In G. Christ, C. Messner, & L. Behar (Eds.), *Handbook of oncology social work* (pp. 673–677). Oxford University Press.

Institute of Medicine. (2008). *Cancer care for the whole patient: Meeting psychosocial health needs*. National Academies Press. https://doi.org/10.17226/11993

Johnson, S., Parsons, M., Dorff, T., Moran, M., Ward, J., Cohen, S., Akerley, W., Bauman, J., Hubbard, J., Spratt, D., Bylund, C., Swire-Thompson, B., Onega, T., Scherer, L., Tward, J., & Fagerlin, A. (2021). Cancer misinformation and harmful information on Facebook and other social media. *Journal of the NCI, 114*(7), 1036–1039. https://doi.org/10.1093/jnci/djab141

Lazard, A., Collins, M., Hedrick, A., Varma, T., Love, B., Valle, C., Brooks, E., & Benedict, C. (2021). Using social media for peer-to-peer cancer support: Interviews with young adults with cancer. *JMIR Cancer*, *7*(3), e28234. https://doi.org/10.2196/28234

Mahajan, S., Lu, Y., Spatz, E. S., Nasir, K., & Krumholz, H. M. (2021). Trends and predictors of use of digital health technology in the United States. *American Journal of Medicine*, *134*(1), 129–134. https://doi.org/10.1016/j.amjmed.2020.06.033

McKinsey & Company. (2021, July 9). *Telehealth: A quarter-trillion-dollar post-COVID-19 reality?* https://www.mckinsey.com/industries/health care-systems-and-services/our-insights/telehealth-a-quarter-trillion-dollar-post-covid-19-reality

Pautex, S., Notaridis, G., Déramé, L., & Zulian, G. B. (2010). Preferences of elderly cancer patients in their advance directives. *Critical Reviews in Oncology/Hematology*, *74*(1), 61–65. https://doi.org/10.1016/j.critrevonc.2009.04.007

Pramesh, C. S., & Badwe, R. A. (2020). Cancer management in India during COVID-19. *New England Journal of Medicine*, *382*(20), e61. https://doi.org/10.1056/nejmc2011595

Redondo-Sama, G., Matulic, V., Munté-Pascual, A., & de Vicente, I. (2020). Social work during the COVID-19 crisis: Responding to urgent social needs. *Sustainability*, *12*(20), 8595. https://doi.org/10.3390/su12208595

Schreyer, A. (2021). A time for transformation. *Social Work: A Journal of the National Association of Social Workers*, *66*(3), 184–185.

Subbiah, I., Hamilton, E., Knoll, M., Shanahan, K., & Meisel, J. (2019). A big world made small: Using social media to optimize patient care. *ASCO Educational Book*, *39*, e212–e218. https://doi.org/10.1200/edbk_246643

Wang, Q., Berger, N., & Xu, R. (2021). Analyses of risk, racial disparity, and outcomes among U.S. patients with cancer and COVID-19 infection. *JAMA Oncology*, *7*(2), 220–227. https://doi.org/10.1001/jamaoncol.2020.6178

Webb, M., Hurley, S. L., Gentry, J., Brown, M., & Ayoub, C. (2021). Best practices for using telehealth in hospice and palliative care. *Journal of Hospice and Palliative Nursing*, *23*(3), 277–285. https://doi.org/10.1097/njh.0000000000000753

26

Leadership Development in Oncology and Palliative Care Social Work

Penelope Damaskos, Linda Mathew, and LaKeisha Jackson

Key Concepts

- Leadership development in palliative and oncology social work needs to be strengthened early on career track, as well as in master's level programs.
- Leadership opportunities are available in macro, mezzo, and micro social work practice.
- Leadership development must include an increased focus on Black, Brown, Latinx, Indigenous, and multiracial (BBLIM); Asian American & Pacific Islander (AAPI); and lesbian, gay, bisexual, transgender, queer, and intersex (LGBTQI) social workers.
- Leadership within a pandemic requires extra attention to multiple use of communication forums.

Keywords: Asian American and Pacific Islander (AAPI), Black, Brown, Latinx, Indigenous, and multiracial (BBLIM); lesbian, gay, bisexual, transgender, queer, and intersex (LGBTQI); macro/mezzo/micro practice, oncology social work, palliative social work, social work leadership

Palliative care services are specifically designed to address the quality-of-life concerns of seriously ill people. When palliative care is integrated into routine oncology services, it can improve symptom burden caused by treatment, quality of life, and patient and caregiver satisfaction (Bosma et al., 2010). Most oncology social workers (OSWs) will assist adults, children, and families who are facing progressive, life-limiting illness, dying, death, or bereavement. OSWs also use palliative skills to alleviate suffering and improve a patient's quality of life and death by addressing physical, psychological, social, spiritual, and practical concerns.

Penelope Damaskos, Linda Mathew, and LaKeisha Jackson, *Leadership Development in Oncology and Palliative Care Social Work* In: *Oncology and Palliative Social Work.* Edited by: Susan Hedlund, Bryan Miller, Grace Christ, and Carolyn Messner, Oxford University Press. © Oxford University Press 2024. DOI: 10.1093/oso/9780197607299.003.0026

Social work leadership can be defined as the ability to work effectively with individuals, families, and groups; to collaborate constructively with organizations and communities to promote social justice; to be advocates for social change; and to address individual and social problems (Sullivan, 2016). The Institute of Medicine (IOM) report, *Cancer Care for the Whole Patient: Meeting Psychosocial Health Needs*, highlights the demand for social work leadership across all aspects of the health care delivery system (Adler et al., 2008; Otis-Green et al., 2015). OSWs are well positioned to take leadership roles in many treatment settings, and they are integral to palliative care teams. OSWs help improve support for people with life-threatening illnesses or those who are dying or bereaved. Oncology social work comes with a broad psychosocial perspective that transcends the illness-based diagnostic and treatment paradigm (Hedlund, 2015; Jones et al., 2014). OSWs bring to the interprofessional team expertise in health and social systems, individual and family dynamics, cultural diversity, grief and loss, communication, advocacy, and ethical considerations. Practicing OSWs can unlock numerous opportunities, from supporting the patient and caregivers to the development of programs and policies with a wide impact on oncology palliative practice. OSWs have comprehensive skills as not only clinicians but also educators, administrators, researchers, and public policymakers.

This chapter describes leadership efforts that promote the unique functions and challenges leaders face in oncology and palliative care social work. We review current oncology and palliative care social work training programs and discuss the challenges and opportunities of developing leadership skills at the macro, mezzo, and micro areas of practice. Finally, we cover leadership training specifically for BBLIM, AAPI, and LBGTQI social workers throughout their professional development.

Leadership Training in Oncology and Palliative Care Social Work

Current Educational Opportunities

For years, scholars within the social work field have noted the essential role OSWs and palliative care social workers (PCSWs) play within the interprofessional team (Hedlund, 2015; Jones et al, 2014; Otis-Green et al, 2015; Zebrack et al, 2022). The focus on the development of leadership skills and training within these two subspecialities has become a goal of such nationally based training programs as ExCEL in Social Work—Excellence in Cancer Education and Leadership (Otis-Green et al., 2015). ExCEL was designed to enhance OSWs' leadership skills and confidence within clinical settings by helping trainees identify opportunities to improve delivery of care within their area practice. This program increased participant awareness to create culturally competent programs and services within the oncology treatment settings and promoted OSW contributions in clinical care (Otis-Green et al., 2015).

Several university-based programs offer pre- and post-masters palliative care training. New York University's (NYU) Silver School of Social Work, Zelda Foster Studies Program, and Smith College's Certificate in Palliative and End-of-Life Program have post-master's programs, while Fordham University's School of Social Service has a fellowship and continuing education program dedicated to palliative care. The Smith and NYU programs provide in-depth training focused on palliative care that includes both mentoring and leadership components. Also available online and in collaboration with the National Association of Social Work is the Educating Social Workers in Palliative and End-of-Life Care (ESPEC), which has a leadership and mentorship component. All these programs have provided valid contributions on multiple levels, for example, increasing OSWs' and PCSWs' exposure to opportunities to take on more leadership roles in their work environments, contributing to the development of current and future leaders through targeted coursework and the development of mentorship structures, continuing OSWs' and PCSWs' professional development and support once they enter the clinical arena through funding to attend national conferences, and establishing online networking forums (Gilliam et al., 2016).

Although these programs provide excellent foundational training in palliative care social work, they could make a clearer connection to the role of oncology social work or the use of palliative practices that are inherent in the clinical approaches highlighted through supervision. Our social work education and training should complement palliative care principles and skills that include but are not limited to support for patient and family autonomy, pain and symptom management, and psychosocial interventions along the continuum of illness and at end of life. The question is whether thousands of health care social workers are maximizing their contributions and assuming the opportunities for leadership this national call demands (Sumser et al., 2015). The need to increase OSWs development of leadership skills across many areas is pressing given changes in health care that have resulted from the COVID-19 pandemic and the increased need for palliative trained social workers. Additionally, leadership voids will result after the wave of retirements that are occurring throughout health care resulting in a profession-wide "brain drain" (Messner, 2010).

Leadership Development Opportunities Across Macro, Mezzo, and Micro Levels in the Clinical Arena

Macro social work practice addresses and initiates changes in the larger sociopolitical systems that impact mental and physical health of the individual. Macro social work practice looks at policy advocacy, community development and organizing, organizational management, and leadership. The call for macro practice and the focus on systemic racism is critical now more than ever, as NASW mandates social workers to act against oppression, racism, discrimination, and inequities, and to acknowledge personal privilege of the social work clinicians (NASW, 2021). Macro embodies all social worker's commitment to social justice and social change regardless of the subspeciality by promoting structural solutions to systemic inequalities along race, class, gender, and gender identity. Despite this increased call to action, master's level social work education historically has had limited focus on macro approaches in social work practice. For example, of the social work students enrolled in graduate programs, only 10% focus on macro social work practice; 3% to 4% focus on administrative social work practice, and 2% to 5% focus on community organizing and planning (Pritzker & Applewhite, 2015; Zippay & Demone, 2011). More coursework that bridges this gap would be a crucial step toward more comprehensive preparation for OSWs to become leaders within the field (Gilliam et al., 2016).

Macro social work also includes leadership and management. In general, management supervises everyday activities of staff, tasks, and routines that are necessary for an organization to remain viable and function smoothly (Sullivan, 2016). By contrast, leadership involves the ability to communicate vision, inspiration, innovation, creativity, and power (Fisher, 2009; Hill et al., 2010). OSWs have multiple opportunities to highlight their leadership skills in the clinical arena and beyond.

Mezzo refers to midlevel social workers or those who have been in the field for many years and have clinical and/or programmatic expertise. Mezzo presents as a phase of professional expansion, where social workers can become supervisors, educators, program managers, researchers, and mentors. In the mezzo phase OSW/PCSWs develop mentorship and skill-building forums and promote programmatic innovation within the clinical settings (Sullivan, 2016). Also during this phase of professional development, OSWs can serve on national professional boards and can influence policies. It is also in this phase that OSWs present at national conferences.

On the micro level, OSWs provide counseling to patients and their families, advocate for patients, and are an integral part of the interdisciplinary medical team (Fobair et al., 2009). It is in this initial phase of professional development that OSWs focus on their clinical development and expertise, while growing their group work and program development skills. The clinical area is ripe with leadership opportunities for OSW/PCSWs, whose excellent communication skills can facilitate difficult yet necessary conversations within complex medical settings. Clinical acumen is an important framework for the development of leadership skills where our training as clinicians underscores our ability to communicate about complex situations at an exceptional level.

Despite the interconnectedness between clinical training and leadership skills all along the professional trajectory, the emphasis and time dedicated to training social workers in administrative systems or macro practice is secondary to clinical or micro social work practice (Pritzker & Applewhite, 2015; Zippay & Demone, 2011). This is evidenced by the disproportionate emphasis placed on micro practice in both social work practice and educational settings (Council on Social Work Education [CSWE], 2015). The development of clinical skills is a valuable foundation for macro or administrative practice; however, the direct link between a clinical foundation with leadership development and communication skills is directly drawn in neither social work education nor many clinical settings.

Challenges and Opportunities for Leadership in Oncology Palliative Care

Fostering collaboration and effective communication between PCSWs and OSWs can be a challenge for leaders of palliative care programs in oncology settings. While they both provide valuable input into each case, PCSWs are usually part of a consulting service whereas OSWs are more often integral members of the clinical or treating teams. This divide can create communication challenges when the interprofessional team (IPT) relies on the PCSW to be the source of psychosocial support to the patient and their caregivers and does not recognize that the team member most familiar with the patient is the OSW. Bridging this divide presents a leadership opportunity where the PCSW can incorporate the OSW into clinical meetings to inform the IPT about the patient's psychosocial issues. The supervisory challenge is helping PCSWs and OSWs recognize not only that they are stronger as a team but that together, they can provide more comprehensive support to patients and their caregivers.

Opportunity for Visibility and Developing Our Voice

A fundamental part of OSWs' and PCSWs' work is maintaining patient privacy. However, this fact can create an inherent struggle between the desire to be recognized for the important services we provide and the confidential nature of our work. Cultivating comfort with visibility by speaking in meetings and case discussions should be an integral aspect of individual supervision as well as an important part of the peer/group meetings. Increased visibility for OSWs/PCSWs should be encouraged by social work department directors and managers by rotating the leadership of staff meetings so that all attendees have the experience of running a nonclinical meeting that is more goal- than process-oriented.

Communicating information across interprofessional areas can either enhance or undermine team building. Too often, social workers cede leadership to administrative colleagues without recognizing that the skills we take for granted (communication about difficult topics, group facilitation, advocacy, or program development) are essential leadership skills. Visibility and assertiveness of social work staff with the interprofessional team should be cultivated by the social work leadership and supervisors within the department. Transparent communication and articulation of clear departmental goals to the senior management team initiates a chain reaction of communication to staff at all levels. Transparency in communication not only is essential for sustaining an agile and committed team but also fosters respectful exchange among all team members; in turn, cultivating interdepartmental transparent communication creates a culture that promotes visibility and is used with interprofessional teams in the clinical setting (Box 26.1).

Box 26.1

During the COVID-19 epidemic many hospital services scrambled to transition to remote work for staff and telehealth for patient care. Drawing on years of experience with remote groups, one social work department was able to quickly transition all patient care and staff support programs to an online platform. This resulted in an enormous increase in patient and caregiver group participation. In addition, through the online format, medical staff were able to access ongoing self-care and support programs. Social work assumed a leadership role in the development of both patient and staff support programs based on our clinical knowledge, program delivery expertise, and group experience.

Challenges of Visibility

Promoting the visibility of social work withing an IPT can pose challenges, as OSWs and PCSWs can be reluctant to communicate their assessments. The task of supervision with OSWs and PCSWs then is to reflect on situations/meetings where they felt silenced because, "No one listens to me anyway." Visibility can have a negative effect on BBLIM, AAPI, and LGBTQI social workers—people who are already constantly navigating multiple identities within inherently White-dominant and heteronormative structures. Private discussion between a supervisor and their supervisee can provide a venue in which to explore these complex situations that operate on multiple levels and require a mutual sense of respect and safety. Since supervisors play a dual role of both clinician and boss (for example, conducting performance reviews and other administrative duties related to human resources), it is important to have clear guidelines around and expectations about these discussions. Supervisors must carefully balance their dual role to allow supervisees to be vulnerable and cultivate self-awareness without fear of repercussions. Promoting self-reflection is also a key component of clinical supervision and fosters continual engagement in the work over time while helping OSWs and PCSWs develop personal resilience (Damaskos, 2011).

Supervisors should recognize when mentoring staff that not everyone will follow the same routes for leadership growth. While we have established professional development paths—public speaking, developing clinical expertise within a defined aspect of work, supervising a student, or developing specific programs such as a bereavement or caregivers—some might be interested in using their social work training to pursue leadership in a related area such as ethics or spirituality. Understanding an individual's interests can lead not only to better staff retention but also to a deeper connection to the meaning of the work.

Effective Leadership in Clinical Settings

Cultivating a productive and collaborative relationship with administrative colleagues is essential for OSWs and PCSWs. Creating leadership opportunities outside the clinical role can begin with the appointment of an OSW or PCSW to key institutional committees and groups, such as ethics, quality, and safety committees; institutional review boards; institution-wide staff support groups; equity, diversity, and inclusion committees; patient and family advisory councils; and employee resource networks (ERNs). ERNs provide opportunities to interact with colleagues from other areas of the hospital or within their affinity groups, which contributes to both professional and personal visibility.

Leadership development can also happen as staff prepare for public speaking engagements at conferences or as guest lecturers. In addition, creating forums to discuss research and scholarship through, for example, writing workgroups can foster mentorship relationships beyond the supervisory dyad. Administrators can facilitate flex hours if a staff member is pursuing training that furthers their professional scope of practice; advanced training and expanded expertise not only increases the quality of service an OSW or PCSW provides to patients and their caregivers but also contributes to increased staff resilience and job satisfaction (Damaskos, 2011).

Promoting interprofessional collaboration among social workers and practitioners in other disciplines such as nursing or medicine can also create leadership opportunities (Blacker et al., 2016). Through engagement with other disciplines, social workers can educate colleagues about the clinical scope of social work. For example, they can provide education about how family dynamics around the illness and caregiving can impact care or model how to discuss emotionally laden concerns, such as delivering bad news. Collaborating with other disciplines also benefits OSWs and PCSWs as they demonstrate expertise, which in turn, increases visibility, institutional value, and leadership development.

Unique Challenges Presented by COVID-19

During the COVID-19 pandemic, working life quickly changed in ways that were previously unimaginable. Working from home, virtual meetings, and limited in-person interactions with patients and department staff presented enormous challenges for practitioners of all disciplines in oncology and palliative care. Virtual platforms provided constant connection if desired, but the nature of the platform also increased a sense isolation and development of burnout and compassion fatigue. Meaningful engagement based on clear communication from departmental leaders to staff members has been necessary to sustain cohesive, collaborative departments that could support OSWs and PCSWs in their work providing important services to patients.

Racial Disparities in Leadership

Cultural awareness and practicing antiracism are necessary components of effective and inclusive leadership in social work. Health care organizations and schools of social work must embrace and actively foster equity, diversity, and inclusion in all aspects of social work, especially leadership positions. Many schools of social work are still working to establish cultural diversity and inclusion in faculty hiring (Ashley & Paez, 2015). In 2019, CSWE research revealed that only 39% of full-time faculty and 42% of part-time faculty identified as BBLIM, AAPI, or LGBTQI (CSWE, 2020). This lack of diversity in higher education can impact the sense of belonging of students from these groups and lead them to question whether there is a place for them in social work leadership.

Unconscious bias and the lack of diversity in health care, including among OSW and PCSW leaders, can have a negative impact on the quality of care OSWs and PCSWs provide to the diverse populations they serve. Despite many initiatives to diversify health care institutions over the past ten years, the lack of BBLIM, AAPI, and LGBTQI representation among OSWs and PCSWs remains significant. Research (and common sense) indicate that a lack of diversity in the workplace has had and will continue to have a deleterious effect on the oncology workforce due in part to a sense of not belonging (Myshko, 2021). Training and mentoring BBLIM, AAPI, and LGBTQI social workers is the responsibility of both schools of social work and oncology organizations. Promoting diversity, equity, and inclusion benefits schools and health care institutions, students and staff, and most important, the populations OSWs and PCSWs serve.

Box 26.2

As a recently promoted Oncology Social Work Manager, my first day revealed how inherent racism is in the health care setting. On my first day, I was asked not once but twice and by two different physicians if I was representing the front desk, and they were surprised when I informed them that I was the manager for the Social Work Department. Being a Black woman, I am used to such micro-aggressions; still, this did not lessen the sting that the assumption my new colleagues made about me based on my race. This bias, be it unconscious or not, was my first introduction to leadership in oncology and what has let me on a path of highlighting the importance of diversity in leadership and specifically, in who is providing oncology care.

—LaKeisha Jackson

Increasing Diversity Through Leadership

Diversity-focused training and career development programs can help address the ongoing racial inequities among OSWs and PCSWs (Association of Oncology Social Workers [AOSW], n.d.; Myshko, 2021). Achieving diversity will require health care organizations to create learning opportunities and safe environments in which to address challenging issues, such as systemic racism and unconscious bias. Organizations should be intentional in attracting, welcoming, and retaining a diverse workforce to address the needs of an increasingly diverse oncology patient population (Myshko, 2021). Providing culturally competent cancer care requires a commitment to addressing the societal factors that contribute to the ongoing disparities in the workforce and in health care. Diverse workforces allow OSWs to demonstrate integrity, compassion, and leadership in oncology practice, while acknowledging the communities served (AOSW, n.d.).

Clinical social workers provide an estimated 65% of all mental health services in the United States (NASW, 2021). As leaders and administrators in health care organizations and education begin to reach retirement age, there is an urgent need to develop and implement succession plans for social work leadership (Messner, 2010). This is a significant moment in our development as a profession to affirmatively allocate resources to professional development of future leaders in oncology social work.

Mentorship and Inclusion

Field instruction and clinical supervision share several aims and characteristics with mentorship (Shulman, 2011; Wayne et al., 2010). Both encourage self-reflection, professional use of self, and transmitting social work's core code of ethics. While field instruction and clinical supervision are primarily concerned with teaching the knowledge, skills, and values that ensure provision of ethical clinical care (NASW, 2021), mentorship promotes professional development in addition to what is received through field instruction and clinical supervision (Gardner et al., 2015).

The lack of racial diversity in oncology social work can be seen in the current membership enrollment of the AOSW (n.d.), whose membership is 90% White and a little over 8% Black and Hispanic combined. The recent appointment of a diversity and inclusion chair on the AOSW board of directors is a meaningful step toward creating stronger connections between BBLIM,

AAPI, and LGBTQI social workers and the professional organization that cultivates OSW leadership nationwide. While it is an encouraging first step, a lot of work remains to be done to cultivate and sustain the truly diverse and integrated workforce needed for current and future leadership development (Box 26.2).

Fostering an inclusive environment involves:

- Including BBLIM, AAPI, and LGBTQI staff in the interview process to provide the opportunity for input into the selection process.
- Creating a mentoring system where new staff can connect to a colleague that can be accessed as a sounding board outside the supervisory dyad.
- Encouraging involvement in ERNs and other institution-based affinity groups to expand networks outside of department.
- Developing department-wide forums to discuss antiracism within the clinical practice.
- Developing training pathways for supervisors and departmental leaders on antiracism work both inside and outside the workplace—if available.
- Include antiracism and social justice topics in departmental educational meetings and smaller group discussion forums.

Given the complexities of our health care systems and the acute psychosocial issues that affect our patients, the need to refocus on leadership development has never been greater. From training in master's and post-master's programs to on-the-job learning, opportunities for leadership development are always present. Department heads, supervisors, managers, and frontline social workers can contribute to forums to help OSWs and PCSWs use their clinical acumen to bring valuable information to IDT meetings and seize other valuable leadership opportunities. Current leaders can help OSWs and PCSWs develop leadership skills through creating peer-led forums in the workplace, leadership development in supervision, strengthening leadership connection in training and master's levels programs and inclusion of BBLIM, AAPI, and LGBTQI social workers.

Guiding Best Practices for the Future

Augmentation of leadership development throughout the professional career should include several best practices:

- **Education:** Educational forums should include leadership development and discussions about connections among clinical expertise, visibility, and leadership. Creating on-the-job opportunities through peer-led forums—for example, researching and writing for professional journals and attendance at clinical case conferences—is important.
- **Supervision:** The one-on-one setting is an excellent opportunity for planning a professional development trajectory consistent with the individual's interests. Creating mentorship opportunities outside the supervisory dyad either within the workplace or beyond should be promoted. Mentorship networks can also be fostered through national conferences, national boards, and involvement in ERNs.
- **Inclusion:** Diversifying social work staff should be prioritized both for leadership opportunities and professional growth. Attracting BBLIM, AAPI, and LGBTQI social workers to oncology and palliative care must start in the master's programs and selection for clinical internships.

Pearls

- Focusing on leadership development is increasingly necessary in the face of complex psychosocial needs of our patients/clients and increased retirements contributing to "brain drain."
- Leadership development is an integral component of professional development.
- Promoting leadership throughout educational and workplace settings is an ever-present opportunity that requires more attention.
- Leadership development must include increased focus on the development of BBLIM, AAPI, and LGBTQI social workers.

Pitfalls

- Current lack of focus in the educational and on-the-job forums available to social workers that support leadership development.
- Lack of training or a focus on the skills social workers bring to the IPT results in social work marginalization in the workplace.
- Persistent territorial issues between OSWs and PCSWs create divisions that weaken rather than strengthen our roles as leaders in the clinical arenas.

- The dearth of BBLIM, AAPI, and LGBTQI social workers in either oncology or palliative care social work is a detriment to inclusive leadership development across all professional trajectories.

Additional Resources

American Association for Cancer Research: https://cancerprogressreport.aacr.org/disparities/chd20-contents/chd20-overcoming-cancer-health-disparities-through-diversity-in-cancer-training-and-workforce/

Fordham University School of Social Service, Palliative Care Fellowship: http://www.palliativecarefordham.com/

National Association of Social Workers. *Educating social workers in palliative and end-of-life care (ESPEC).* https://www.socialworkers.org/espec

New York University, Silver School of Social Work, Zelda Foster Studies: https://socialwork.nyu.edu/faculty-and-research/faculty-initiatives/zelda-foster-studies.html

Smith College School of Social Work, Palliative/ELC Certificate Curriculum: https://ssw.smith.edu/academics/continuing-education/graduate-certificate-programs/certificate-palliative-and-end-life

References

Adler, N. E., Page, A., & Institute of Medicine (U.S.) Committee on Psychosocial Services to Cancer Patients/Families in a Community Setting. (Eds.). (2008). *Cancer care for the whole patient: Meeting psychosocial health needs.* National Academies Press.

Ashley, W., & Paez, J. (2015). Enhancing strengths-based social work pedagogy: From cultural competence to critical race theory. *International Journal of Interdisciplinary Educational Studies, 10*(4), 15–25. https://doi.org/10.18848/2327-011X/CGP/v10i04/53291

Association of Oncology Social Workers. (n.d.). *Diversity and* inclusion *statement and goals.* Retrieved December 23, 2022, from https://aosw.org/about-aosw/diversity-inclusion-statement/

Blacker, S., Head, B. A., Jones, B. L., Remke, S. S., & Supiano, K. (2016). Advancing hospice and palliative care social work leadership in interprofessional education and practice. *Journal of Social Work in End-of-Life and Palliative Care, 12*(4), 316–330. https://doi.org/10.1080/15524256.2016.1247771

Bosma, H., Johnston, M., Cadell, S., Wainwright, W., Abernethy, N., Feron, A., Kelly, M., & Nelson, F. (2010). Creating social work competencies for practice in hospice palliative care. *Palliative Medicine, 24*(1), 79–87.

Council on Social Work Education. (2015). *2014 Statistics on social work education in the United States.* https://www.cswe.org/getattachment/7a5c0198-7164-4e7f-96e4-5ee2a87b9cbc/2014-statistics-on-social-work-education-in-the-united-states.pdf/

Council on Social Work Education. (2020). *2019 Statistics on social work education in the United States.* https://www.cswe.org/getattachment/215ee172-3f6e-464a-b435-7dd795f80129/cswe_rpt_19-m.pdf/

Damaskos, P. (2011). *The presence of resilience in oncology social workers* (Doctoral dissertation). Yeshiva University. ProQuest Dissertations & Theses.

Fisher, E. A. (2009). Motivation and leadership in social work management: A review of theories and related studies. *Administration in Social Work, 33*(4), 347–367.

Fobair, P., Stearns, N. N., Christ, G., Dozier-Hall, D., Newman, N. W., Zabora, J., Schnipper, H. H., Kennedy, V., Loscalzo, M., Stensland, S. M., Hedlund, S., Lauria, M. M., Fife, M., Herschl, J., Marcusen, C. P., Vaitones, V., Brintzenhofeszoc, K., Walsh, K., Lawson, K., & Desonier M. (2009). Historical threads in the development of oncology social work. *Journal of Psychosocial Oncology, 27*(2), 155–215.

Gardner, D. S., Gerbino, S., Walls, J. W., Chachkes, E., & Doherty, M. J. (2015). Mentoring the next generation of social workers in palliative and end-of-life care: The Zelda Foster studies program. *Journal of Social Work in End-of-Life & Palliative Care, 11*(2), 107–131. https://doi.org/10.1080/15524256.2015.1074142

Gilliam, C. C., Chandler, M. A., Al-Hajjaj, H. A., Mooney, A. N., & Vakalahi, H. F. (2016). Intentional leadership planning and development: The collective responsibility to educate more social work leaders. *Advances in Social Work, 17*(2), 330–339. https://doi.org/10.18060/18606

Hedlund, S. (2015). Oncology social work: Past, present, and future. In G. Christ, C. Messner, & L. Behar (Eds.), *Handbook of oncology social work: Psychosocial care for people with cancer* (pp. 9–13). Oxford University Press.

Hill, K. M., Ferguson, S. M., & Erickson, C. (2010). Sustaining and strengthening a macro identity: The association of macro practice social work. *Journal of Community Practice, 18*(4), 513–527.

Jones, B., Phillips, F., Head, B. A., Hedlund, S., Kalisiak, A., Zebrack, B., Killburn, L., & Otis-Green, S. (2014). Enhancing collaborative leadership in palliative social work in oncology. *Journal of Social Work in End-of-Life and Palliative Care, 10*(4), 309–321. https://doi.org/10.1080/15524256.2014.975319

Messner, C. (2010). Impending oncology social worker shortage? *Oncology Issues, 9*, 46–47. https://www.accc-cancer.org/docs/documents/oncology-issues/articles/2003-2016/2010/so10/so10-impending-oncology-social-worker-shortage.pdf?sfvrsn=c3f7d758_2

Myshko, D. (2021). Diversity gap persists for racial and ethnic minorities in oncology. *Oncology Live, 22*(5), 59. https://www.onclive.com/view/diversity-gap-persists-for-racial-and-ethnic-minorities-in-oncology

National Association of Social Workers. (2021). *Code of ethics*. https://www.socialworkers.org/About/Ethics/Code-of-Ethics/Code-of-Ethics-English

Otis-Green, S., Jones, B., Zebrack, B., Kilburn, L., Altilio, T. A., & Ferrell, B. (2015). ExCEL in social work: Excellence in cancer education & leadership: An oncology social work response to the 2008 Institute of Medicine report. *Journal of Cancer Education, 30*(3), 503–513. https://doi.org/10.1007/s13187-014-0717-8

Pritzker, S., & Applewhite, S. R. (2015). Going "macro": Exploring the careers of macro practitioners. *Social Work, 60*(3), 191–199. https://doi.org/10.1093/sw/swv019

Shulman, L. (2011). *The skills of helping individuals, families, groups, and communities* (7th ed.). Brooks-Cole.

Sullivan, W. P. (2016). Leadership in social work: Where are we? *Journal of Social Work Education, 52*(Suppl.1), S51–S61.

Sumser, B., Remke, S., Leimena, M., Altilio, T., & Otis-Green, S. (2015). The serendipitous survey: A look at primary and specialist palliative social work practice, preparation, and competence. *Journal of Palliative Medicine, 18*(10), 881–883. https://doi.org/10.1089/jpm.2015.0022

Wayne, J., Bogo, M., & Raskin, M. (2010). Field education as the signature pedagogy of social work education. *Journal of Social Work Education*, *46*(3), 327–339.

Zebrack, B., Schapmire, T., Otis-Green, S., Nelson, K., Miller, N., Donna, D., & Grignon, M. (2022). Establishing core competencies, opportunities, roles, and expertise for oncology social work. *Journal of Social Work*, *22*(121). https://doi.org/10.1177/14680173211051983

Zippay, A., & Demone, H. (2011). Initial macro-level job responsibilities among MSW graduates. *Administration in Social Work*, *35*(4), 412–424.

27 Creating Partnerships

Fostering Collaboration and Managing Conflict

Stephanie Fooks-Parker, Barbara Jones, and Tara Schapmire

Key Concepts

- Social workers face challenges in interprofessional collaboration, managing conflict, and partnering with the team.
- Social work leadership is critical in interprofessional collaboration.
- Social workers can be encouraged and mentored to find their voice to fully contribute their skills and knowledge to interprofessional teams.
- Social work can foster collaboration by using and expanding profession-specific competencies for interprofessional collaborative practice.
- Social work leadership has implications for research, policy, and education.

Keywords: Competencies, health care, interprofessional collaboration, leadership, social work

One of the biggest challenges for health care providers is attaining what has come to be known as the "quintuple aim" of care: improving population health, enhancing the care experience, reducing costs, reducing professional burnout, and improving health equity (Nundy et al., 2022). The social work profession offers unique skill sets that can inform, contribute to, and enhance each of these aims. For over 100 years, social workers have been working in health care settings as part of interprofessional teams, bringing unique perspective to health care environments (Ambrose-Miller & Ashcroft, 2016; Cleak & Turczynski, 2014). As outlined in Standard 8 (Interdisciplinary and Interorganizational Collaboration [IIC]) of the National Association of Social Work (NASW) *Standards of Social Work Practice in Health Care Settings*, social workers practicing in health care settings shall "promote collaboration among health care team members, other colleagues, and organizations to

Stephanie Fooks-Parker, Barbara Jones, and Tara Schapmire, *Creating Partnerships* In: *Oncology and Palliative Social Work*. Edited by: Susan Hedlund, Bryan Miller, Grace Christ, and Carolyn Messner, Oxford University Press.
 DOI: 10.1093/oso/9780197607299.003.0027

support, enhance, and deliver effective services to clients and client support systems" (NASW, 2016, p. 31). However, we must remember that successful collaboration is not a given but rather, an ongoing process that requires conscious planning and active organizational and induvial support.

The World Health Organization (WHO) defines interprofessional collaborative practice (IPCP) as "multiple health workers from different professional backgrounds working together with patients, families, caregivers and communities to deliver the highest quality of care" (2010, p. 4). The 2019 National Academies of Sciences, Engineering, and Medicine (NASEM) report, *Integrating Social Care into the Delivery of Health Care*, highlights the importance of social workers in interprofessional teams. Social workers play a key role in understanding these concepts; they have excellent insights into social determinants of health and the patient/family perspective and can effectively communicate these insights to everyone involved in the care process. However, collaborating with people from varied disciplines with different perspectives and goals can lead to conflicts within an interprofessional care team. This chapter explores how social workers face unique challenges when engaging in interprofessional collaboration. We also highlight how the leadership skills and strategies social workers bring to a team can help all members of the team manage potential conflict and embrace collaboration for the larger benefit of patients and families. Finally, we argue that as social workers continue to promote our unique value and demonstrate our contributions to our teams, the opportunities for education, research, and policymaking are ever present and expanding.

Social workers face challenges with interprofessional collaboration that can affect the effectiveness of the entire health care team. Among these are imbalanced power dynamics or a lack of equal representation among the professions during care planning and implementation. Karam et al. (2018) reviewed the qualitative literature of IPCP and found that power imbalances among interprofessional team members based on social and organizational structure were potential roadblocks to successful IPCP. Trust, understanding, and respect promoted by open communication were crucial to overcoming these potential barriers and balancing power dynamics among team members. In addition, Karam et al. (2018) found that focusing on shared goals and patient-centeredness can improve IPCP. Participants of a study conducted by Ambrose-Miller and Ashcroft (2016) recommended the need for organizational leadership to foster a collaborative workplace culture focused on client care and clear communication of team members' roles in decision-making processes.

The advocate role is ingrained within the social work profession. The insights and advocacy social workers bring on behalf of patients and families can sometimes create or exacerbate interprofessional tensions (e.g., if one professional feels that their authority or expertise is being called into question by an issue a social worker raises). However, in most cases, a social worker's insights help educate other professionals on the team and elevate communication both among the team and with the patient and family. For example, the following case study illuminates how other professionals on the team may become frustrated with or make judgments about patients and families due to their behaviors or the family's perceived lack of concern. Social workers can bridge this gap in ways that minimize frustration or judgment and prioritize respectful understanding (Box 27.1).

Box 27.1

J is a 4-month-old baby boy with infant leukemia whose only chance of cure is a bone marrow transplant. J lives with his mother, father, and 7-year-old brother. J and his family live about 3 hours from the transplant center. J's family has been in the country for many years; however, English is not their first language. J's father is a delivery man who uses the family car for work; this means that J's parents can only visit J on the father's days off (1 or 2 days per week). Some members of the team expressed frustration about the family not being at bedside more often. When mom or dad would call for updates, some team members would also express frustration because they were calling at "inconvenient" times. The social worker was able to help the team understand the financial and logistical barriers the family faced and clarify that these barriers in no way reflected negatively on their devotion to their child. The social worker also shared with the team the emotional toll not being at bedside was having on the mother. The social worker found it necessary to develop strategies to support both the family and the interprofessional team and to ensure follow-through among all participants. A team member began to call the family daily with updates and share pictures via the electronic medical record. When parents visited, a team member would spend time with the family; eventually, they started the education process in preparation for future discharge. During rounds, the social worker would share information or updates about the family and let the team members know when the family was expected to be at bedside. Over time and through getting to know the family and better understanding their challenges, team members became less frustrated.

Lack of role clarity and task ambiguity may hinder interprofessional collaboration. Practitioners in different disciplines may not understand one another's lexicons, scopes of practice, or procedures. Health professionals have unique training, education, and perspectives toward practice. Physicians, nurses, pharmacists, and social workers (along with other members of the interprofessional team) view and frame patient problems and their solutions through separate lenses (Gehlert & Browne, 2019). Patient care conferences with the team can help improve role definitions and allow members of each discipline to participate equally in the team and educate one another on their perspectives. Ultimately, open communication will help the patient receive the best possible treatment (Box 27.2).

Box 27.2

M, a 4-year-old girl who was diagnosed with cancer in 2020, is the second youngest of five children. M's family had been involved with the Department of Human Services, and the day of her diagnosis was the day M's mother regained physical custody of her. Prior to this, M was living with the maternal grandmother. Once M started to feel better from her emergent round of chemotherapy, the care team observed her exhibiting numerous behavioral concerns, including hitting, biting, and scratching both staff and her caregivers. Her problem behaviors amplified around invasive procedures and hands-on care. With the support of her interdisciplinary team and the members of the team working effectively together, M was able to successfully get through surgery, metaiodobenzlguanidine (MIBG) therapy, and cycles of chemotherapy. During M's final chemotherapy session and prior to a planned stem cell transplant, M's social situation drastically changed, which unfortunately correlated with a major regression of her behavior. The team was concerned that M might struggle with the transplant due to the regimented treatment it required. On the first day of the admission for stem cell transplant, M had several episodes of agitation, demonstrated that she was at risk for harming herself, and bit a staff member's arm. Due to these concerning behaviors, the team put pretransplant conditioning chemotherapy on hold and initiated interprofessional collaboration with the first of many weekly patient care conferences. Some team members worried that M would not be able to endure the stem cell transplant and that chemotherapy should be continued instead. With the social worker taking the lead, the conferences included the FLOC (front line ordering clinician), inpatient nurse leads, child life specialist, a BCBA (board-certified behavior analyst), a psychologist, a psychiatrist, and creative arts therapists. The purpose of the meetings was to develop strategies to ensure M's and her family's success during transplant. The primary caregivers participated in the initial planning meeting and were updated as the team developed strategies. After over 2 months in the hospital, M successfully received her stem cell transplant without injuring herself or staff.

Organizational structure and philosophy can pose another challenge to interprofessional collaboration. Health care leaders unfamiliar with the advantages of interprofessional team care remain entrenched in a "that's not the way *we* do things" mindset. Promoting true collaborative practice requires a shift—to a "bottom up/top down" approach change in practice that honors multiple perspectives including those of the patient and family (Blacker et al., 2016). With a top-down approach all decisions are made only by the leadership at the top. Shared decision-making including all voices can lead to better collaboration. When decisions are made without collective and varied input, IPCP fails (Box 27.3).

Box 27.3

P was a pediatric oncology social worker at a large teaching hospital on the East Coast. P and the oncology child life specialist decided to write and produce an educational video about childhood cancer and the psychosocial issues patients face. The oncology division's faculty invited the social worker and the child life therapist to present and discuss the project at the faculty meeting and ultimately agreed to support the project. P and the child life specialist felt it necessary and appropriate to include a nurse, a psychologist, and a physician as part of the team to plan and complete the video. As planning continued, P's boss requested a meeting with her. At the meeting, P received a reprimand for attending the faculty meeting and orders to discontinue the project. The boss felt attending the faculty meeting was inappropriate, since social workers had never attended or been asked to attend those meetings; there was no need to collaborate with others disciplines on a project like this and that social work should be the only discipline involved. The video was completed without any social work involvement.

Importance of Social Work Leadership in Interprofessional Collaboration

The NASEM report, *Integrating Social Care into Health Care* (2019), highlights the essential roles social workers occupy in providing whole-person care for individuals, families, and communities. Specifically, the report recommends that health care organizations take steps to integrate social care into health care, including but not limited to hiring and promoting social workers with unique and specific skill sets aligned with caring for the whole person and promoting value-based care (NASEM, 2019). Social workers' skills in empathy, listening, care coordination, understanding people in their environments, advocacy, and respecting and honoring cultural and spiritual influences on health make them uniquely qualified to contribute to the care delivery system and interprofessional teams. In fact, social workers' expertise in collaboration and communication situates them as not just qualified to contribute to but also essential to IPCP. Social workers not only contribute to IPCP through their specific training but also can step into active leadership roles in care planning, interprofessional education (IPE), palliative care, family meetings, and organizational structures (Gehlert & Browne, 2019; Jones & Phillips, 2016; Otis-Green et al., 2015).

When social workers take a leadership role in health care settings, they can provide a coordinated, compassionate response to crisis that is otherwise lost when they are undervalued or disempowered and do not have the authority to offer their practice wisdom and evidence-based interventions collectively (Jones et al., 2020). Social workers can assume leadership roles in health care settings as directors, team leaders, and chairs as well as take charge of patient care activities. In practice, social workers may lead by hosting and facilitating family meetings and conferences (Fineberg & Bauer, 2011), teaching interprofessional teams (Jones et al., 2020), leading palliative care initiatives (Blacker et al., 2016), and identifying and responding to social determinants of health (de Saxe Zerden et al., 2020).

Specifically, social workers need to step into leadership roles and know our own worth in the interprofessional health care setting. Many health social workers proactively and vocally work to improve patient care every day, but others may need mentorship, education, coaching, and support to find their voice in health care. Because power differentials still exist among health care professions, it is important for social workers in educational programs to receive training in interprofessional models that honor social work expertise and provide direct skills training in IPCP. Social workers bring an important equity and justice lens to our work that needs to be integrated into all of health care, especially in settings that have not traditionally been focused on justice in the provision of services.

Finding Our Voice

Social workers can employ specific strategies to train ourselves, our colleagues, and our students to find our voices within interprofessional teams. First, we must acknowledge that a historical barrier to an equal seat at the table among other health care professions has been the lack of formal power and influence social workers have had in our hierarchical, often physician-centric, health care systems. Traditional hierarchies and entrenched notions of the supremacy of medicine to social dynamics, however, are shifting as more social workers assume formal leadership roles in their institutions and people in other professions come to value more highly the contribution of our profession. Some strategies for finding our voice include:

- participate in interprofessional education initiatives
- review and remind ourselves of our own skill set
- become a field instructor and mentor students
- stay current on social work literature and medical literature in our practice area (e.g., NASEM reports)
- meet with other social workers in similar settings for support
- practice speaking up
- identify and nurture relationships with allies on our interprofessional teams (e.g., physicians, nurses, child life therapists, psychologists)
- publish and present our work
- partner with the local university and schools of social work
- claim our knowledge
- take leadership roles in our settings and professional organizations
- join regional or national organizations for exposure and collegiality and engage in related listserv discussions and conferences
- continue education in leadership or IPCP
- take risks (e.g., volunteer to serve on ethics or search committees)
- engage in research and education
- practice self-compassion and patience
- connect with mentors, colleagues, and coaches
- seek funding for our work
- elevate others with intentionality

While these are all strategies that we can take in our individual settings, it is important that we also have structural supports in our institutions and in local and national policy. This requires leadership from both health care systems and policymakers to consider new ways to employ, recognize, reimburse, and support social workers and social work leadership. Some of the ways that social work can be supported structurally include:

- faculty appointments
- appropriate reimbursement for services
- having agency of defining scope of practice

- being supervised by other social workers
- departments of social work
- participating in research and education
- being included in decision-making
- having flexible time to participate in research, education, scholarship, program development
- participating in decision-making related to patient care
- sitting on committees throughout systems
- being included in leadership at all levels

Core Competencies for Interprofessional Collaboration

Once social workers more strongly assert our leadership abilities and find our social work voice, we can seek additional resources that promote IPCP by distinguishing *professional* from *interprofessional* competencies in health care. One of the barriers to IPCP remains the fact that students in the numerous health professions learn in professional silos (Head et al., 2016; Institute of Medicine, 2014; Schapmire et al., 2021; Schapmire et al., 2018) yet are expected to collaborate well once they enter the working world. Following the best practices of professional and interprofessional competencies can help address all the challenges to collaboration highlighted earlier (lack of role clarity, power imbalances, and organizational/structural support for IPCP). Professional competencies in health care are the "integrated enactment of knowledge, skills, values, and attitudes that define the areas of work of a particular health profession applied in specific care contexts" (Interprofessional Education Collaborative [IPEC], 2016, p. 8).

While useful and necessary for practicing within one's professional scope, professional competency is not as helpful when one considers the necessity of interprofessional collaboration to achieving the quintuple aim of health care (Nundy et al., 2022). To facilitate the overall goals of health care and create a more collaborative environment, each team members should also focus on interprofessional competencies, which are an "integrated enactment of knowledge skills, values, and attitudes that define working together across professions, with other health care workers, and with patients, along with families and communities, as appropriate to improve health outcomes in specific contents" (IPEC, 2016, p. 8). In 2009, the Interprofessional Educational Collaborative (IPEC) was formed with the stated goal of helping prepare future health professionals for enhanced team-based care of patients and improved

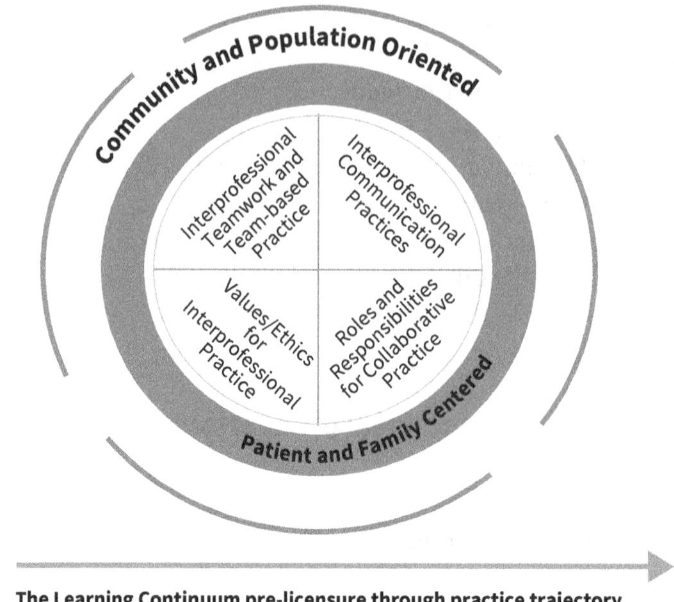

Figure 27.1 IPEC interprofessional collaboration competency domain (2016).

population health outcomes. Notably, social work was absent from this initial formation; however, IPEC later expanded membership to encompass several other professions essential to interprofessional collaborative practice, including social work. As of 2022, IPEC comprised 21 member organizations, including but not limited to the American Association of Colleges of Nursing, American Association of Colleges of Pharmacy, American Association for Respiratory Care, American Council of Academic Physical Therapy, American Dental Education Association, American Occupational Therapy Association, American Psychological Association, American Speech-Language Hearing Association, Association of American Medical Colleges, and Council on Social Work Education.

In response to the WHO call for coordinated interprofessional education where health professionals can learn about, from, and with each other (2010), IPEC has developed and maintained core competencies for interprofessional collaborative practice, building on each profession's expected disciplinary competencies. The IPEC core competencies were first published in 2011, updated in 2016, and currently under review for update in 2023. The competencies can be useful to social workers in taking the lead to improve IPCP in their settings and creating IPCP-specific learning opportunities for practicum students in master of social work programs as well as other clinical learners.

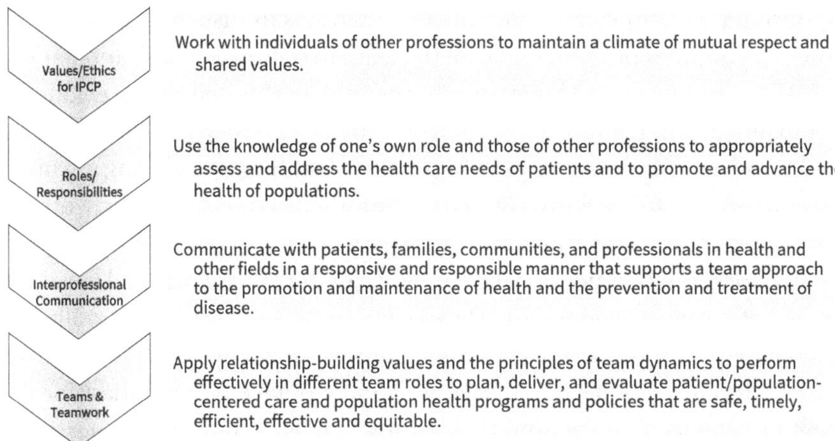

Figure 27.2 IPEC core competencies for interprofessional collaborative practice (2016).

Available at www.ipecollaborative.org, the IPEC core competencies highlight interprofessional collaboration (Figure 27.1) and the importance of health care professionals using a shared taxonomy across the disciplines.

The competencies (Figure 27.2) and their associated subcompetencies help institutions and teams focus on shared values and ethics, shared roles and responsibilities, interprofessional communication, and improving teams and teamwork. In both educational and practice settings at the micro level, these competencies can be used to coordinate efforts across the health professions to embed essential content in all health professions education curricula from prelicensure throughout the practice trajectory. The competencies also guide professional and institutional development of learning approaches, curriculum, and assessment strategies to achieve productive outcomes. They provide a foundation for a learning continuum in interprofessional competency development across the professions, as well as a lifelong learning trajectory. They can be used to prompt dialogue to evaluate the fit between educationally identified core competencies for interprofessional collaborative practice and practice needs/ demands. They allow opportunities to integrate essential interprofessional education content consistent with current accreditation expectations for each health professions' education program (IPEC, 2016). On a macro level, they provide accreditors a common set of interprofessional standards and assist professional licensing and credentialing bodies in defining testing content in IPCP.

In each of the case descriptions above, these competencies could be used. The teams in each scenario could commit to using 10 minutes of team time each week to reviewing at least one subcompetency and developing shared goals for improvement in that area. For example, under the IPEC Roles and

Responsibilities competency, one subcompetency is to "use unique and complementary abilities of all members of the team to optimize health and patient care" (IPEC, 2016, p. 12). This is specific and measurable and can be evaluated by individuals and teams on a scale from novice to expert. The team could spend time thinking about ways to improve their rating by ensuring a whole-person approach to care through educating themselves about each other's scopes of practice, thus optimizing future patient care.

Social workers face unique challenges when finding their voice and engaging in interprofessional collaboration. Developing social work leadership skills and implementing specific strategies will ensure that all health care professionals manage internal and external conflict well and embrace collaboration for the benefit of patients, families, and their teams. Implementing interprofessional collaborative practice competencies will improve successful collaborations, thereby facilitating the quintuple aim of health care (Nundy et al., 2022). As social workers continue to promote their value and engage with their teams, the opportunities for education, research, and policymaking are ever present. In educational realms, it is imperative to recognize the WHO mandate for coordinated interprofessional education where health professionals can learn about, from, and with each other (2010). Educators can ensure this by creating such learning opportunities. Research on the effectiveness of IPE and IPCP is growing and must continue. At the policy level, accrediting, credentialing, and licensing bodies can use the shared nomenclature in the IPEC Competencies to create standards and test content. Social workers have a responsibility to step into leadership in collaborative practice and education to contribute to enhancing care for patients, families, and communities.

Guiding Best Practices for the Future

Implementing the IPEC Core Competencies for Interprofessional Care can improve collaboration and move teams and institutions toward attaining the quintuple aim of health care: improving population health, enhancing the care experience, reducing costs, reducing professional burnout, and improving health equity (Nundy et al., 2022).

Pearls

- Be willing to step out of your comfort zone by seeking and accepting leadership opportunities. This will promote confidence building and improve your IPCP.

- Find mentors/leaders in your specific social work area and those with expertise in IPCP for guidance as you move into leadership roles.
- Be willing to challenge authority and the status quo to improve care and health care delivery.

Pitfalls

- Avoid training, practicing, and researching in professional silos.
- Avoid not claiming our authority, our voice, our leadership, and our expertise in social determinants of health at the micro, mezzo, and macro levels.
- Avoid focusing only on social work professional competencies without expansion to interprofessional competencies.

Additional Resources

Interprofessional Curriculum for Oncology Palliative Education (iCOPE): http://icopeproject.org/

Interprofessional Education Collaborative (IPEC): https://www.ipecollaborative.org/ipec-core-competencies

Interprofessional Education eXchange (IPEX): https://www.ipexproject.org/

References

Ambrose-Miller, W., & Ashcroft, R. (2016). Challenges faced by social workers as members of interprofessional collaborative health care teams. *Health and Social Work*, *41*(2), 101–109. https://doi.org/10.1093/hsw/hlw006

Blacker, S., Head, B. A., Jones, B. L., Remke, S. S., & Supiano, K. (2016, October–December). Advancing hospice and palliative care social work leadership in interprofessional education and practice. *Journal of Social Work in End-of-Life and Palliative Care*, *12*(4), 316–330. https://doi.org/10.1080/15524256.2016.1247771

Cleak, H. M., & Turczynski, M. (2014). Hospital social work in Australia: Emerging trends or more of the same? *Social Work in Health Care*, *53*(3), 199–213. https://doi.org/10.1080/00981389.2013.873516

de Saxe Zerden, L., Cadet, T. J., Galambos, C., & Jones, B. (2020). Social work's commitment and leadership to address social determinants of health and integrate social care into health care. *Journal of Health and Human Services Administration*, *43*(3), 309–323. https://doi.org/10.37808/jhhsa.43.3.5

Fineberg, I. C., & Bauer, A. (2011). Families and family conferencing. In T. Altilio & S. Otis-Green (Eds.), *Oxford textbook of palliative social work* (pp. 235–250). Oxford University Press. https://doi.org/10.1093/med/9780199739110.003.0022

Gehlert, S., & Browne, T. A. (Eds.). (2019). *Handbook of health social work* (3rd ed.). Wiley. https://doi.org/10.1002/9781119420743

Head, B. A., Schapmire, T., Earnshaw, L., Faul, A., Hermann, C., Jones, C., Martin, A., Shaw, M. A., Woggon, F., Ziegler, C., & Pfeiffer, M. (2016, June). Evaluation of an interdisciplinary curriculum teaching team-based palliative care integration in oncology. *Journal of Cancer Education*, *31*(2), 358–365. https://doi.org/10.1007/s13187-015-0799-y

Institute of Medicine. (2014). *Dying in America: Improving quality and honoring individual preferences near the end of life*. National Academies Press. http://www.nap.edu/catalog/18748/dying-in-america-improving-quality-and-honoring-individual-preferences-near

Interprofessional Education Collaborative. (2016). *Core competencies for interprofessional collaborative practice: 2016 Update*. https://nebula.wsimg.com/2f68a39520b03336b41038c370497473?AccessKeyId=DC06780E69ED19E2B3A5&disposition=0&alloworigin=1

Jones, B., Currin-McCulloch, J., Petruzzi, L., Phillips, F., Kaushik, S., & Smith, B. (2020). Transformative teams in health care. *Advances in Social Work*, *20*(2), 424–439. https://doi.org/10.18060/23671

Jones, B., & Phillips, F. (2016). Social work and interprofessional education in health care: A call for continued leadership. *Journal of Social Work Education*, *52*(1), 18–29. https://doi.org/10.1080/10437797.2016.1112629

Karam, M., Brault, I., Van Durme, T., & Macq, J. (2018). Comparing interprofessional and interorganizational collaboration in health care: A systematic review of the qualitative research. *International Journal of Nursing Studies*, *79*, 70–83. https://doi.org/10.1016/j.ijnurstu.2017.11.002

National Academies of Sciences, Engineering Medicine. (2019). *Integrating social care into the delivery of health care: Moving upstream to improve the nation's health*. National Academies Press. http://www.ncbi.nlm.nih.gov/books/NBK552597/

National Association of Social Work. (2016). *Standards for social work practice in health care settings*. Retrieved from https://www.socialworkers.org/LinkClick.aspx?fileticket=fFnsRHX-4HE%3D&portalid=0

Nundy, S., Cooper, L. A., & Mate, K. S. (2022). The quintuple aim for health care improvement: A new imperative to advance health equity. *Journal of the American Medical Association*, *327*(6), 521–522. https://doi.org/10.1001/jama.2021.25181

Otis-Green, S., Jones, B., Zebrack, B., Kilburn, L., Altilio, T. A., & Ferrell, B. (2015). ExCEL in social work: Excellence in cancer education and leadership: An oncology social work response to the 2008 Institute of Medicine report. *Journal of Cancer Education*, *30*(3), 503–513. https://doi.org/10.1007/s13187-014-0717-8

Schapmire, T. J., Head, B. A., Furman, C. D., Jones, C., Peters, B., Shaw, M. A., Woggon, F., Ziegler, C., & Pfeifer, M. P. (2021). The interprofessional education exchange: The impact of a faculty development program in interprofessional palliative oncology education on trainee competencies, skills, and satisfaction. *Palliative Medicine Reports*, *2*(1), 1–9. https://doi.org/10.1089/pmr.2021.0045

Schapmire, T. J., Head, B. A., Nash, W. A., Yankeelov, P. A., Furman, C. D., Wright, B. R., Gopalraj, R., Gordon, B., Black, K. P., Jones, C., Hall-Faul, M., & Faul, A. C. (2018). Overcoming barriers to interprofessional education in gerontology: The interprofessional curriculum for the care of older adults. *Advances in Medical Education and Practice*, *9*, 109–118. https://doi.org/10.2147/AMEP.S149863

World Health Organization. (2010). *Framework for action on interprofessional education & collaborative practice*. Retrieved from http://www.who.int/hrh/resources/framework_action/en/index.html

28
Capturing the Contribution of International Oncology and Palliative Social Work

Geok Ling Lee and Cecilia Lai Wan Chan

Key Concepts

- Cultural sensitivity is essential to working with patients from different ethnic or religion backgrounds.
- A person-centered approach to patient care requires communication in the context of the cultural and religious background of patients and family members.
- The concept of suffering and pain and end-of-life care decisions is culturally contextualized, as illustrated by Chinese, Indian, and Muslim religious perspectives.
- Creative services and innovations by oncology and palliative social workers are being implemented in different parts of the world.

Keywords: autonomy, Buddhist/ism, Chinese, culturally safe care, communication, culture, decision-making, empowerment, end-of-life care, family orientation, Indian, Hindu/ism, Islam/Muslim, pain and suffering, palliative care, person-centered care, respect, rituals

An estimated 19.3 million new cancer cases and almost 10 million cancer deaths occurred worldwide in 2020. Of these, half of all new cancer cases and 58.3% of cancer deaths occurred in Asia (Sung et al., 2021). Asia's population consists of approximately 4.7 billion people, accounting for more than half of the world's population (7.9 billion) (World Population Review, n.d.). Yet, the practice of oncology and palliative social work is mainly based on the Western model of health care (Choong, 2015).

Geok Ling Lee and Cecilia Lai Wan Chan, *Capturing the Contribution of International Oncology and Palliative Social Work*
In: *Oncology and Palliative Social Work.* Edited by: Susan Hedlund, Bryan Miller, Grace Christ, and Carolyn Messner,
Oxford University Press. © Oxford University Press 2024. DOI: 10.1093/oso/9780197607299.003.0028

Hinduism, Islam, Buddhism, and Chinese traditional religions are the major religions practiced in Asia. Each of these religions prescribes unique teachings and has expectations about the rituals and practices that must occur for a person to have a good death. Interestingly, Indians, Malays, and Chinese are also three of the key immigrant groups to major cities of the world. The general ethos of palliative care is compassionate care, which includes safeguarding patients from excruciating pain and suffering through modern methods of pain control and management. However, the experiences of cancer patients, especially those at the advanced stages, and their end-of-life decisions are closely associated with their familiar cultural and religious practices. The much-emphasized dignified patient care, with the goal to honor and protect the dying and their surviving family, can only be conveyed by words and actions coherent with their worldviews and cultural, religious, and philosophical practices (Gustafson & Lazenby, 2019).

This chapter focuses on understanding pain and suffering and their relationship with end-of-life decisions, as well as life and death outlooks from the Asian cultural-religious perspectives. It also showcases culturally sensitive practices by oncology and palliative social workers in different parts of the world, all with the intention to deliver care that preserves dignity at the end of life. Taboos on discussing death-related issues, ambivalence about proper death preparation, support that can also feel like pressure from members of the immediate and extended families, and conflicts between traditional Eastern cultural practices and Western medical care are examples of topics around which oncology and palliative social workers should be mindful or discerning. By being aware of, curious about, and respectful of cultural differences, oncology and palliative social workers can contribute to fostering more peaceful deaths among the many various cultures of people of Asian descent.

The Concept of Pain and Suffering

A well-established approach to palliative and end-of-life care is Dame Cicely Saunders's "total pain" concept, which she defined as suffering that encompasses all aspects of a person's physical, psychological, social, and spiritual life (Mehta & Chan, 2008). One of the principles of palliative care is to manage pain using a total pain management perspective that aims to improve quality of life for patients and families. Yet, other cultural groups—for example, the Chinese—perceive the physical and mental aspects of pain and suffering as being "welded" to each other. In Chinese language and culture, the physical and mental aspects of pain and suffering are interrelated and not distinctively differentiated, which reflects the holistic concept of health prevalent in Asian societies (Lee et al., 2016).

In the second wave of positive psychology (PP 2.0), suffering is proposed as the necessary foundation for well-being, which can only be achieved through the dialectical process of dual-system (approach-avoidance system) model, or yin-yang interactions. Wong and Yu argue that suffering is an inevitable aspect of life, and that painful experiences have adaptive values that can help enhance one's resilience and meaning. Through the dual-system process, one has a higher chance of success of transforming suffering into well-being (Wong & Yu, 2021).

Religious Perspectives on Human Suffering and End-of-Life Care

The value of suffering in the form of pain associated with cancer can also be examined from the different perspectives of Asian-based religions, namely Buddhism, Islam, and Hinduism. People who practice these religions may not perceive suffering as a problem in need of alleviation. In fact, they may be quite distressed by the notion that their pain must be prevented or relieved because for them suffering is a fundamentally important element of lived human existence.

One's spiritual beliefs about suffering affect one's concept of appropriate end-of-life care. For example, Buddhists view pain and suffering as an intrinsic part of being alive and believe that the source of suffering lies within our subjective minds. To a Buddhist, suffering (e.g., enduring the pain of illness) provides an opportunity for one to contemplate the meaning of cyclical existence and to cultivate compassion for others' hardships. Generally, Buddhists tend to be psychologically prepared to accept impending death with calmness, peace, and dignity (Fitzpatrick et al., 2016).

Hindus believe suffering is the inevitable result of past actions—a combination of cosmic and moral cause and effect (also known as karma). Some Hindus welcome the endurance of pain as a way to ward off even more bad karma, which could intensify future suffering. Hindus are not fatalists, however; rather, they take responsibility for their actions and accept the resultant karma (Fitzpatrick et al., 2016). Belief in reincarnation may bring great comfort to dying patients and their surviving families as they know that their loved ones will be reborn into a new, possibly better life if they have accumulated good karma and atoned for bad karma. Thus, in end-of-life care, what may seem to be unnecessary endurance of pain to non-Hindu health professionals may in fact simply reflect a Hindu patient's determination to meet death with a clear and conscious mind to "pay" past "debts."

Muslims believe that suffering is divinely ordained, temporary, and has a purpose, such as an opportunity for repentance to avoid Allah's wrath and seek His approval (Choong, 2015). When a child dies from a life-threatening disease, Muslim parents can be as devastated as any other parents. However, they also believe that a child's death is a test of calamity from God that elicits two important Islamic themes: intercession and substitution. Intercession refers to "the ability of a person to plead for additional mercy and succor from God when judging a person's deeds and determining if they should go to heaven or hell" (Hedayat, 2006, p. 1286). This means that not only does a deceased child automatically receive entry to heaven as an innocent soul and without standing for judgment but so do the child's parents. Substitution refers to the bereaved parents who will be blessed by Allah with another virtuous child (Hedayat, 2006).

Culturally and Religiously Sensitive Social Work Practice in Oncology and Palliative Care

In the West, spirituality and religion are often defined as different but interrelated concepts. However, in Asian societies, religion is often embedded in spirituality. For example, in the Islamic context, "there is no spirituality without religious thoughts and practices, because religion provides the spiritual path for salvation and is regarded as a way of life" (Cheraghi et al., 2005, p. 474).

Among many Asian religions, sanctity of life supersedes quality of life because life originates from God or one's higher power. If end-of-life choices in palliative care are deemed as possible last opportunities to exercise self-determination and preserve human dignity, a dying Asian patient may weigh these choices equally as their last opportunity for repentance to avoid wrath and seek approval from their God or higher power (Engelhardt, 2012). In a way, people in Asian societies embrace dignity differently—for example, Chinese people believe in the human capacity to endure pain and in "the intrapsychic attributes of moral transcendence and spiritual surrender" (Ho et al., 2013, p. 460). If a person can endure the pain and suffering of a serious illness, then they may find a spiritual and moral development that seeks forgiveness, atones for one's sins, and purifies the soul. Depending on their religious background, this process can lead to eternal life or a good rebirth (Choong, 2015).

Muslims believe that health is a gift from Allah and that illness can only occur through Allah's will. An illness may be seen as a divinely ordained test and means to actualize Allah's plan, which is often intertwined with human experiences deemed necessary for one's spiritual development (Rouzati, 2018). Moreover, others are expected to care for the sick, especially a child, elderly parent, or spouse. When this happens in the end-of-life care context, the aim of caregiving is to encourage and support the dying person in cementing their relationship with Allah firmly before death (Choong, 2015). An essential virtue for a Muslim patient to have at the end of life is patience—an important theme in Islam (Hedayat, 2006). In the Islamic context, life is a journey through the embodied world, and death (which should not be hastened or shortened through assisted dying) is a journey through the spiritual world. Islamic faith counsels Muslim patients to bear tribulations with fortitude, to continue to praise Allah in both good and bad times, and to be patient while waiting for judgment day (Box 28.1).

Box 28.1

Mr. Ali was 65 years old when he received a diagnosis of end-stage lung cancer. He was initially shocked to learn of his illness, as his family had no history of cancer. As he reflected on the past and recognized the mischief he had gotten into in his younger years, he returned to Allah and his Islamic faith. Soon, he was able to accept his diagnosis, believing that Allah had given him the disease out of love and a desire to teach him the right values. Mrs. Ali, Mr. Ali's primary caregiver, also encouraged him not to fret about worldly matters but to be patient and focus on the afterlife. Seeking forgiveness, Mr. Ali prayed five times a day, thanking Allah for giving him a healthy body, for His goodness and greatness, for correcting his values, and for letting him die as a Muslim.

As his condition deteriorated, Mr. Ali prayed more diligently to obtain peace. He said his prayers to Allah whenever he could not sleep. Every morning upon awakening, he looked up at the sky and prayed, thanking Allah for keeping him alive. Every day, he switched on the television and watched religious talks.

Besides religious practice, Mr. Ali also tried to lead a life as normal as possible. He shopped with his wife, received visits from relatives and friends, participated in simple household chores, and spent quality time with his son. In sum, Mr. Ali worked hard to continue living while also accepting his diagnosis and waiting patiently for his death with the presence of family and social support.

Dying is also seen as a time for reflection for practicing Buddhists—the period in which one may engage in contemplating death as a means through which to grasp the impermanence of life. This time allows one to be closer to the Higher Power by engaging in religious activities such as prayers (mantra) or recitation of religious scriptures (sutra). As such, Buddhist patients may wish to practice mindfulness instead of focusing on their physical complaint. While there is no single way for an oncology or palliative care social worker to help every patient, they must take care to help patients achieve their preferred state of mind at end of life without compromising quality of life for either the patient or their family caregiver(s) (Box 28.2).

Box 28.2

Mrs. Ong was a 70-year-old patient with end-stage colon cancer admitted to an inpatient hospice. She was a practicing Buddhist who followed the teaching of Four Noble Truths. Remembering the first of these truths—"all existence is suffering"—Mrs. Ong refused to receive opioids even though her pain score was high at 7. She insisted on staying mindful of the pain and refused sedation. This created a sense of sadness and even anxiety in Mr. Ong, her husband and main caregiver. The situation was made worse when the medical team thought that Mr. Ong had prevented Mrs. Ong from receiving opioids. Upon learning about Mrs. Ong's religious practice, the palliative social worker intervened and encouraged Mrs. Ong to consider the Middle Path—another of Buddha's teachings—as a possible way to relieve suffering. The social worker quoted the sutra of a string instrument: if the string is too tight, it will break when struck; if the string is too loose, the music will sound unharmonious. However, if the string is neither tight nor loose, the music is the clearest. Upon hearing the story, Mrs. Ong agreed to receive opioids to reduce her pain score to 4. This enabled her to continue practicing mindfulness and simultaneously, reduced Mr. Ong's overwhelming concern for his wife.

Palliative and end-of-life care philosophy aligns well with Hindu values, which hold that death is part of life and should be neither prolonged nor hastened. A dying Hindu patient may feel the need to alleviate his past karma by resolving conflicts (e.g., seeking forgiveness), fulfilling all known responsibilities (e.g., as a son, husband, or father), fasting, repenting through religious ceremonies, making sacrifices (e.g., shaving one's head), performing good deeds or donating money to charitable causes, making pilgrimages, or enduring pain even when pain medication is available (Thrane, 2010). Participating in the abovementioned activities can be critical for patients' spiritual well-being, but the ability to do so is largely dependent on the place of care and the patient's physical condition. Because Asian societies remain as collective entities generally, family members almost always play an active and crucial role in decision-making, particularly when it comes to medical and treatment decisions. Even though a particular patient is seriously ill, they still reside within a wider network of family relationships. For example, in an Indian Hindu family, a senior male family member is seen as the head figure (or even "god") of the family and primary decision-maker. Thus, a wife will listen to a husband and a widowed mother will listen to the eldest son. As such, creating opportunities and assisting the patient and family to complete prayers, repentance, or other religious ceremonies at home will be very helpful (Box 28.3).

Box 28.3

Mr. Shiva was an 80-year-old Hindu man with end-stage liver cancer, a widower with two children and four grandchildren. He received a terminal discharge as he saw artificial prolongation of life (e.g., intubation) as interfering with karma.

Once Mr. Shiva returned home, he was visited by relatives who sought forgiveness or to resolve conflicts. Even though Mr. Shiva was prescribed with fentanyl patch for pain relief, he insisted on bearing the pain to "pay for" his past bad deeds. Family members assisted Mr. Shiva in performing religious ceremonies, saying prayers, and doing penance for his spiritual well-being.

At his deathbed, Mr. Shiva was surrounded by family members and relatives who sang sacred hymns and chanted mantra. A temple priest came to perform religious ceremonies and prayers. Holy ash was applied to Mr. Shiva's forehead, and a tulsi leaf and few drops of sacred water were placed in the mouth for purity and a peaceful transition to another new life.

After his death, all the deities' pictures were turned to face the wall. Mr. Shiva's body was in turn placed in the home's hall with the head facing south, indicating a return to the Mother Earth. Mr. Shiva's eldest son then led and performed ritual bathing and dressing with the temple priests' assistance. Relatives and friends said their last farewells to Mr. Shiva before the body was sent for cremation. The sending off was performed only by the male family members.

Among Hindus, the period immediately following death (which may last up to a year) is seen as a period of impurity. During this time, Mr. Shiva's surviving family was supported by and received food from the community. They also refrained from participating in festivals or celebrations and did not visit the temple.

Added Challenges in End-of-Life Care During the Pandemic

Since the onset of COVID-19, many countries across the globe have experienced third and fourth waves of the disease, and some countries have even faced a fifth wave. By May 2022, the world had recorded over 520 million cases and more than 6 million deaths (Worldometer, n.d.). The COVID-19 pandemic brought to oncological and palliative social work not only an unprecedented global health crisis but also an unmatched challenge.

COVID-19 health care policies and protocols meant to keep staff, patients, and families safe from the disease have greatly changed the way providers approach oncological and palliative social work. For example, infection control measures and social distancing have restricted and even prohibited family visits at hospitals, hospices, and nursing homes. In turn, this has prevented the presence of loved ones during a person's final hours or at the moment of death. The idea of a loved one dying alone may produce fears of the patient not being cared for, suffering due to physical or existential pains, and being treated as a "number" (Yardley & Rolph, 2020). The one or two nominated family members who are allowed to visit the dying patient in hospital or hospice may themselves have to be socially isolated and subsequently unable to attend the physical funeral. The principles of providing dignified care and death are disrupted, added with the absence of cultural practices and significance of dying during the end of life. For many, praying, hugging, kissing, saying "good-bye," or even simply being present is not possible.

During such trying periods, social workers can model best-practice psychosocial care or even guide ethically difficult situations for dying patients and their family members by facilitating communications among them and seeking an understanding of all the perspectives they bring to the table. For example, a social worker can provide comfort, reduce distress, and help a patient and their relatives prepare for end of life by involving them in a discussion and decision-making using a culturally appropriate approach through an online platform. Doing so can empower the family in decision-making that is culturally safe and may prevent family members from feeling unprepared for death, which studies have shown to be associated with higher levels of complicated grief after the patient dies (Hebert et al., 2006). By adopting a compassionate approach, social workers can also support and accept without judgment difficult decisions made by the family. In essence, social workers should accommodate and even encourage a patient and their family to engage in culturally or religiously significant practices so long as they do not directly undermine medical care plans or health care policies. Doing so, is as integral to the delivery of high-quality, patient-centered care as the administering of chemotherapy, radiation, or surgical procedures.

During COVID, many families were forced to hold remote or severely restricted in-person celebration of life events, funerals, memorials, and burials. Complicated grief, secondary traumatic stress, guilt, and even moral distress can emerge if bereaved families lack access to the social networks that would normally support them during these important grieving and celebratory transition rituals. COVID-19 has forced social workers to be creative in developing culturally appropriate and personalized rituals to support family members in celebrating the life of their loved one and reducing the impact of their circumstances of death. One example is to host an online *puja* (ceremonial worship) for a Hindu family where guests can join the family in singing, praying, and lighting incense at the funeral. However, social workers should follow up with and support the bereaved family at the next contact since the emotions and reactions that may arise after a video call are unknown.

Death may be a universal endpoint, but beliefs and practices surrounding how people respond to and interact with the dying process, the death event, and what happens to the body after death vary across cultural and religious contexts. Cultures have uniquely ritualized expressions of grief and understandings of bereavement. Practicing person-centered holistic care and empowerment of patients requires one to take cultural-religious practices into consideration. Oncological and palliative social workers thus need to be aware of cross-cultural and cross-religious sensitivity care provision when patients and their families are facing the host of challenges that life-threatening diseases create (not to mention the grief surrounding the impending death of a loved one) and when they are at their most vulnerable. Culturally safe care is particularly critical when a dying patient and their family members come from cultural or religious groups with unique cultural and religious needs. Oncological and palliative social workers must understand and respect cultural and religious differences around disease, death, and dying and foster the ability of each patient and their family to receive care that preserves not only the patient's but their family members' dignity at the end of life.

Guiding Best Practices for the Future

Social workers must always try to understand pain, suffering, and end-of-life decisions from the cultural-religious perspectives of patients and their families. In Asian societies, suffering may not be seen as a problem in need of eradication but an inevitable aspect of life that contributes in positive ways to one's moral and spiritual developments. To provide care that truly honors and protects dying patients and their surviving families, one needs to meet the client where they are—that is, to think, feel, and act with respect toward the cultural-religious philosophical beliefs and practices of the dying patients and their families.

Pearls

- Religious and cultural beliefs have a significant influence on patients' lives, especially during the dying process. Therefore, cultural competency is essential to social work practice.
- Cultural competency and patient-centered care is best achieved when a social worker has a basic understanding of (or willingness to learn) and genuine respect for the rituals and customs of major world religions.
- Culturally safe care requires recognizing the spiritual and religious needs of a dying patient and their larger family.
- Many cultures and religions maintain the primacy of sanctity of life over quantity or quality of life.

Pitfalls

- Focusing too much on cultural or religious practices without acknowledging the uniqueness of each individual may limit professional practice. Oncological and palliative social workers must approach every patient and family as unique rather than assume they will follow a set "checklist" of cultural or religious practices attributed to their culture and religion.
- Harm may occur if social workers are unaware of their own cultural and religious beliefs and neglect to consider how their personal subject position might influence their interactions with patients from differing cultural or religious groups.

Additional Resources

Readings

Ho, R. T. H., Wan, A. H. Y., Chan, J. S. M., Ng, S. M., Chung, K. F., & Chan, C. L. W. (2017). Study protocol on comparative effectiveness of mindfulness meditation and qigong on the psychophysiological outcomes of patients with colorectal cancer: A randomized controlled trial. *BMC Complementary and Alternative Medicine*, *17*(1), 390–397. https://doi.org/10.1186/s12906-017-1898-6

Lau, B. H.-P., Chow, A. M. Y., Ng, T.-K., Fung, Y.-L., Lam, T.-C., So, T.-H., Chan, J. S. M., Chan, C. H. Y., Zhou, J., Tam, M. Y. J., Tsang, M.-W., Cheng, N. S. Y., Lim, P. F. M., Chow, S.-F., Chan, C. L. W., & Wong, D. F. K. (2020). Comparing the efficacy of integrative body-mind-spirit intervention with cognitive behavioural therapy in patient-caregiver parallel groups for lung cancer patients using a randomized controlled trial. *Journal of Psychosocial Oncology*, *38*(4), 389–405. https://doi.org/10.1080/07347332.2020.1722981

Xiu, D., Fung, Y.-L., Lau, B. H.-P., Wong, D. F. K., Chan, C. H. Y., Ho, R. T. H., So, T.-H., Lam, T.-C., Lee, V. H.-F., Lee, A. W. M., Chow, S.-F., Lim, F. M., Tsang, M. W., Chan, C. L. W., & Chow, A. Y. M. (2020). Comparing dyadic cognitive behavioral therapy (CBT) with dyadic integrative body-mind-spirit intervention (I-BMS) for Chinese family caregivers of lung cancer patients: A randomized controlled trial. *Supportive Care in Cancer*, *28*, 1523–1533. https://doi.org/10.1007/s00520-019-04974-z

Websites

Chan, I. K. N., Fong, C. H. C., Wong, E. Y. W., Lou, V. W. Q., & Chan, C. L. W. (Eds.). (2019). *Innovation. Impact: The foundation of community-based end-of-life care in Hong Kong*. Jockey Club End-of-life Community Care Project. http://www.socsc.hku.hk/JCECC/case_book/HKU_SS_JCECC_book.pdf

Crossroads Hospice and Palliative Care. (2015, December 30). The culture connection: Hindu end-of-life practices. *Healthcare Professionals Blog*. https://www.crossroadshospice.com/hospice-palliative-care-blog/2015/december/30/the-culture-connection-hindu-end-of-life-practices-healthcare-professionals-blog/

Sultan, M. (2017, November 13). Pulling the plug: The Islamic perspectives on end-of-life care. *Nature and Science/Health*. https://yaqeeninstitute.org/read/paper/pulling-the-plug-the-islamic-perspectives-on-end-of-life-care

References

Cheraghi, M. A., Payne, S., & Salsali, M. (2005). Spiritual aspects of end-of-life care for Muslim patients: Experiences from Iran. *International Journal of Palliative Nursing*, *11*(9), 468–474. https://doi.org/10.12968/ijpn.2005.11.9.19781

Choong, K. A. (2015). Islam and palliative care. *Global Bioethics*, *26*(1), 28–42. https://doi.org/10.1080/11287462.2015.1008752

Engelhardt, H. T. (2012). Suffering, dying, and death: Palliative care ethics "after God." *European Journal of Science and Theology*, *8*(2), 5–13.

Fitzpatrick, S. J., Kerridge, I. H., Jordens, C. F. C., Zoloth, L., Tollefsen, C., Tsomo, K. L., Jensen, M. P., Sachedina, A., & Sarma, D. (2016). Religious perspectives on human suffering: Implications for medicine and bioethics. *Journal of Religion and Health*, *55*, 159–173. https://doi.org/10.1007/s10943-015-0014-9

Gustafson, C., & Lazenby, M. (2019). Assessing the unique experiences and needs of Muslim oncology patients receiving palliative and end-of-life care: An integrative review. *Journal of Palliative Care*, *34*(1), 52–61. https://doi.org/10.1177/0825859718800496

Hebert, R. S., Dang, Q., & Schulz, R. (2006). Preparedness for the death of a loved one and mental health in bereaved caregivers of patients with dementia: Findings from the REACH study. *Journal of Palliative Medicine*, *9*, 683–693. https://doi.org/10.1089/jpm.2006.9.683

Hedayat, K. (2006). When the spirit leaves: Childhood death, grieving, and bereavement in Islam. *Journal of Palliative Medicine*, *9*(6), 1282–1291. https://doi.org/10.1089/jpm.2006.9.1282

Ho, A. H. Y., Chan, C. L. W., Leung, P. P. Y., Chochinov, H. M., Neimeyer, R. A., Pang, S. M. C., & Tse, D. M. W. (2013). Living and dying with dignity in Chinese society: Perspectives of older palliative care patients in Hong Kong. *Age and Ageing*, *42*(4), 455–461. https://doi.org/10.1093/ageing/aft003

Lee, G. L., Pang, G. S. Y., Akhileswaran, R., Ow, M. Y. L., Fan, G. K. T., Wong, C. F., Wee, H. L., & Cheung, Y. B. (2016). Understanding domains of health-related quality-of-life concerns of Singapore Chinese patients with advanced cancer: A qualitative analysis. *Supportive Care in Cancer*, *24*(3), 1107–1118. https://doi.org/10.1007/s00520-015-2886-3

Mehta, A., & Chan, L. S. (2008). Understanding of the concept of "total pain": A prerequisite for pain control. *Journal of Hospice and Palliative Nursing*, *10*(1), 26–32. https://nursing.ceconnection.com/ovidfiles/00129191-200801000-00008.pdf

Rouzati, N. (2018). Evil and human suffering in Islamic thought: Toward a mystical theodicy. *Religions*, *9*(2), 47. https://doi.org/10.3390/rel9020047

Sung, H., Ferlay, J., Siegel, R. L., Laversanne, M., Soerjomataram, I., Jemal, A., & Bray, F. (2021). Global cancer statistics 2020: GLOBOCAN estimates of incidence and mortality worldwide for 36 cancers in 185 countries. *CA: A Cancer Journal for Clinicians*, *71*, 209–249. https://doi.org/10.3322/caac.21660

Thrane, S. (2010). Hindu end of life: Death, dying, suffering, and karma. *Journal of Hospice and Palliative Nursing*, *12*(6), 337–342. https://nursing.ceconnection.com/ovidfiles/00129191-201011000-00003.pdf

Wong, P. T. P., & Yu, T. T. F. (2021, September 1). Existential suffering in palliative care: An existential positive psychology perspective. *Medicina*, *57*(9), 924. https://doi.org/10.3390/medicina57090924

Worldometer. (n.d.). *COVID-19 coronavirus pandemics*. Retrieved May 18, 2022, from https://www.worldometers.info/coronavirus/

World Population Review. (n.d.). *Asia population 2022*. Retrieved May 16, 2022, from https://worldpopulationreview.com/continents/asia-population

Yardley, S., & Rolph, M. (2020). Death and dying during the pandemic. *BMJ*, *369*, m1472. https://doi.org/10.1136/bmj.m1472

Epilogue

Oncology Social Work Leadership: Innovators in a Changing World

Susan Hedlund, Bryan Miller, Grace Christ, and Carolyn Messner

> For all of us both hurting & healing who choose to carry on.
>
> **(Gorman, 2021, p. v)**

Innovation

Throughout this book, we have attempted to emphasize the value of early integration of palliative care principles into routine cancer care. Early integrated palliative care improves quality of life and is recognized by oncologists as a standard of cancer care for all patients. However, not all patients have the same access to palliative care, particularly outside the hospital setting. As there are not enough palliative care specialists in the United States, there is currently a movement to train all clinicians in "primary palliative care," intended to align with patient preferences and whole-person care.

Resilience

Living in and practicing during the pandemic reinforced the need for earlier integration of palliative care principles into standard cancer care. The pandemic further revealed the enormous disparities in care that continue to exist for our vulnerable populations. A long-standing history of systemic racism in health care and provider bias are significant problems that all oncology and palliative social workers should work to eliminate. Understanding our own biases and creating partnerships within communities of color or other underserved populations and agencies who work with the most vulnerable should

Susan Hedlund, Bryan Miller, Grace Christ, and Carolyn Messner, *Epilogue* In: *Oncology and Palliative Social Work*. Edited by: Susan Hedlund, Bryan Miller, Grace Christ, and Carolyn Messner, Oxford University Press.
DOI: 10.1093/oso/9780197607299.003.0029

be priorities for health care systems moving forward. Many professional organizations are prioritizing strategies of outreach for health equity. Together, it is imperative to share our collective wisdom and energy to change access to health care nationally, while also prioritizing the health and well-being of the health care workforce.

Creativity

In many ways, as we find ourselves at the end of the COVID-19 public health emergency, oncology and palliative social workers are in uncharted territory. We don't know what to expect or what lies ahead in our health care systems or in our world. Innovations in care are evolving, and as our patients experience new approaches to treatment (including the growing prevalence of oral medications to treat cancer), we must work to evolve systems of support to help patients and their loved ones navigate care. For those who are more vulnerable and/or for whom English is not their first language, it will be crucial to develop services that are responsive to their specific needs.

Hope

As we write this epilogue, we reflect on how the "trifecta" of COVID-19, the flu, and the respiratory syncytial virus occurring simultaneously stressed an already distressed health care system. Many people chose to leave the health care workforce during the pandemic, and those left behind are experiencing greater stress and job dissatisfaction. How do we take care of the workforce and one another during these times? Strategies such as psychological first aid and employee wellness initiatives are important first steps. As we anticipate the "silver tsunami" of an aging population combined with the growing challenges of workforce shortages and the rising cost of cancer care, more than ever, oncology and palliative social work perspectives will be needed. Teaching and mentoring the next generation of oncology and palliative social workers will be vital. Using research to guide best practices and fostering the growth of creative leadership will help ensure that oncology social workers continue to have a seat at the table to promote strategies of equity, inclusiveness, and affirming patient-centered care.

Many have suggested that the times we are in are "unprecedented." At the same time, we are watching resilience, adaptability, and innovation evolve, and oncology and palliative social workers are at the heart of these endeavors.

We hope the ideas offered in this book will encourage you to reflect, to grow, and to carry on. Thank you, for all you do for our patients and those who love them.

Reference

Gorman, A. (2021). *The miracle of morning: Call us what we carry*. Viking.

Index

For the benefit of digital users, indexed terms that span two pages (e.g., 52–53) may, on occasion, appear on only one of those pages.

Tables, figures, and boxes are indicated by *t*, *f*, and *b* following the page number

AAMC (Association of American Medical Colleges), 43, 391
Abrams, Ruth, 8–9
academic training programs, 323–26
Academy of Oncologic Physical Therapy, 79
acceptance and commitment therapy (ACT), 111, 116–17, 131–32, 207*t*
access to care, 12–13, 36, 219, 302–3
  case studies, 303*b*
  during COVID-19, 311–12
access to information, 113–14
accountability, 40
Accountability for Cancer Care Through Undoing Racism and Equity (ACCURE) project, 104–5
accreditation, 326–27, 332
ACCURE (Accountability for Cancer Care Through Undoing Racism and Equity) project, 104–5
ACHP-SW (Advanced Certified Hospice and Palliative Social Work) certification, 342–43, 348–49
ACS. *See* American Cancer Society
ACT (acceptance and commitment therapy), 111, 116–17, 131–32, 207*t*
action alerts, 306
activities of daily living (ADLs), 216
acute cancer pain syndromes, 126
ADA (Americans with Disabilities Act), 230–31
adaptation
  for children, adolescents, and young adults, 242*t*
  as a way of life during COVID-19, 363–64
ADEI (antiracism, diversity, equity, and inclusion), 325, 326
adjustment disorders, 10–11, 100–1
ADLs (activities of daily living), 216
adolescents and young adults (AYAs), 240–48
  best practices for work with, 256–58
  case studies, 241, 256
  developmental issues, 242*t*, 252–53
  end-of-life conversations, 253–55
  facts and figures, 248
  interventions for, 282*t*
  medical care for, 251
  practice models for work with, 282*t*
  questions, 251*t*
  reflections on working with, 255
  resources for, 259
  special programs for, 250
  support networks for, 248–50
  survivorship, 253
Adriamycin, 75
adults
  middle age, 227–39
  older, 215–26
  patients with children and teenagers, 229–30, 230*b*
  sandwich generation, 230
  young, 240–60
advance care planning, 185–86
  case studies, 298*b*
  for LGBTQI persons, 271
Advanced Certificate of Oncology Social Work Practice (University of Pennsylvania), 328*t*, 345–46
Advanced Certified Hospice and Palliative Social Work (ACHP-SW) certification, 342–43, 348–49
advance directives, 294
Advanced Palliative Care and Hospice Social Work Certification (APHSW-C), 343–45, 348–49
advocacy, 100–1, 301, 304–6, 332–33, 386
  developing our voice, 374

advocacy (*cont.*)
- ethical issues, 306
- finding our voice, 389–91
- history of, 304–5
- legal issues, 306
- social work, 304–5
- strategies for finding our voice, 390
- ways to engage in, 305–6

affirming care environments, 263–64
affirming communication, 265–66, 265*t*
Affordable Care Act, 12–13
African Americans. *See* Black people/African Americans
ageism, 217
agnosticism, 269
Alameda County Care Alliance (California), 87
Alaska Native Tribal Health Consortium, 86
Alex's Lemonade Stand Foundation for Childhood Cancer, 259
alignment, 100–1
allyship, 78
alternative therapy, 89–90
ambulance agencies, 85–86
ambulatory care, 8
Amedisys, 83
American Academy of Hospice and Palliative Medicine, 187, 305
American Academy of Social Work and Social Welfare, 51–52
American Association for Cancer Research, 381
American Association for Respiratory Care, 391
American Association of Colleges of Nursing, 391
American Association of Colleges of Pharmacy, 391
American Cancer Society (ACS), 10, 117, 331–32
- cancer-related information, 113
- resources, 54, 66, 238, 367

American Cancer Society Cancer Action Network, 305
American Childhood Cancer Organization, 259
American College of Surgeons, 9–10, 25, 98, 331
American Council of Academic Physical Therapy, 391
American Dental Education Association, 391
American Hospital Association, 319
American Indians/Alaska Natives, 276
- cancer health disparities, 33
- COVID-19 case rates and mortality, 311
- social workers, 324–26
- U.S. population, 277–78

American Journal of Bioethics, 307
American Medical Association (AMA), 317, 319
American Occupational Therapy Association, 391
American Psychological Association, 391
American Psychosocial Oncology Society (APOS), 117, 331
- opportunities for professional development, 328*t*, 335
- resources, 119
- website, 337

American Public Health Association, 315
American Society of Clinical Oncology (ASCO), 187, 219
- Commission on Cancer, 341–42
- guidelines for best practices, 183–84, 219
- guidelines for depression, 131–32
- guidelines for palliative care, 184
- Policy Statement on Cancer Care Disparities, 34
- resources, 54, 119, 367
- vision for access to palliative care, 302

American Society of Preventive Oncology, 337
American Speech-Language-Hearing Association, 391
Americans with Disabilities Act (ADA), 230–31
anchor institutions, 100–1
anger/irritability, 199*t*, 200
anorgasmia, 132
anticipatory grief, 195–97
antiemetics, 132
antihistaminergic medications, 132
antiracism, 347–48
antiracism, diversity, equity, and inclusion (ADEI), 325, 326
anxiety, 10–11, 111, 132, 248
- evidence-based therapies for, 116–17
- in grief, 199*t*, 200

AOSW. *See* Association of Oncology Social Work
APHSW-C (Advanced Palliative Care and Hospice Social Work Certification), 343–45, 348–49

APOS. *See* American Psychosocial Oncology Society
APOSW (Association of Pediatric Oncology Social Work), 328*t*, 337
Ariadne Labs, 192
aromatase inhibitors, 75
ASCO. *See* American Society of Clinical Oncology
Asia, 397
Asian religions, 400, 405–6
Asians/Asian Americans, 276
  cancer health disparities, 33
  case studies, 287, 330–31
  COVID-19 case rates and mortality, 311, 316
  social workers, 324–26, 330–31
  U.S. population, 278
assessment
  of bereft individuals, 199–205
  biopsychosocial, 114
  biopsychosocial-spiritual, 127–28, 154, 159*b*
  cultural, 204–5
  geriatric assessment (GA), 217
  as intervention, 114–15
  of older adults, 219–20
  pain, 127–28
  in palliative care, 219–20
  physical/somatic, 199–200
  psychological/relational, 200–2
  social/societal, 202–3
  spiritual, 157–58, 204
  spirituality-focused questions, 158*b*
assistance, 100–1
Association of American Medical Colleges (AAMC), 43, 391
Association of Community Cancer Centers, 337
Association of Oncology Social Work (AOSW), 34, 117, 305, 306, 325–26, 331, 340
  certification, 341–42
  membership, 378–79
  opportunities for professional development, 328*t*, 331, 335
  resources, 119, 307, 349
  Scope and Standards of Practice, 322, 327
  Social Work Oncology Research Group, 332
  website, 290, 337
Association of Pediatric Oncology Social Work (APOSW), 328*t*, 337
atezolizumab, 20–21
atheism, 269
attachment theory, 198
autonomy, 297*b*
  at end of life, 364–66
  respect for, 296–98
Awake to Woke to Work model (Equity in the Center), 40
awareness, 100–1, 185–86
AYAs. *See* adolescents and young adults
Ayurvedic medicine, 74

bachelor of social work (BSW) degree, 324–25
Beatson, George Thomas, 18–19
Bendheim Integrative Medicine Center (Memorial Sloan Kettering), 89–90
beneficence, 297*b*, 298–99
benzodiazepines (BZDs), 132
bereavement
  assessment of, 199–205
  definition of, 195–96
  examples, 200, 201, 203, 204
  spirituality in, 204
  theoretical models of, 197–98
bereavement care, 195–200
  best practices for, 208–9
  examples, 205
  interventions, 205–8, 207*t*, 235–36
  for middle-aged adults, 235–36
  resources, 209
  self-care strategies, 206
bereavement groups, 204–5, 206–8
best practices
  for affirming communication, 265–66
  for bereavement care, 208–9
  for cancer care for middle-aged adults, 236–37
  for cancer care for older adults, 223–24
  for end-of-life care, 191–92
  for ethical and legal issues, 306–7
  for the future, 64–66
  guidelines for, 183–84
  guiding, 12–14, 27–28, 40, 52–54, 78–79, 90–91, 106–7, 136–37, 151–52, 162–64, 175–77, 191–92, 208–9, 223–24, 236–37, 256–58, 272–73, 287–89, 288*f*, 306–7, 318–19, 335–37, 347–49, 366–67, 379–81, 394–95
  for informal caregivers, 175–77
  for integrating cultural humility, 40

best practices (*cont.*)
for leadership development, 379–81
for mitigating negative social determinants of health (SDOH) impacts, 52–54
for pain, symptom, and toxicity management, 136–37
for palliative care, 183–84
for palliative care for LGBTQI persons, 272–73
for spiritual care, 162–64
for working with children and AYAs, 256–58
for working with multicultural groups, 287–89, 288*f*
bias
implicit, 103, 325, 377*b*, 377
provider, xxi
bile duct cancer, 33
biomedicine
challenges, 88–90
conventional, 88–90
ethical principles and theory, 296
Western worldview toward palliative care, 278–79
biopsychosocial assessment, initial, 114
biopsychosocial-spiritual assessment, 127–28, 154, 159*b*
Black, Indigenous, people of color (BIPOC), 216, 276–77
Black Lives Matter, 358
Black people/African Americans, 276
breast cancer survivors, 76–77
cancer care for, 62–63, 223*b*
cancer-related health disparities, 32–33, 60
case studies, 222*b*, 223*b*, 235–36
COVID-19, 218, 221, 311, 316
end-of-life care for, 203
faith-based programs for, 87
health disparities, 32–33, 60
hospice care for, 223*b*
LGBTQI, 265–66
medical mistrust, 221–23, 222*b*
oncology social workers (OSWs), 325–26, 378–79
palliative care for, 217, 220–21
racism against, 62–63 (*see also* racism)
social workers, 324–25
social work perspective, 218
underserved populations, 187
U.S. population, 277–78
Bladder Cancer Advocacy Network, 361
Board of Oncology Social Work (BOSW) Certification, 334, 337, 341–42, 345, 348–49
body image, 228, 252
bone marrow transplants, 5
Bo's Place, 259
BOSW (Board of Oncology Social Work) Certification, 334, 337, 341–42, 348–49
BRAF/MEK/MAP kinase, 19
breakthrough pain, 126
breast cancer
case studies, 75, 124, 168–69, 223*b*, 235–36, 284, 357
inequities in incidence specific to race, ethnicity, and demographics, 33
informal caregivers for people with, 168–69
social determinants of health (SDOH) and, 49–50
targeted therapy for, 18–20
Bridge model, 143–44, 144*f*
Brief FOCUS Program, 176*t*
Bright IDEAS: Problem-Solving Skills Training, 176*t*
BSW (bachelor of social work) degree, 324–25
Buddhism, 269, 398, 399, 402*b*, 402
burnout, 303–4, 309
BZDs (benzodiazepines), 132

cachexia, 129–31
California State University, 336
campaigns, letter-writing, 303*b*, 305
Camp Kesem, 230*b*
Canada, 85
cancer, 3, 4
accepting and adapting as a way of life, 363–64
advanced, 185
as biopsychosocial illness, 119
case studies, 111, 149
as chronic disease, 17–18
diagnosis of, 4–5
as dread disease, 359
financial toxicity of, 11
in middle age, 227–39
older persons with, 215–26
palliative care experiences in, 49
physical symptoms of, 125–26
prevalence of, 3–4
prevention of, 48–49

psychosocial aspects of, 110–22, 228–33
psychosocial needs in, 10–11
symptoms associated with, 129–34
Cancer Alley, 104
Cancer and Aging Research Group, 217
Cancer and Careers, 238
Cancer and Mental Health Collaborative, 152
cancer care
for adolescents and young adults (AYAs), 251
best practices for, 223–24
case history, 13
case studies, 386, 387
collaborative care, 143–44
in COVID-19, xxi, 13
disparities in, 12–13, 279–80, 280*f*
ethical issues, 302
highlights from Mumbai, 361-66
inequities in, 143
interprofessional spiritual care, 154–66
interventions, 362–63
leadership challenges and opportunities, 373
for middle-aged adults, 233–36
for older adults, 217, 223–24
on-the-job training in, 363
overview, 3–16
in pandemics, disasters, and other traumatic events, xxi, 57–68
for people with serious mental illness (SMI), 143–44
Policy Statement on Cancer Care Disparities (ASCO), 34
psychosocial care, 361-66
psychosocial support services, 302
racism in, 62–64
social determinants of health (SDOH) outcomes in, 62–63
symptoms after, 70–71
team-based, 14
treatment landscape, 17–31
treatment options, 4, 5–8
vectors of, 356–58
Cancer*Care,* 10, 117
cancer-related information, 113
resources, 79, 119, 238, 259, 367
website, 230*b*, 337
Cancer Care for the Whole Person: Meeting Psychosocial Health Needs (IoM), 9
cancer caregivers. *See also* caregivers
informal, 167–80
cancer detection, 48–49
cancer-directed therapy
ethical issues, 300–1
toxicities, 134–35
Cancer Family Caregiving Experience, 172*t*
Cancer.gov, 79
cancer health disparities, 32–37
Cancer Health Equity Institute (CHEI), Morehouse School of Medicine 66
Cancer Legal Resource Center, 238
Cancer.Net, 337
cancer pain, 125–26
cancer pain syndromes, 126
cancer-related health disparities, 45–56
cancer support. *See* cancer care
Cancer Support Community, 117
resources, 28, 79, 230*b*, 238, 367
website, 337
cancer vaccines, 20–22
Cannon, Ida, 98–99
CAPC. *See* Center to Advance Palliative Care
CARE (Caregiver Advise Record Enable) Act, 175–77
caregivers, 169
case vignette, 168
of children with cancer, 251*t*
guided questions to ask, 168
helpful questions to ask, 148–49
informal, 167–80
involvement in care, 100
in middle adulthood, 229
of people with serious mental illness (SMI) and cancer, 147–48
psychosocial support for, 170
questions of, 251*t*
social work role with, 129
support for, 100, 170
Caregiver Speaks, 176*t*
caregiving, 169–71
competencies in, for clinicians, 171
conceptual frameworks related to, 172*t*
general principles of social work related to, 169–70
hours of care per week, 168, 169
interprofessional competencies, 171
interventions for related psychosocial issues, 174–75, 176*t*
positive aspects, 173–74
principles and foundations of, 171–72
psychosocial assessments of, 174
psychosocial challenges, 172–73

Caring Bridge, 238
CAR-T cells (chimeric antigen receptor T cells), 7–8, 20–22
case history, 13
case studies
  from COVID-19 pandemic, 364, 365
  end-of-life care, 189, 190, 401*b*–3*b*
  hospice care, 189, 190, 224*b*, 402*b*
  in interprofessional collaboration, 386–88
  medical mistrust, 222*b*
  older adults, 223*b*
CBT. *See* cognitive-behavioral therapy
CDC. *See* Centers for Disease Control and Prevention
Cedars-Sinai Health System, 84
cellular immunotherapy, 7–8
Center for Spirituality, Theology, and Health, 164
Centers for Disease Control and Prevention (CDC), 43, 79, 104–5
Centers for Medicare and Medicaid Services (CMS)
  Accountable Health Communities Health-Related Social Needs Screening Tool, 107
  accreditation, 332
  resources, 92, 107
Center to Advance Palliative Care (CAPC)
  resources, 28, 87, 91, 137, 192, 259
  Social Work Serious Illness Designation Foundational Skills, 137
certification, 340, 344–46
  Advanced Certificate of Oncology Social Work Practice (University of Pennsylvania), 328*t*, 345–46
  Advanced Certified Hospice and Palliative Social Work (ACHP-SW), 342–43, 348–49
  Advanced Palliative Care and Hospice Social Work Certification (APHSW-C), 343–45, 348–49
  best practices for, 347–49
  Board of Oncology Social Work (BOSW) Certification, 334, 337, 341–42, 345, 348–49
  Oncology Social Work Certificate, 341–42
  Online Post-Master's Certificate Program (New York University), 345–46
  opportunities for, 327*t*
  Palliative/End-of-Life Care Certificate (Smith College School of School Work), 327*t*, 336, 371, 381
  Post-MSW Palliative Care Social Work Certificate Program (California State University), 336
cervical cancer, 33
chemotherapy, 6–7
  case studies, 75, 387
  side effects, 134
chemotherapy-induced peripheral neuropathy, 126
chemotherapy toxicity calculator (Cancer and Aging Research Group), 217
chemsex, 262–63
children
  best practices for work with, 256–58
  case studies, 241, 249, 387–88
  developmental issues, 242*t*, 252–53
  end-of-life conversations, 253–55
  facts and figures, 248
  interventions for, 282*t*
  pain assessment tools for, 128
  practice models for working with, 282*t*
  questions of parents/caregivers of, 251*t*
  reflections on working with, 255
  resources for, 259
  special programs for, 250
  support networks for, 248–50
  survivorship, 253
  symptom management for, 133–34
  websites for patients with, 230*b*
Children's Oncology Camping Association, International, 259
Children's Oncology Group (COG), 251
Children's Treehouse Foundation, 230*b*
chimeric antigen receptor T cells (CAR-T cells), 7–8, 20–22
Chinese, 398–99, 400
Christianity, 269
chronic cancer pain syndromes, 126
chronic disease, 17–18
chronic myelogenous leukemia, 19
chronic stress, 35–36
client meetings, initial, 114
clinical cases, 75, 124
clinical depression, 110–11, 112
clinical interventions, 116–17
  self-exploration of one's own spirituality, 160–61
  spiritual care, 159–60
clinical practice
  case studies, 111, 149
  implicit bias, 103

innovations, 87–90
issues and interventions, 95–211
leadership, 375–76
Clinical Practice Guidelines for Quality Palliative Care (National Consensus Project [NCP] for Quality Palliative Care [NCP]), 205
clinical trials, 7
clinicians
competencies in caregiving, 171
ethical issues, 296–300
closed-captioning, 361
coaching, health and wellness, 77–78
COC (Commission on Cancer), 9–10, 11, 98
Code of Ethics (NASW), 41–42, 57, 62–63, 64, 170, 277, 295, 296–97, 306–7, 322, 326–27, 332
cognitive-behavioral therapy (CBT), 111, 116–17
for anxiety, 132
for depression, 131–32
for middle-aged cancer patients, 233–34
for prolonged grief disorder (PGD), 207*t*, 208
spiritually modified, 160
cognitive disabilities, 282*t*
cognitive grief symptoms, 199*t*, 200
Coley, William Bradley, 20
Coley toxins, 20
collaboration
core competencies for, 391–94
interprofessional, 376, 384, 385, 386, 388–89, 391–94 (*see also* interprofessional collaborative practice)
medical-legal partnerships (MLPs), 299–300
collaborative care
cancer care, 143
for people with serious mental illness (SMI) and cancer, 143–44
person-centered, 143–44, 144*f*
colon cancer, 19–20, 189, 402*b*
colorectal cancer, 19, 33
comfort care, 123–40
Commission on Cancer (COC), 9–10, 11, 98
committees, 331
communication
affirming, 265–66, 265*t*
best practices for, 265–66
developing our voice, 374
elderspeak, 217
end-of-life conversations, 253–55
person-centered language, 151
spiritual language, 158
transparent, 374
community-based exercise programs, 77
community-based knowledge transfer, 77–78
community engagement, 334–35, 360–61
community health navigators, 147
community organizing, 104–6
community outreach, 264, 360–61
Compassionate Friends, 259
compassion fatigue, 303–4, 309, 329–30
compensation, 333–34
complementary medicine, 89–90
complicated grief therapy, 207*t*
comprehensive palliative care services, 266–70
Conference on Medicine and Religion, 164
conferences, 327, 328*t*
conflict management, 384–96
Confucianism, 269
connection
in grief, 199*t*
sharing support, 357
vectors of cancer support, 356–58
constipation, 129–31
constructivism, 198
Contessa, 83–84
Contessa/Mt. Sinai, 83
continuing education (CE), 326–27, 335, 340, 344
best practices for, 347–49
organizations that offer, 327, 328*t*
coping, 242*t*
Council on Social Work Education (CSWE), 322, 324–26, 391
Council on Spiritual Practices, 164
counseling
individual, 116
supportive, 206–8
Courageous Parents Network, 259
COVID-19, long, 13
COVID-19 pandemic, xxi, 60–61, 110–11, 205–6, 309, 310, 318, 359
accepting and adapting as a way of life, 363–64
access and care issues, 311–12
cancer care, 13
case narratives, 364, 365
death toll, 221, 310–11
end-of-life care, 404–5

COVID-19 pandemic (*cont.*)
impact on communities of color, 311
institutional responses, 313–17
leadership development, 374*b*
in Mumbai, 363–64
racial inequity in, 61, 62
resources for, 319
social work during, 327–30
social work perspective, 218
supervision during, 330
unique challenges, 376
unique features, 310–13
COVID-19 vaccines, 313
CREATE: Compassion, REsilience, And TEam building, 316–17
creativity, 410
credentialing, 344–46, 347–49
crisis management, 319
crisis standards of care (CSC), 314–16
CRS (cytokine release syndrome), 21
CSC (crisis standards of care), 314–16
CSWE (Council on Social Work Education), 322, 324–25, 391
CTLA-4 (cytotoxic T lymphocyte antigen 4), 20–21
cultural competence, 257, 280–81, 406
definition of, 37
five essential steps, 64–65
models, 38, 290
resources, 290
Standards for Cultural Competence (NASW), 40, 277
Uses Sue's model for developing, 290
cultural humility, 89–90, 257, 258, 280–81
best practices for integrating, 40
definition of, 257, 280–81
emergence of, 37–40
cultural responsiveness, 257
cultural sensitivity, 400–3, 405–6
culture, 187, 204–5
cutaneous symptoms, 131
cytokine release syndrome (CRS), 21
cytotoxic T lymphocyte antigen 4 (CTLA-4), 20–21
Cytoxan, 75

Dallas Pain Questionnaire (DPQ), 128
DBT (dialectical behavior therapy), 116–17
Dear Jack Foundation, 259
decathexis, 197–98
decision-making, 242*t*, 248, 249
delirium, 133
delivery of care
5As model, 100–1
innovations in, 82
demographics, 277–78
depression, 131–32
clinical, 110–11, 112
guidelines for, 131–32
interventions for, 208
major, 111
depressive disorders, 10–11
despair, 199*t*, 200
developmental issues
for children, teens, and young adults, 252–53
differences in sex development (DSD), 265–66
diagnosing cancer, 4–5
Diagnostic and Statistical Manual of Mental Disorders (DSM), 87–88, 112, 201
dialectical behavior therapy (DBT), 116–17
differences in sex development (DSD), 265–66
digital disparities, 358, 367
digital interactions, 366
digital platforms, 82–83
dignity, 400
dignity therapy, 131–32
disaster management
cancer care amid, 57–68
duty to plan, 315
history of postdisaster response and recovery, 310
professional issues, 309–21
racial inequity and, 61
resources for, 319
disaster management plans, 314
disasters, 310
disbelief, 199*t*, 200
discrimination, 35–36
effects on grief experience, 203, 209
forms of, 76–77
LGBTQI, 262–63
nondiscrimination policy, 263–64
disease (concept), 88–89
disorganization, 200
distress
existential, 110–11
moral, 298, 303–4, 314–16
psychosocial, 110–11
distress management (DM), 97–98, 111

best practices for, 106–7, 136–37
evidence-based therapies, 116–17
NCCN Guidelines
Version 2.2022, 114–15
diversity
increasing, 378
in leadership, 377*b*, 377
multicultural populations, 275–91
DM. *See* distress management (DM)
do-not-resuscitate (DNR) orders, 249
double-strand breaks (DSBs), 19–20
Dougy Center: The National Grief Center for Children and Families, 259
DPM (dual process model), 197–98
DPQ (Dallas Pain Questionnaire), 128
dry mouth (xerostomia), 130
DSBs (double-strand breaks), 19–20
DSD (differences in sex development), 265–66
dual process model (DPM), 197–98
Duke University Center for Spirituality, Theology and Health, 164
duloxetine, 132
dumping, 36–37
Dyadic Cancer Outcomes Framework, 172*t*
dyadic interventions, 174–75
dysphagia, 129–31
dyspnea, 129

e-action alerts, 306
Edmonton Symptom Assessment Scale, 184
Educating Social Workers in Palliative and End-of-Life Care (ESPEC) program, 371
education
academic training programs, 323–26
best practices for, 347–49, 380
and cancer health disparities, 32–33
cancer patient, 358–59
continuing education (CE), 326–27, 328*t*, 335, 340, 344
current opportunities, 370–71
interprofessional education (IPE), 388–89, 394
Interprofessional Educational Collaborative (IPEC), 392*f*, 392–94, 393*f*, 395
for leadership development, 380
organizations that offer national conferences/continuing education, 327, 328*t*
Palliative Care Hospice Education and Training Act (PCHETA), 303*b*, 305
patient, 358–59
with technology, 358–59
educational policies and accreditation standards (EPAS), 326
EGFR (epidermal growth factor receptor), 19
elderspeak, 217
electronic medical records (EMRs), 354
elitism, 76–77
emergency care, 84–85
emerging therapies, 7–8
emotional support, 112
employee resource networks (ERNs), 375–76
employment, 230–31
employment policy, 264
EMRs (electronic medical records), 354
endocrine therapy, 134–35
end-of-life care, 181–94
autonomy in, 364–66
best practices for, 191–92
case studies, 189, 190, 249, 401*b*, 402*b*, 403*b*
for children, 249
during COVID-19, 404–5
for LGBTQI individuals, 270–71
for middle-aged adults, 234
religious perspectives on, 399–400
resources, 406
spiritual support, 159*b*
Standards for Palliative and End of Life Care (NASW), 326–27
telehealth impact on, 356
end-of-life conversations, 253–55
end-of-life planning, 270–71
Engage Initiative (Cancer and Mental Health Collaborative), 152
EPAS (educational policies and accreditation standards), 326
epidermal growth factor receptor (EGFR), 19
epistemological pluralism, 88–90
equity, 32–44
Equity in the Center, 40
ERNs (employee resource networks), 375–76
ERT-C, 176*t*
escitalopram, 132
ESPEC (Educating Social Workers in Palliative and End-of-Life Care) program, 371
ethical climate, 303–4

ethical issues, 295–308
in advocacy, 306
best practices for, 306–7
biomedical, 296
for clinicians, 296–300
Code of Ethics (NASW), 41–42, 57, 62–63, 64, 170, 277, 296–97, 306–7, 322
in Mumbai, 363
organizational, 300–3
policy, 304
principles and theory, 296, 297*b*
ethical practice, 156
ethical responsibility, 304
euthanasia, 159*b*
Evidence-Based Cancer Control Programs, National Cancer Institute (NCI), 177
evidence-based procedures, 84
evidence-based therapies, 116–17
ExCEL in Social Work—Excellence in Cancer Education and Leadership, 370–71
exercise
community-based programs, 77
lifestyle medicine, 71–72
existential distress, 110–11
existentialism, 269
Experience Camps, 259
Eye Movement Desensitization and Reprocessing Therapy, 207*t*

faith-based programs, 87
family, 118–19
affirming care environments for LGBTQI patients and families, 263–64
definition of, 248
involvement and support for, 100
family advisory councils, 13–14
family caregivers. *See also* caregivers
conceptual frameworks related to, 172*t*
domains of preparedness, 171
family-centered care, 257
family-centered care policy, 103–4
Family Medical Leave Act (FMLA), 175–77, 230–31
FDA (Food and Drug Administration), 19, 315
fee-for-service, 85–86, 182–83
fellowships, 328*t*, 381
fertility
in middle adulthood, 228
preservation of, 253
FICA (faith/belief, importance, community, and address in care), 127
financial issues
compensation, 333–34
with digital platforms, 82–83
fee-for-service payments to ambulance agencies, 85–86
lower income populations, 32–33
in middle adulthood, 230–31
reimbursement discounts for telehealth, 355
Financial navigation program, 176*t*
financial toxicity, 11, 50–51, 53, 54
First Nations people, 269
5As model, 100–1
FLACC (face, legs, activity, cry, consolability) scale, 128
Floyd, George, Jr., 35
FMLA (Family Medical Leave Act), 175–77, 230–31
Food and Drug Administration (FDA), 19, 315
Fordham University School of Social Service, 371, 381
friends, 118–19
frontline workers, 312–13
fundamental tenets, 114

GA (geriatric assessment), 217
gastric cancer, 33, 256
gastrointestinal (GI) symptoms, 129–31, 132
GCSW (Grand Challenges for Social Work), 51–52
gender (term), 263–64
gender identity, 262, 265*t*
gender minorities, 76–77, 276
Generalized Anxiety Disorder Questionnaire (GAD-7), 132
genetic alterations, 18–20
genetic testing, 256
Georgetown University National Center on Cultural Competency, 290
George Washington Institute for Spirituality and Health, 164
geriatric assessment (GA), 217
Gilman, Alfred, 6
Gleevec (imatinib), 19
Goodman, Louis, 6
government-driven palliative care models, 84–85

Grand Challenges for Social Work (GCSW), 51–52
grassroots-based models, 85–87
grassroots-based palliative care, 84–87
gratitude, 199*t*
Greensboro Health Disparities Collaborative, 104–5
grief, 209
  anticipatory, 195–97
  assessment of, 199–205
  decathexis, 197–98
  definition of, 195–96
  examples, 200, 201, 203, 205
  interventions for, 207*t*, 208, 235–36
  predeath, 195–96
  prolonged grief disorder (PGD), 200–2, 207*t*, 208
  symptoms of, 199–200, 199*t*
  theoretical models of, 197–98
"grief brain," 199*t*
grief resources, 259
group-thinking behavior, 313
guardians, 248
guilt, 199*t*, 200

haloperidol, 133
Hamer, Fannie Lou, 57
The Hastings Center, 307
health: social determinants of (SDOH). *See* social determinants of health (SDOH)
health and wellness coaching, 77–78
health care, 311–12
health care disparities, xxi, 12–13
  in cancer care, 279–80, 280*f*
  determinants of, 279–80, 280*f*
  in middle adulthood, 232–33
  in palliative care, 220, 279–80, 280*f*
  racism, 36–37, 377*b*
health care enterprises, 354
health care providers, xxi
health care systems, 390–91
health care workers
  COVID-19 cases, 316
  health threats during COVID-19, 312–13
  models for staff support, 316–17
  moral distress, 314–16
  recommended steps to care for, 317
  staff shortages, 312
health disparities, 47
  cancer-related, 32–37, 45–56, 279–80, 280*f*
  determinants of, 279–80, 280*f*
  LGBTQI, 262–63
  populations at risk, 276
  social determinants of health (SDOH) and, 47–50
  social work and, 47–48
  social work roles in addressing, 41–42, 51–52
health equality, 33–34
health equity, 33–34
Health Insurance Portability and Accountability Act (HIPAA), 355
health-related quality of life (HR-QOL), 26–27
Healthy People 2030, 47, 76
HeLa (Henrietta Lacks) cells, 221
hematologic cancers, 4, 5
hematopoietic stem cell transplants, 5
hepatitis B vaccine (HBV), 21
HER2 (human epidermal growth factor receptor 2), 18–19
Heterogeneity of Caregiving Model, 172*t*
heterosexism, 265*t*
Hinduism, 269, 398, 399–400, 402–3, 403*b*, 407
Hispanic/Latinx, 276
  COVID-19 case rates and mortality, 311, 316
  health disparities, 33
  palliative care for, 217
  social workers, 324–26, 378–79
  underserved populations, 187
  U.S. population, 277–78
history
  of oncology social work, 8–9
  of postdisaster response and recovery, 310
  roots of mistrust, 221–23
  of social work advocacy, 304–5
home care, 83, 190
homeless persons, 282*t*
home services, 83–84
homophobia, 76–77
hope, 410–11
HOPE (hope, organized religion, personal spirituality/ practices, and effects), 127
hormonal therapy, 6
hospice care, 262
  case studies, 189, 190, 223*b*, 402*b*
  home services, 83, 190
  Medicaid benefits, 188
  Medicare benefits, 188
  on Native American lands, 86–87

hospice care (*cont.*)
Palliative Care Hospice Education and Training Act (PCHETA), 303*b*, 305
spiritual care, 160*b*
transitioning to, 188–90
hospital care
rural emergency hospitals (REHs), 84–85
staff shortages, 312
HPV (human papillomavirus) vaccine, 21, 262–63
Huberman Labs, 209
human epidermal growth factor receptor 2 (HER2), 18–19
humanism, 269
human papillomavirus (HPV) vaccine, 21, 262–63

IADLs (instrumental activities of daily living), 216
Ibrance (palbociclib), 75
ICD *(International Classification of Diseases)*, 201
ICIs (immune checkpoint inhibitors), 7–8, 20–22
iCOPE (Interprofessional Curriculum for Oncology Palliative Education), 395
identity, gender, 262, 265*t*
identity/sense of self, 252
illness (concept), 88–89
imatinib (Gleevec), 19
Imerman Angels, 238
immigrants, 398
case vignettes, 284
interventions for, 282*t*, 284–86, 285*f*
practice models for work with, 282*t*
U.S. population, 278
immune checkpoint inhibitors (ICIs), 7–8, 20–22
immunotherapy, 6, 20–22
cellular, 7–8
emerging therapies, 7–8
side effects, 135
Implicit Association Test (IAT), 290
implicit bias, 103, 325, 377*b*, 377
IMRT (intensity-modulated radiation therapy), 22–23
incarcerated people, 282*t*
inclusion, 378–79, 380
Indians, 398
Indigenous Americans
Black, Indigenous, people of color (BIPOC), 216, 276–77
COVID-19 death rates, 221
social workers, 325
underserved populations, 187
Indigenous ways, traditional, 269
individual counseling, 116
infants, 242*t*, 251*t*
informal caregivers, 167–80
best practices for, 175–77
case vignette, 168
hours of care each week, 168
population, 167–68
information access, 113–14, 364–66
misinformation, 366
opportunity for visibility and developing our voice, 374
vectors of cancer support, 356–58
initial client meeting and biopsychosocial assessment, 114
innovation, 409
innovative models, 81–93
Institute for Healthcare Improvement, 105
Institute of Medicine (IOM), 9, 219–20
institutional racism, 36–37
institutions
ethical issues, 300–3
responses to COVID-19, 313–3
structural supports for social work, 390–91
instrumental activities of daily living (IADLs), 216
intake practices, 264
integrative programs, 69–80, 89–90
integrative strategies, 73–75
intensity-modulated radiation therapy (IMRT), 22–23
Intensive Care Society (UK), 317
interdisciplinary care, 26–27, 119
internalized racism, 37
International Association for the Study of Pain, 124
International Classification of Diseases (ICD), 201
International Society of Geriatric Oncology (SIOG), 219
International Waldenstrom's Macroglobulinemia Foundation, 361
international work, 397–408
internships, 328*t*
interpersonal racism, 37
interprofessional care

competencies in, 171
for symptoms after cancer care, 70–71
interprofessional collaboration, 376, 388–89
interprofessional collaborative practice (IPCP)
barriers to, 391
best practices for, 394–95
case studies, 75, 386–88
challenges, 384, 385–88
core competencies, 391–94, 392*f*, 393*f*
definition of, 385
resources, 395
Interprofessional Curriculum for Oncology Palliative Education (iCOPE), 395
interprofessional education (IPE), 388–89, 394
Interprofessional Educational Collaborative (IPEC), 391–94, 392*f*, 393*f*, 395
Interprofessional Education eXchange (IPEX), 395
interprofessional practice (IPP), 161–62
interprofessional teams (IPTs), 373, 388
intersex people, 265–66, 265*t*
intimacy, 228
Intimacy and Relationship Process Model, 172*t*
intrapersonal racism, 37
IOM (Institute of Medicine), 9, 219–20
IPCP. *See* interprofessional collaborative practice
IPE (interprofessional education), 388–89, 394
IPEC (Interprofessional Educational Collaborative), 391–94, 392*f*, 393*f*, 395
IPEX (Interprofessional Education eXchange), 395
ipilimumab, 20–21
IPP (interprofessional practice), 161–62
IPTs (interprofessional teams), 373, 388
Islam, 269, 398, 399, 400–1, 407

John Templeton Foundation, 164
Joint Commission, 332
Journal of the American Medical Association, 6, 315
Judaism, 269
Judi's House/JAG Institute, 259
justice, 297*b*, 299–300

Kaiser Family Foundation, 43
Kleinman, Arthur, 88–89

Lacks, Henrietta, 221
Lakota people, 86
Lambda Legal Tools for Life, Burial, and Financial Planning, 272*t*
language
elderspeak, 217
end-of-life conversations, 253–55
person-centered, 151
spiritual, 158
Latinas. *See also* Hispanic/Latinx
health disparities, 33
leadership
challenges and opportunities, 373
in clinical settings, 375–76
during COVID-19 pandemic, 374*b*
definition of, 370
diversity in, 377*b*, 377
importance of, 388–89
increasing diversity through, 378
in interprofessional collaboration, 388–89
racial disparities, 377
social work, 370, 388–89, 409–11
leadership development, 335–36, 369–83
best practices for, 379–81
education, 370–71
opportunities for, 328*t*, 369, 370–73
resources for, 381
training, 370–73
learning exercise, 235–36
legacy work, 190
legal issues, 295–308
in advocacy, 306
best practices for, 306–7
case studies, 298*b*
medical-legal partnerships (MLPs), 299–300
lesbian, gay, bisexual, transgender, queer, and intersex (LGBTQI) persons, 261
advance care planning, 271
affirming care environments for, 263–64
best practices for, 272–73
cancer disparities, 262–63
cancer survivors, 76–77
discrimination against, 262–63
end-of-life planning, 270–71
interventions for, 282*t*
palliative care for, 261–74
practice models for work with, 282*t*
resources for, 272*t*
social determinants of health (SDOH), 262–63
spiritual considerations, 269–70
terminology, 265*t*

lethality, synthetic, 19–20
letrozole, 75
letter-writing campaigns, 303*b*, 305
leukemia, 4, 386
Leukemia and Lymphoma Society, 10
LGBT Community Centers, 272*t*
LGBTQI persons. *See* lesbian, gay, bisexual, transgender, queer, and intersex persons
liberation-informed care, 101–3, 106
liberation psychology, 102–3
libido, low, 132
licensing, 344
lifelong learning, 344
life review, 160*b*
lifestyle medicine, 72–73
liver cancer, 33, 403*b*
Livestrong, 238
lobby days, 305
long COVID, 13
long-term care, 267
loss and bereavement, 195–211
lower income and education populations, 32–33
lung cancer, 33, 190, 401*b*
lymphedema, 127, 131
lymphomas, 4
Lynch syndrome, 19–20

macro/mezzo/micro social work, 369, 372–73
major depressive disorder (MDD), 200–1
Malays, 398
marginalized populations, 187
marketing, 264
Massachusetts General Hospital, 98–99
master of social work (MSW) degree, 324–26, 328*t*
MBSR (mindfulness-based stress reduction), 74
McGill Pain Questionnaire (MPQ), 128
MDD (major depressive disorder), 200–1
meaning-centered psychotherapy (MCP), 160*b*, 160
meaning-making, 185–86, 198
media
  narrative-based, 357
  new, 356–58
Medicaid, 82, 188
medical care
  for AYAs with cancer, 251
  technology and, 353–56
medical-legal partnerships (MLPs), 299–300
medical mistrust, 221–23, 222*b*
medical pluralism, 88–90
medical racism and neglect, 203
Medicare, 82, 85–86, 182–83, 188, 216–17
meetings, client, 114
melanoma, 20–21
Memorial Sloan Kettering, 89–90
mental health therapy, 206–8
mental illness. *See* serious mental illness (SMI)
mentorships, 327–30, 328*t*, 378–79
men who have sex with men (MSM), 262–63, 267
Mexican immigrants, 278, 284
mezzo social work, 369, 372–73
MI (motivational interviewing), 116–17
micro social work practice, 369, 372–73
middle adulthood, 227, 237
  best practices for work with middle-aged cancer patients, 236–37
  cancer in, 227–39
  case scenario, 235–36
  interventions for middle-aged cancer patients, 233–36
  psychosocial factors, 228–33
  systemic factors in, 228–33
mindfulness, 73–75
mindfulness-based stress reduction (MBSR), 74
minority populations, 76–77, 216, 217, 276–77
misinformation, 366
Mississippi River, 104
mistrust, 221–23, 222*b*
MLPs (medical-legal partnerships), 299–300
Model of Culture and Social Class for Families Facing Cancer, 172*t*
molecular alterations, 18–20
monoclonal antibodies (mAbs), 6, 135
moral distress, 298, 303–4, 314–16
Morehouse School of Medicine Cancer Health Equity Institute (CHEI), 66
motivational interviewing (MI), 116–17
mountain-top experiences, 160*b*
mourning, 195–96
MPQ (McGill Pain Questionnaire), 128
MSM (men who have sex with men), 262–63, 267
MSW (master of social work) degree, 324–26, 328*t*

multiculturalism, 277, 289
multicultural populations, 275–91
best practices for work with, 287–89
future priorities, 287, 288*f*
interventions for, 281–86, 282*t*
practice models for work with, 281–86, 282*t*
resources for, 289
terminology, 289
multiple myeloma, 4, 33
multiprofessional teams, 364
multiracial populations, 277–78
Mumbai, India
ethical and professional considerations, 363
psychosocial cancer care highlights from, 361–66
way of life, 363–64
Murray-Garcia, Jann, 37–38
Muslims, 399, 400, 401*b*, 401
myeloproliferative neoplasms, 4
MyPal, 83

NAMI (National Alliance on Mental Illness), 152
narrative-based media, 357
NASW. *See* National Association of Social Workers
National Academies of Sciences, Engineering, and Medicine (NASEM), 98–99, 100–1, 385
National Advisory Committee on Rural Health and Human Services, 92
National Alliance for Children's Grief, 259
National Alliance on Mental Illness (NAMI), 152
National Association of Social Workers (NASW), 34, 41, 325, 340
Advanced Certified Hospice and Palliative Social Work (ACHP-SW) certification, 342–43, 348–49
advocacy arm, 306
Code of Ethics, 41–42, 57, 62–63, 64, 170, 257, 277, 295, 296–97, 306–7, 322, 326–27, 332
curriculum model, 344
definition of multiculturalism, 277
Educating Social Workers in Palliative and End-of-Life Care (ESPEC) program, 371
resources, 349, 381
Standards for Cultural Competence, 40, 277
Standards for Palliative and End of Life Care, 326–27
Standards for Practice in Health Care Settings, 326–27, 384–85
website, 337
National Cancer Institute (NCI), 13–14, 104–5, 331–32
cancer-related information, 113
Evidence-Based Cancer Control Programs, 177
resources, 28, 54, 177
Surveillance, Epidemiology, and End Results (SEER) program, 33
National Center for Complementary and Integrative Health, 119
National Center on Cultural Competency, 290
National Comprehensive Cancer Network (NCCN), 9–10, 185
Clinical Practice Guidelines in Oncology—Supportive Care, 137
Guidelines for Patients, 367
Guidelines Version 2.2022, Distress Management, 114–15
national conferences, 327, 328*t*
National Consensus Project for Quality Palliative Care (NCPQPC), 205, 341
National Health Center for Complementary and Integrative Health, 113
National Helpline, Substance Abuse and Mental Health Services Administration (SAMHSA), 152
National Hospice and Palliative Care Organization, 34, 87, 192, 342
National Institutes of Health (NIH), 259
National Library of Medicine (NLM), 290
National Resources Center on LGBT Aging to Find LGBT-Affirming National and Local Resources, 272*t*
Native American lands, 86–87
Native Americans. *See* Indigenous Americans
Native Hawaiians and other Pacific Islanders, 276, 324–26
nausea and vomiting, 124, 129–31
NCCN. *See* National Comprehensive Cancer Network
NCP (National Consensus Project), 205
needs assessment, 148–49, 269
neglect, medical, 203
neuropathic pain, 125–26

neuropathy, peripheral, 126
new media, 356–58
New Mexico, 86
New York University (NYU) Silver School of Social Work
  Online Post-Master's Certificate Program, 345–46
  opportunities for professional development, 328*t*
  Zelda Foster Studies Program, 328*t*, 336, 371, 381
nivolumab, 20–21
nociceptive pain, 125
nondiscrimination policy, 263–64
nonmaleficence, 297*b*, 298–99
nonprofit organizations, 361
non–small cell lung cancer (NSCLC), 19
NORD (National Organization of Rare Diseases), 361
Not Alone with Cancer (Abrams), 8–9
NTRK/ROS1, 19
numbness, 199*t*, 200
nutrition, 71–72
NYU. *See* New York University

olanzapine, 133
olaparib, 19–20
older adults, 215–16
  assessment of, 219–20
  cancer care for, 217, 223–24
  interventions for, 217, 282*t*
  LGBTQI elders, 262, 267, 270, 272*t*
  long-term care for, 267
  palliative care for, 219–21
  population, 215
  practice models for work with, 282*t*
  psychosocial needs, 216–17
  resources for, 272*t*
  societal perceptions, 217
  U.S. population, 278
OncoLink, 137
oncology care. *See* cancer care
Oncology Nursing Society, 117
oncology social work. *See also* social work
  during COVID-19, 327–30
  history of, 8–9
  international, 397–408
  leadership training in, 370–73
  professional development, 322–39
  psychosocial needs of patients, 10–11
  telehealth impact on, 356
Oncology Social Work Certificate, 341–42
oncology social workers (OSWs), 322–24, 325–26, 327, 369–71. *See also* social workers
  Certified Oncology Social Worker (OSW-C), 337, 345
  compensation, 333–34
  leadership opportunities, 372–73
  mentorships, 327–30, 328*t*
  opportunities for visibility, 374
  professional development activities, 327–30
  professional development opportunities, 327, 328*t*, 335
  racial diversity of, 378–79
  resources for, 337
  role in organizing patient education workshops, 360
  self-care, 333
  supervision of, 327–31
on-the-job training, 363
opioid crisis, 135–36
opioids, 301*b*
organizations
  ethical issues, 300–3
  professional, 331
  responses to COVID-19, 313–3
oropharynx cancers, HPV-mediated, 23
OSW-C (Certified Oncology Social Worker), 337, 345
OSWs (oncology social workers), 322–24, 325–26, 327. *See also* social workers
outpatient care, 8
ovarian cancer, 19–20, 287

pain
  breakthrough, 126
  cancer, 125–26
  concept of, 398–99
  definitions of, 124–27
  measurement of, 127–28
  nature of, 124–27
  neuropathic, 125–26
  nociceptive, 125
  postradiation syndromes, 127
  postsurgical syndromes, 127
  somatic, 125
  total, 125, 184–85, 398–99
  as treatment-related toxicity, 126–27
  visceral, 125
pain assessment, 127–28

pain assessment tools, 128, 185
Pain Disability Index, 129
pain management, 71–72, 123–40
  best practices for, 136–37
  case studies, 301*b*, 402*b*
  clinical cases, 75, 124
  ethical issues, 301
  opioid crisis, 135–36
  resources, 137
  social work role in, 129
palbociclib (Ibrance), 75
palliative care, 262
  access to services, 219, 302–3, 303*b*
  assessment in, 219–20
  best practices, 183–84, 191–92
  for Black people, 220–21
  cancer and experiences of, 49
  case narratives, 189
  comprehensive services, 266–70
  core competencies, 341
  during COVID-19, 327–30
  definition of, 182
  delivery innovations, 82
  disparities in, 220
  at end of life, 181–94
  ethical issues, 295–308, 301*b*, 303*b*
  example interventions, 284–86, 285*f*
  government-driven models, 84–85
  grassroots-based models, 84–87
  guidelines for, 184
  home-based, 83–84
  innovative models, 81–93
  leadership challenges and opportunities, 373
  for LGBTQI persons, 261–74
  models, 182–83
  on Native American lands, 86–87
  for older adults, 219–20
  primary, 409
  social determinants of health (SDOH) and, 49
  spirituality and, 156
  Standards for Palliative and End of Life Care (NASW), 326–27
  standards of practice, 341
  telehealth impact on, 356
  for undocumented immigrants, 284–86, 285*f*
  worldviews toward, 278–79
Palliative Care Hospice Education and Training Act (PCHETA), 303*b*, 305
Palliative Care Outcome Scale (PCOS), 128
Palliative Care Research Cooperative Group Caregiver Core, 178
palliative care social work (PCSW), 81–82. *See also* social work
palliative care social workers (PCSWs), 370–71, 372–74. *See also* social workers
palliative sedation, 133
PANCAN (Pancreatic Cancer Action Network), 358
pancreatic cancer, 19–20
pandemics
  cancer care amid, xxi, 57–68
  professional issues in, 309–21
Paramedics Providing Palliative Care at Home program, 85
parents and parenting, 229–30
  questions of parents of children with cancer, 251*t*
  websites for patients with children and teenagers, 230*b*
PARPis (poly[ADP-ribose] polymerases inhibitors), 19–20
partners and partnerships
  creating partnerships, 384–96
  medical-legal partnerships (MLPs), 299–300
  in middle adulthood, 229
patient- and family-centered care policy, 103–4
patient-centered care, 406
patient-centered care model, 217–18
patient education, 358–59
patient education workshops, 360–61
patient/family advisory councils (PFACs), 13–14
Patient Health Questionnaire-9 (PHQ-9), 127, 131–32
patient-reported outcomes (PROs), 83, 97–98
Patient Reported Outcomes Measurement Information System (PROMIS), 178
Patient Self-Determination Act, 296–97
PCHETA (Palliative Care Hospice Education and Training Act), 303*b*, 305
PCOS (Palliative Care Outcome Scale), 128
PCSW (palliative care social work), 81–82. *See also* social work
PCSWs (palliative care social workers), 370–71, 372–74. *See also* social workers
pediatric pain assessment tools, 128

pediatric symptoms, 133–34
pembrolizumab, 20–21
peripheral neuropathy, chemotherapy-induced, 126
personal protective equipment (PPE), 310
person-centered approach, 397
person-centered collaborative care, 143–44, 144*f*
person-centered language, 151
perspectives, 1–93
PFACs (patient/family advisory councils), 13–14
PGD (prolonged grief disorder), 200–2, 207*t*, 208
PHQ-9 (Patient Health Questionnaire-9), 127, 131–32
physical care, 267
physical pain, 126–27. *See also* pain
physical symptoms
  in cancer, 125–26
  in grief, 199–200, 199*t*
physical therapy (PT)
  clinical case, 75
  psychologically informed, 71–72
podcasts, 367
policy issues, 304
poly(ADP-ribose) polymerases (PARP) inhibitors (PARPis), 19–20
polytheism, 269
positive thinking, 113
postdisaster response and recovery, 310
postradical neck dissection syndrome, 127
postsurgical pain syndromes, 127
post-thoracotomy pain syndrome, 127
post-traumatic growth (PTG), 235
post-traumatic stress, 132–33
post-traumatic stress disorder (PTSD), 10–11, 87–88, 111, 117–18
  in cancer, 132–33
  in grief, 200–1
  interventions for, 207*t*, 208
PPE (personal protective equipment), 310
PQRST mnemonic, 128
PRAPARE (Protocol for Responding to and Assessing Patient Assets, Risks, and Experiences), 107
precision medicine, 18, 19–20
predeath grief, 195–96
preschoolers, 242*t*, 251*t*
preteens, 242*t*
prevention, 300
primary palliative care, 25
Princess Margaret Cancer Centre, 316–17
Priselac, Thomas, 84
professional considerations, 363
professional development, 322–39
  case example, 330–31
  opportunities for, 327, 328*t*, 335
professional organizations, 331
professional psychosocial oncology assistance, 117
professional responsibility, 304
prognostic awareness, 185–86
prolonged grief disorder (PGD), 200–2, 207*t*, 208
PROs (patient-reported outcomes), 83
prostate cancer, 19–20, 33
Protocol for Responding to and Assessing Patient Assets, Risks, and Experiences (PRAPARE), 107
psychiatric symptoms, 131–34
psychiatrists, 145–47
psychological factors, 114–15
psychologically informed physical therapy, 71–72
psychological symptoms
  in cancer, 131–34
  in grief, 200–2
psychology, liberation, 102–3
psychosocial assessments, 174
psychosocial care
  cancer-related, 9, 110–22
  for caregiving-related issues, 174–75, 176*t*
  case #1, 111
  challenges, 172–73, 362–63
  current trends, 9–10
  dyadic interventions, 174–75
  ethical issues, 302
  future directions, 100–1
  highlights from Mumbai, 361–66
  interventions, 115–16, 174–75, 176*t*, 177, 362–63
  for LGBTQI people, 267–69
  models of support, 10
  on-the-job training in, 363
  palliative care, 267–69
  professional, 117
  support for caregivers, 170
psychosocial distress
  among cancer survivors, 70
  among LGBTQI persons, 110–11
psychosocial needs

in middle adulthood, 228–33
of older adults, 216–17
of oncology patients, 10–11
psychosocial oncology research, 331–32
psychotherapy, 136
for anxiety, 132
meaning-centered (MCP), 160*b*, 160
PTG (post-traumatic growth), 235
PTSD. *See* post-traumatic stress disorder
public health, 35–36, 38*f*
pulmonary symptoms, 129

quality of life, health-related (HR-QOL), 26–27
quetiapine, 133

race-based traumatic stress (RBTS), 87–88, 91
Race IAT—Project Implicit, 290
racial disparities, 377
Racial Equity Tools, 43
racial inequity, 61
racism, xxi, 32–44
effects on grief experience, 203, 209
in health care settings, 377*b*
institutional, 36–37
internalized, 37
interpersonal, 37
intrapersonal, 37
medical, 203
as public health crisis, 35–36, 38*f*
as social determinants of health (SDOH), 62–63, 76–77
structural, 36
systemic, 36–37, 38*f*, 63–64, 358
racism fatigue, 61–62
radiation therapy, 5–6, 22–24
intensity-modulated (IMRT), 22
postradiation pain syndromes, 127
side effects, 129–30, 134
stereotactic body (SBRT), 23–24
stereotactic radiosurgery (SRS), 23–24
RAISE (Recognize, Assist, Include, Support, and Engage) Family Caregivers Act, 175–77
RAS mitogen-activated protein kinase (RAS-MAPK), 19
RBTS (race-based traumatic stress), 87–88, 91
Red Crescent, 310
Red Cross, 310
refugees & asylum seekers, 282*t*
regret, 199*t*
rehabilitation, 69–80
REHs (rural emergency hospitals), 84–85
relational symptoms, 200–2
relief, 199*t*
religious beliefs, 154, 155, 399–400, 406
religious sensitivity, 400–3, 405–6
remdesivir, 315
remote work, 374*b*, 376
research, psychosocial oncology, 331–32
resilience, 409–10
resources
additional, 15, 28, 42, 54, 66, 79, 91, 107, 119, 137, 152, 164, 177, 192, 209, 238, 259, 289, 307, 319, 337, 349, 367, 381, 395, 406
employee resource networks (ERNs), 375–76
for LGBTQ elders, 272*t*
websites for patients with children and teenagers, 230*b*
respect for autonomy, 296–98
responsibility, professional and ethical, 304
responsiveness, cultural, 257
risperidone, 133
rituals, 235
rucaparib, 19–20
rural emergency hospitals (REHs), 84–85
rural populations, 32–33, 276

sadness, 199*t*, 200
SAGE: Services and Advocacy for GLBT Elders, 272*t*
The Samfund, 259
SAMHSA (Substance Abuse and Mental Health Services Administration), 92, 152, 290
sandwich generation, 230
Santeria, 269
SARS-CoV-2 (severe acute respiratory syndrome coronavirus 2), 310
Saunders, Cicely, 184–85, 398–99
SBRT (stereotactic body radiation therapy), 23–24
school-age children, 242*t*, 251*t*
screening
ethical issues, 300
social-risk, 99–100
structural vulnerability, 98–99
SDOH. *See* social determinants of health
seasons of survival, 69

sedation, palliative, 133
selective serotonin-reuptake inhibitors (SSRIs), 132
self-care, 206, 319, 333, 374*b*
self-exploration, 160–61
self-identity, 252
Serious Illness Conversation Guide, 192
serious mental illness (SMI), 141–42
  best practices for, 151–52
  cancer care for people with, 143
  caregivers for people with cancer and, 147–48
  case study, 149
  collaborative care for people with cancer and, 143–44, 144*f*
  helpful questions to ask patients and caregivers, 148–49
  patient assessment, 148–49
  person-centered collaborative care for people with cancer and, 143–44, 144*f*
serotonin-norepinephrine reuptake inhibitors (SNRIs), 132
sertraline, 132
Sesame Street in Communities, 259
severe acute respiratory syndrome coronavirus 2 (SARS-CoV-2), 310
sexism, 76–77
sexual activity, 262–63
sexuality, 228
sexual minorities, 76–77, 276
sexual orientation or gender identity (SOGI), 262, 263–64, 265*t*, 266
sexual side effects, 132
shamanism, 269
sharing support, 357
Shirley Haynes Institute for Palliative Care (California State University), 336
shock, 199*t*, 200
siblings, 250, 251*t*, 258
Silver School of Social Work (New York University)
  Online Post-Master's Certificate Program, 345–46
  opportunities for professional development, 328*t*
  Zelda Foster Studies Program in Palliative and End-of-Life Care (PELC), 328*t*, 336
single-strand breaks (SSBs), 19–20
SIOG (International Society of Geriatric Oncology), 219
Sisters Network® Inc., 361
SMI. *See* serious mental illness
Smith College School of School Work Palliative/End-of-Life Care Certificate, 328*t*, 336, 371, 381
SNRIs (serotonin-norepinephrine reuptake inhibitors), 132
social connectivity, 356–58
Social Determinants Framework for Cancer Equity, 76
social determinants of health (SDOH), 20, 22, 33, 45–56, 78, 334–35
  best practices for mitigating negative impacts of, 52–54
  in cancer care, 76–77
  in cancer prevention and detection, 48–49
  definition of, 46, 76
  determinants of cancer and palliative care disparities, 279–80, 280*f*
  determinants of health disparities, 47–50
  LGBTQI, 262–63
  racism as, 62–63
  social work roles in addressing, 51–52
  terminology, 46–47
social factors, 114–15
social-risk screening and referral, 99–100
Social Security Disability Insurance (SSDI), 230–31
social/societal assessment, 202–3
social support, 112
social work
  for at-risk multicultural groups, 281–86, 282*t*, 285*f*
  core values, 170–71
  during COVID-19, 327–30
  culturally sensitive, 400–3
  ethical practice, 156
  5As model, 100–1
  fundamental tenets, 114
  general principles related to caregiving, 169–70
  health disparities and, 47–48
  history of, 8–9, 304–5
  international, 397–408
  interventions, 282*t*, 284–86, 285*f*
  leadership, 409–11
  leadership training in, 370–73
  macro/mezzo/micro, 369, 372–73
  oncology, 8–9
  professional development, 322–39
  religiously sensitive, 400–3

role in addressing social determinants of health (SDOH) and health disparities, 51–52
role in eliminating health inequities, 41–42
role in support of caregivers, 170
role with patients and caregivers, 129
social determinants of health (SDOH) and, 47–48
standards of practice, 326–27
structural support for, 390–91
Social Work, Hospice and Palliative Care Network (SWHPN), 34, 325, 331, 340, 343
opportunities for professional development, 328*t*
resources, 337, 349
social work advocacy, 304–5. *See also* advocacy
social workers, 145
case example, 330–31
compensation, 333–34
core competencies, 341
finding our voice, 389–91
leadership development, 369–83
oncology social workers (OSWs), 322–24, 325–26, 327–30, 333–34, 335, 337, 369–71, 372–74, 378–79
opportunities for visibility, 374
palliative care social workers (PCSWs), 370–71, 372–74
professional development opportunities, 327, 328*t*, 335
and psychiatrists, 146
racial diversity of, 378–79
resources for, 337
roles, 145, 360
self-care, 333
standards of practice, 341
visibility challenges, 375
social work leadership, 388–89, 409–11
Social Work Oncology Research Group, Association of Oncology Social Work (AOSW), 332
Society for Social Work and Research (SSWR), 328*t*, 337
Society for Social Work Leadership in Healthcare (SSWLHC), 328*t*, 335
Society for Spirituality and Social Work, 164
socioeconomically disadvantaged populations, 276
socioeconomic status (SES), 48–49
SOGI (sexual orientation or gender identity), 262, 263–64, 265*t*, 266
solid tumor cancers, 4, 5
somatic pain, 125, 199–200
South Dakota, 86
spiritual assessment, 127–28, 157–58, 204
spiritual care, 163*b*, 164
best practices for, 162–64
clinical interventions, 159–60
end-of-life care, 159*b*
hospice care, 160*b*
interprofessional practice (IPP), 161–62
for LGBTQI people, 269–70
palliative care, 269–70
resources, 164
Spiritual Competency Academy, 164
spiritual history assessment tools, 127
spirituality, 154, 163*b*, 163–64, 187, 269
acknowledging and addressing, 156
assessment questions focused on, 158*b*
in bereavement, 204
case studies, 223*b*
clients' desires and experiences about integration of care, 156–57
clinician self-exploration of one's own, 160–61
definition of, 155, 269–70
dimensions of, 204
examples, 204
in middle adulthood, 231–32
relevance of, 156
in social work practice, 156–57
spiritual language, 158
spiritual needs assessment, 269
spiritual practices, 269
SRS (stereotactic radiosurgery), 23–24
SSDI (Social Security Disability Insurance), 230–31
SSRIs (selective serotonin-reuptake inhibitors), 132
SSWLHC (Society for Social Work Leadership in Healthcare), 328*t*, 335
SSWR (Society for Social Work and Research), 328*t*, 337
staff shortages, 312
staff support, 316–17
standards of practice, 326–27, 341
crisis standards of care, 314–16
Scope and Standards of Practice (AOSW), 322, 327
Standards for Cultural Competence (NASW), 40, 277

standards of practice (*cont.*)
  Standards for Palliative and End of Life Care (NASW), 326–27
  Standards for Practice in Health Care Settings (NASW), 326–27, 384–85
state licensing, 344
stem cell transplants, 5, 387
stereotactic body radiation therapy (SBRT), 23–24
stereotactic radiosurgery (SRS), 23–24
stomach cancer, 33, 256
strength assessment, 148–49
stress
  chronic, 35–36
  mindfulness-based stress reduction (MBSR), 74
  moral distress, 298, 303–4
  post-traumatic, 132–33
  race-based traumatic, 87–88, 91
stress-related disorders, 10–11
structural support, 390–91
Structural Vulnerability Assessment Tool, 107
structural vulnerability screening, 98–99
Stupidcancer, 259
Substance Abuse and Mental Health Services Administration (SAMHSA), 92, 152, 290
suffering
  concept of, 398–99
  religious perspectives on, 399–400
suicide risk, 117–18
supervision, 327–30, 375
  best practices for leadership development, 380
  case example, 330–31
support groups, 118
supportive care, 8
  need for social and emotional support, 112
  vectors of cancer support, 356–58
supportive counseling, 206–8
supportive psychotherapy, 132
support networks, 118–19, 248–50
surgery, 5, 24–26
  postsurgical pain syndromes, 127
  stereotactic radiosurgery (SRS), 23–24
survivors and survivorship, 26–27, 69–70
  for children and AYAs, 253
  clinical case, 75
  post-traumatic growth (PTG), 235
  seasons of survival, 69
  side effects, 23
sustainability, 322–39
SWHPN. *See* Social Work, Hospice and Palliative Care Network
symptoms
  best practices for management of, 136–37
  in cancer, 125–26, 129–34
  cancer treatment-associated, 129–34
  cutaneous, 131
  gastrointestinal (GI), 129–31, 132
  in grief, 199–202, 199*t*
  management of, 123–40
  pediatric, 133–34
  physical, 125–26, 199–200, 199*t*
  psychiatric, 131–34
  psychological, 131–34, 200–2
  pulmonary, 129
  relational, 200–2
synthetic lethality, 19–20
systemic racism, 36–37, 38*f*, 63–64
systemic therapy, 6–7

tai chi, 73–75
talazoparib, 19–20
tamoxifen, 18–19
targeted therapy, 6, 18–20, 135
Task Force for Mass Critical Care, 315
Tata Memorial Hospital (Mumbai, India)
  multiprofessional teams, 364
  psychosocial cancer care highlights from, 361–66
Taxol, 75
T cells, 7–8, 20–22
team-based care
  building a team for, 144–47
  interprofessional teams (IPTs), 373, 388
  key staff, 144
  leadership challenges and opportunities, 373
  multiprofessional teams, 364
  need for, 14
technology, 352–68
  best practices for, 366–67
  impact on medical care, 353–56
  patient education with, 358–59
teenagers (teens)
  adolescents and young adults (AYAs), 240–48, 242*t*, 251*t*
  case scenarios, 241
  websites for patients with, 230*b*
Teen Cancer America, 259
teleconferences, 358–59, 360

telehealth, 83, 86, 113–14, 353–56
case studies, 374*b*
definition of, 353–54
encounters, 354
impact on health care enterprises, 354
impact on oncology and palliative care, 356
pros and cons, 355–56
rapid emergence of, 353–54
reimbursement discounts for, 355
telemedicine. *See* telehealth
telemonitoring programs, 86
terminology, 265*t*, 289
Tervalon, Melanie, 37–38
Theory of Dyadic Illness Management, 172*t*
therapeutic alliance, 114
thoracotomy, 127
TIC. *See* trauma-informed care
toddlers, 242*t*, 251*t*
total pain, 125, 184–85, 398–99
toxicity
of cancer-directed therapy, 134–35
financial, 50–51, 53, 54
treatment-related, 123–40
traditional Chinese medicine, 74
traditional Indigenous ways, 269
training
academic programs, 323–26
end-of-life (EOL), 86
leadership, 370–73
on-the-job, 363
Palliative Care Hospice Education and Training Act (PCHETA), 303*b*, 305
transgender individuals, 262, 265*t*, *See also* lesbian, gay, bisexual, transgender, queer, and intersex (LGBTQI) persons
transparency, 374
transphobia, 265*t*
trastuzumab, 19
trauma-informed care (TIC), 87–88, 101–3, 117–18
traumatic events
cancer care amid, 57–68
professional issues in, 309–21
racial inequity and, 61
treatment(s)
for advanced cancer, 185
challenges of new approaches, 11
changing landscape, 17–31
options for, 4, 5–8
symptoms associated with, 129–34
treatment-related toxicity, 123–40
TRiadic Interactions in Oncology (TRIO) Framework, 172*t*
Triage Cancer Center, 238
trust
building, 148
medical mistrust, 221–23, 222*b*
Tuskegee syphilis experiments, 221
tyrosine kinase inhibitors, 19

underrepresented populations, 213–91
underserved populations, 187–88, 213–91
undocumented immigrants. *See also* immigrants
case vignettes, 284
interventions for, 282*t*, 284–86, 285*f*
practice models for work with, 282*t*
United States
cancer health disparities, 32–37
caregivers, 167–68, 169
health care system, 311–12
older adults, 215
populations, 215, 275–91
University of North Carolina, 104–5
University of Pennsylvania, 328*t*, 345–46
U.S. Department of Health and Human Services, 47, 54, 76, 263–64, 319
U.S. Food and Drug Administration (FDA), 19, 315

vaccines, 20–22, 313
values, core, 170–71
values, needs, and strength assessment, 148–49
VAS (visual analog scale), 128
vascular endothelial growth factor (VEGF), 19
venlafaxine, 132
veterans, 282*t*
victims of human trafficking, 282*t*
victims of violence and sexual abuse, 282*t*
virtual care, 367
virtual platforms, 363, 366, 374*b*, 376
visceral pain, 125
visibility
challenges of, 375
opportunities for, 374
visual analog scale (VAS), 128
vodun, 269
voice
developing our voice, 374
finding our voice, 389–91

Votive Health, 82
vulnerability screening, structural, 98–99
vulnerable populations, 213–91

Washington State Department of Public Health, 319
webcasts, 360
Well Beings Studio, 230*b*
wellness coaching, 77–78
Western biomedicine, 89–90, 278–79
WHO (World Health Organization), 46, 201, 385
whole-person perspective, 27–28
Winters Group, 43
women
- caregivers, 169
- case studies, 235–36, 284–87
- double burden of, 230
- health disparities, 33
- social workers, 324–25

women who have sex with women (WSW), 267
Wong-Baker FACES scale, 128
workshops, patient education, 360–61
World Health Organization (WHO), 46, 201, 385
worldviews, 278–79
WSW (women who have sex with women), 267

xerostomia (dry mouth), 130

yearning/longing, 199*t*, 200
yoga, 73–75
Yoruba religion, 269
young adults. *See also* adolescents and young adults (AYAs)
- case stories, 241, 256
- development, disruption, and coping, 242*t*
- LGBTQI, 265–66
- questions, 251*t*

Zelda Foster Studies Program (NYU Silver School of Social Work), 328*t*, 336, 371, 381
Zuni people, 86

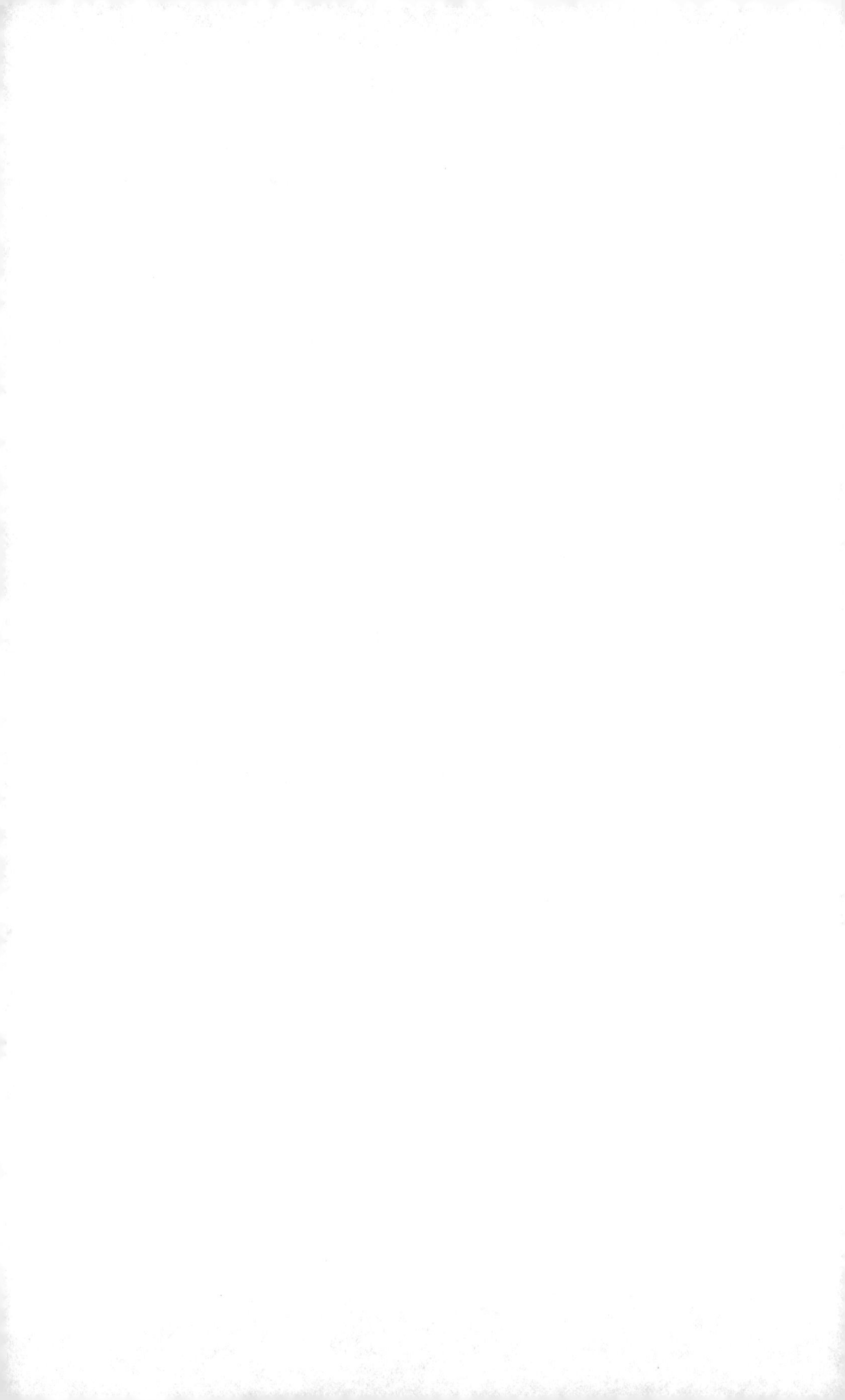